Substance Use and Older People

Addiction Press aims to communicate current ideas and evidence in this expanding field, not only to researchers and practising health professionals, but also to policy makers, students and interested non-specialists. These publications are designed to address the significant challenges that addiction presents to modern society.

Other books in the Addiction Press series

Understanding Hard to Maintain Behaviour Change:
A Dual Process Approach
Ron Borland
9781118572931

Theory of Addiction
Robert West and Jamie Brown
9780470674215

Clinical Handbook of Adolescent Addiction
Edited by R. Rosner
9780470972342

Harm Reduction in Substance Use and High-Risk Behaviour
Edited by R. Pates & D. Riley
9781405182973

Neuroimaging in Addiction
Edited by B. Adinoff & E. Stein
9780470660140

Injecting Illicit Drugs
Edited by R. Pates, A. McBride & K. Arnold
9781405113601

Treating Drinkers and Drug Users in the Community
T. Waller & D. Rumball
9780632035755

Addiction: Evolution of a Specialist Field
Edited by G. Edwards
9780632059768

Substance Use and Older People

Edited by

Ilana Crome, MA MD MPhil FRCPsych
Li-Tzy Wu, ScD MA
Rahul (Tony) Rao, MD MSc FRCPsych
Peter Crome, MD PhD DSc FRCP FFPM FBPharmacolS

WILEY Blackwell

This edition first published 2015 © 2015 by John Wiley & Sons, Ltd

Registered Office
John Wiley & Sons, Ltd, The Atrium, Southern Gate, Chichester, West Sussex,
PO19 8SQ, UK

Editorial Offices
9600 Garsington Road, Oxford, OX4 2DQ, UK
The Atrium, Southern Gate, Chichester, West Sussex, PO19 8SQ, UK
1606 Golden Aspen Drive, Suites 103 and 104, Ames, Iowa 50010, USA

For details of our global editorial offices, for customer services and for information about how
to apply for permission to reuse the copyright material in this book please see our website at
www.wiley.com/wiley-blackwell

Library of Congress Cataloging-in-Publication Data

Substance use and older people / edited by Ilana Crome, Li-Tzy Wu, Rahul (Tony) Rao, Peter Crome.
  p. ; cm.
 Includes bibliographical references and index.
 ISBN 978-1-119-97538-0 (cloth)
I. Crome, Ilana B., editor.   II. Wu, Li-Tzy., editor.   III. Crome, Peter, editor.   IV. Rao, Rahul, editor.
[DNLM: 1. Substance-Related Disorders. 2. Aged. 3. Middle Aged. WM 270]
  HV5824.A33
  362.29084′9–dc23
                                        2014020561

A catalogue record for this book is available from the British Library.

Wiley also publishes its books in a variety of electronic formats. Some content that appears in print may not
be available in electronic books.

Set in 10/12.5pt Sabon by SPi Publisher Services, Pondicherry, India
Printed and bound in Malaysia by Vivar Printing Sdn Bhd

1 2015

This book is dedicated to our families – past, present and future.

CONTENTS

Contributors	xvii
Foreword	xxi
Introduction	xxiv
List of Abbreviations	xxvi

Section 1   Legal and ethical aspects of care for older people with substance misuse   1

1 Negotiating capacity and consent in substance misuse	3
Kritika Samsi	
Introduction	3
Substance abuse and capacity	3
Mental capacity legislation	4
Mental Capacity Act 2005	4
Capacity assessment	5
Capacity and unwise decisions	6
Consent, barriers to decision making and substituted decision making	6
Best interest decisions	8
Independent decision makers	8
Conclusion	9
References	9
2 Elder abuse	11
Jill Manthorpe	
Introduction	11
Defining elder abuse	11
Main reviews	12
Alcohol and substance misuse risk factors	12
Risk factors among older people	13
The effects of elder abuse	14
Discussion	15
Conclusions and next steps	15
References	16

3 **The United States perspective**   18
Cynthia M.A. Geppert and Peter J. Taylor
The ageing of the baby boomers and its impact
on substance abuse   18
Ethical and legal aspects of substance misuse
in older adults   19
    Confidentiality   19
    Informed consent   20
    Capacity   21
    Coercion   24
Conclusion   25
References   25

4 **The European perspective**   27
Abdi Sanati and Mohammed Abou-Saleh
Introduction   27
Use and possession   28
Crime   28
European Convention of Human Rights   28
Delivering services for the elderly with substance
misuse – ethical aspects   29
Research and development   30
Policy making   31
Some differences between Europe and the USA   31
Ethical issues regarding treatment   32
Stigma   32
Underprescribing controlled drugs   32
Summary   33
References   34

5 **Clinical medicine and substance misuse: research, assessments
and treatment**   35
*Amit Arora, Andrew O'Neill, Peter Crome
and Finbarr C. Martin*
Introduction   35
Why is clinical medicine important?   36
    Identification   37
    The health effects of substance abuse   39
Challenges for the future   46
    Research   47
    Identification tools   47
    Training and support   48
Conclusions   49
References   49

Section 2   Epidemiology and demography   57

6 **Cigarette smoking among adults aged 45 and older in the
   United States, 2002–2011**   59
   Shanta R. Dube and Li-Tzy Wu
   Introduction   59
   Evaluation methodology   61
   Results   62
     Sociodemographic characteristics of older adults: 2002 versus 2011   62
     National trend in current smoking prevalence: 2002–2011   65
     Current smoking prevalence by socioeconomic status: 2002 versus 2011   66
     Adjusted odds ratios of correlates of current smoking:
     2002 versus 2011   66
   Discussion   71
   Conclusion   72
   References   73

7 **Epidemiology and demography of alcohol and the older person**   75
   Stephan Arndt and Susan K. Schultz
   Introduction   75
   Main reviews   76
     Epidemiological estimates of prevalence of alcohol use   76
     Estimates of alcohol problems based on amount of drinking   76
     Importance of threshold selection for defining problem use   80
     Estimating problem use from survey samples   80
     Summary of epidemiological estimates   81
     Specific problematic drinking behaviours: binge drinking   81
     Diagnoses of abuse or dependence   83
     Older substance abuse treatment populations   84
     Special populations of older substance users   85
     Demographic correlates of problem use   86
   Discussion   87
   Conclusions and next steps   87
   References   88

8 **Epidemiology and demography of illicit drug use and
   drug use disorders among adults aged 50 and older**   91
   Shawna L. Carroll Chapman and Li-Tzy Wu
   Introduction   91
   Survey studies   92
   Studies of treatment-seeking or clinical patients   101
   Health implications   104
   Discussion   105
   Next steps   106
   References   106

9 Epidemiology and demography of nonmedical prescription
   drug use   109
   Jane Carlisle Maxwell
   Introduction   109
   Findings   110
      National surveys   110
      Emergency department cases   112
      Treatment admissions   113
      Drug poisoning deaths   114
   Discussion   116
   Conclusions   118
   Acknowledgement   118
   References   118

Section 3   Longitudinal studies of ageing
and substance abuse   121

10 Ageing and the development of alcohol use and misuse   123
   Marja Aartsen
   Background   123
   Results   124
      Differences in alcohol use across cohorts   125
      Developments in alcohol use within people   126
      Gender differences   126
      Different trajectories   126
      Age and onset of problem drinking   127
   Discussion   127
      Explanations for age differences in alcohol use   127
   Conclusions   128
   References   129

11 Progression from substance use to the development of
   substance use disorders   133
   Carla L. Storr and Kerry M. Green
   Introduction   133
   Substance use progression process   134
   Risk factors influencing substance use progression   137
      Individual factors   137
      Substance properties   139
      Environmental influences   140
   Future direction   141
   Conclusions   143
   Acknowledgement   144
   References   144

12 **Psychopharmacology and the consequences of alcohol
and drug interactions** 149
*Vijay A. Ramchandani, Patricia W. Slattum, Ashwin A. Patkar,
Li-Tzy Wu, Jonathan C. Lee, Maitreyee Mohanty,
Marion Coe and Ting-Kai Li*
The extent of alcohol and drug misuse among older adults 149
  Substance misuse in the general population 149
  Substance misuse or addiction in clinical settings 150
  Co-morbidities among older substance misusers 151
Psychopharmacology of alcohol and drug misuse in older people 152
  Neurocircuitry of abused substances 152
Alcohol–drug interactions in older adults 155
  Mechanisms of alcohol–medication interactions 156
  Significance of the problem 156
  Concurrent use of alcohol and potentially interacting
  medications 157
  Consequences of concurrent use of alcohol and
  medications 158
Clinical presentation and evaluation of substance
use disorders in the elderly 158
  Clinical presentations (case vignettes) 159
  Medical co-morbidities 161
  Screening for substance use disorders 161
  Evaluation of substance use disorders 162
  Cognitive impairment in the elderly with substance use disorders 163
  Safety assessment of the elderly with substance use disorders 164
  Medications for individuals with substance use disorders 164
Conclusions 166
References 166

**Section 4   Comprehensive geriatric assessment
and special needs of older people** 171

13 **Comprehensive geriatric assessment and the special needs of older people** 173
*Dan Wilson, Stephen Jackson, Ilana B. Crome, Rahul (Tony) Rao
and Peter Crome*
Background 173
Assessment 175
  Setting 176
  Barriers to assessment 176
  High-risk groups 177
  Presenting problems 177
  Collateral information 178
  General principles of assessment 179

Screening 182
Psychiatric assessment 183
Case presentations 184
Driving and substance misuse 184
Older women and alcohol misuse 184
Polysubstance misuse 185
The frequent attender 185
Alcohol and cognitive impairment 186
Pain and substance misuse 187
Discussion 187
Conclusion 187
References 188

Section 5   Screening and intervention in health care settings   193

14 Screening and brief intervention in the psychiatric setting 195
M. Shafi Siddiqui and Michael Fleming
Overview 195
Screening and assessment for alcohol use disorders 197
Single question screen for an alcohol use disorder 197
Quantity and frequency questions 198
Proxy questions such as CAGE 198
Symptoms of abuse or dependence 199
Alcohol biomarkers 199
Illicit drugs 202
Rationale for screening older adults for marijuana,
cocaine and other illicit drugs 202
Screening for illegal drugs in the psychiatric setting 202
Recommended screening questions to detect drug use 202
Screening for drug abuse/dependence 203
Screening for illicit drug use with toxicology screening 203
Prescription drug abuse 204
Rationale for screening older adults 204
Screening for prescription drug abuse 205
Brief intervention for alcohol, prescription drug abuse
and illegal drug use 206
Summary 208
References 209

15 Tobacco use cessation 212
Daniel J. Pilowsky and Li-Tzy Wu
Introduction 212
Smoking cessation interventions among older adults 214
Multimodal interventions 214
Medication-based interventions 216

Counselling and behavioural interventions 217
Physician-delivered interventions 217
Other interventions 218
Conclusions 218
References 219

Section 6 Use of substance abuse treatment services among older adults 223

16 Epidemiology of use of treatment services for substance
use problems 225
Shawna L. Carroll Chapman and Li-Tzy Wu
Introduction 225
Tobacco cessation service use and characteristics 225
Alcohol treatment use and characteristics 230
Trend in substance abuse treatment admissions 238
Drug abuse treatment use and outcomes 243
Substance abuse treatment in general health
care settings 245
Discussion and conclusion 246
References 247

17 Implications for primary care 249
Devoshree Chatterjee and Steve Iliffe
Background 249
Implications for primary care 249
Different populations at risk 250
Screening in primary care 251
Scale of benefit 252
Co-morbidities and social context 252
Conclusions 253
References 253

18 Addiction liaison services 255
Roger Bloor and Derrett Watts
Introduction 255
Organizing an addiction liaison service to a general hospital 256
Case vignette 1 256
Addiction liaison services for older adults 257
Essential elements of liaison service provision for older adults 258
Screening for alcohol problems in older adults 259
Screening for drug use problems 260
Case vignette 2 260
Summary 261
References 262

19 Current healthcare models and clinical practices   265
Rahul (Tony) Rao, Ilana B. Crome, Peter Crome
and Finbarr C. Martin
Introduction   265
An ageing population   265
Service development and provision   266
Integrated care and workforce development   267
Conclusions and recommendations   269
References   269

Section 7   Age-specific treatment interventions and outcomes   271

20 Pharmacological and integrated treatments in older adults
with substance use disorders   273
Paolo Mannelli, Li-Tzy Wu and Kathleen T. Brady
Introduction   273
Tobacco   274
Alcohol   275
Opioids   277
Benzodiazepines   278
Other substances of abuse   280
   Stimulants   280
   Cannabis   281
Integrated treatments   281
Conclusion and future directions   284
References   285

21 The assessment and prevention of potentially inappropriate
prescribing   295
Denis O'Mahony
Introduction   295
Inappropriate psychotropic use in elderly patients   296
Implicit IP criteria   297
Explicit IP criteria   298
Applying STOPP/START criteria as an intervention   299
Other methods of detection and prevention
of IP in older people   307
   Comprehensive Geriatric Assessment (CGA)   307
   Pharmacist review and intervention   308
   Prescriber education, audit and feedback   308
   Computerized provider order entry with clinical
   decision support   309
Conclusions   309
References   310

22 Age-sensitive psychosocial treatment for older adults
   with substance abuse   314
   Kathleen Schutte, Sonne Lemke, Rudolf H. Moos and Penny L. Brennan
   Introduction   314
   Seven characteristics of age-sensitive treatment   316
       1 – Supportive and nonconfrontational   316
       2 – Flexible   316
       3 – Sensitive to gender differences   317
       4 – Sensitive to cultural differences   317
       5 – Focus on client functioning   318
       6 – Holistic   319
       7 – Focus on coping and social skills   319
   Six components of age-sensitive psychosocial treatment   320
       1 – Biopsychosocial assessment   320
       2 – Treatment planning   321
       3 – Attention to co-occurring conditions   322
       4 – Referrals and care coordination   325
       5 – Empirically-supported psychosocial interventions   325
       6 – Adjuncts to psychosocial interventions   328
   Age-segregated or mixed-age treatment   329
   Future directions   330
   Acknowledgements   331
   References   332

23 Integrated treatment models for co-morbid disorders   340
   Rahul (Tony) Rao
   Introduction   340
   Methodological approach to examining SMCD in older people   341
       A. Current systems of care for substance misuse and mental disorders 341
       B. Service implications   342
       C. Principles underlying integrated treatment models
          for SMCD in older people   342
       D. Developing integrated treatment models for older people
          with substance misuse and co-morbid psychiatric disorders   344
       E. Research evidence for integrated treatment models   346
   Future direction and challenges   347
   References   347

Section 8   Policy: proposals for development   351

24 Proposals for policy development: drugs   353
   Susanne MacGregor
   Introduction   353
   Recognition of a need or problem and arguments made to
   justify the development of policy   354

Policy options 356
Policy design and implementation 359
Conclusion 360
References 360

25 Proposals for alcohol-related policy development
United States 364
Ralph Hingson and Ting-Kai Li
Recommended low-risk alcohol consumption levels 364
Traffic crash risks among the elderly 365
Driving policy questions 365
Factors to consider when contemplating legal policies 365
Summary and conclusions 369
References 370

26 Proposals for policy development: tobacco 372
Michael Givel
Introduction 372
Past and present approaches to reduce tobacco consumption 372
Phase three anti-tobacco efforts 373
Legal approach 373
Regulatory and tobacco tax approaches 374
Anti-tobacco counter-marketing campaigns 376
Recent anti-tobacco proposals 376
Product modification and 'safer' cigarettes 376
Harm reduction 377
Cigarette neo-prohibitionism 377
Smoke-free movies 377
Policy proposals to further reduce tobacco prevalence 378
References 378

27 Recommendations 383
Ilana B. Crome, Peter Crome, Rahul (Tony) Rao and Li-Tzy Wu
Background 383
Epidemiology 384
Clinical presentations 384
Education and training 385
Who gets treatment – treatment interventions 386
Concluding remarks 386

Index 388

CONTRIBUTORS

Marja Aartsen, PhD
Assistant Professor Sociology and
Social Gerontology,
Faculty of Social Sciences,
VU University Amsterdam,
Amsterdam, The Netherlands

**Mohammed Abou-Saleh, MPhil
FRCPsych**
Professor of Psychiatry, St George's,
University of London,
London, UK

Stephan Arndt, PhD
Director, Iowa Consortium for
Substance Abuse Research;
Professor, Departments of Psychiatry
and Biostatistics, University of Iowa,
Iowa City, IA, USA

Amit Arora, MD FRCP MSc
Consultant Physician and Geriatrician,
University Hospital of North
Staffordshire, Stoke-on-Trent, UK;
Honorary Clinical Lecturer,
Keele University,
Keele, UK

**Roger Bloor, MD MPsyMed
FRCPsych Cert Med Ed**
Consultant in Addiction Psychiatry,
North Staffordshire Combined
Healthcare NHS Trust,
Teaching Fellow,
School of Medicine,
Keele University,
Keele, UK

Kathleen T. Brady, MD PhD
Associate Provost of Clinical and
Translational Research,
and Director of South Carolina
Clinical and Translational Research
Institute, Medical University of South
Carolina, Charleston, SC, USA

Penny L. Brennan, PhD
Research Health Science Specialist,
Center for Health Care Evaluation,
Veterans Affairs Palo Alto Health Care
System, Menlo Park CA, USA

Shawna L. Carroll Chapman, PhD
Postdoctoral Researcher,
Department of Psychiatry and
Behavioral Sciences,
School of Medicine,
Duke University Medical Center,
Durham, NC, USA

Devoshree Chatterjee, MRCGP
Department of Primary Care &
Population Health,
University College London,
London, UK

Marion Coe, BA
Intramural Research Training
Award Fellow, Section on Human
Psychopharmacology, Laboratory of
Clinical and Translational Studies,
National Institute on Alcohol Abuse
and Alcoholism,
National Institutes of Health,
Bethesda, MD, USA

Ilana B. Crome, MA MD MPhil FRCPsych
Senior Research Fellow, Imperial College, London, UK
Emeritus Professor of Addiction Psychiatry, Keele University, Keele, UK
Honorary Consultant Psychiatrist, South Staffordshire and Shropshire Healthcare NHS Foundation Trust, Stafford, UK
Honorary Professor, Queen Mary University of London, London, UK

Peter Crome, MD PhD DSc FRCP FFPM FBPharmacolS
Honorary Professor, Department of Primary Care and Population Health, University College London, London, UK
Emeritus Professor of Geriatric Medicine, Keele University, Keele, UK

Shanta R. Dube, PhD MPH
Associate Professor, Division of Epidemiology and Biostatistics, School of Public Health, Georgia State University, Atlanta, GA, USA

Michael Fleming, MD MPH
Professor, Department of Psychiatry and Family Medicine, Northwestern University, Chicago, IL, USA

Cynthia M.A. Geppert, MD MA PhD MPH MSBE
Chief, Consultation Psychiatry and Ethics, New Mexico Veterans Affairs Health Care System, Albuquerque, NM, USA
Associate Professor of Psychiatry and Director of Ethics Education, University of New Mexico School of Medicine, Albuquerque, NM, USA

Michael Givel, PhD
Professor, Department of Political Science, The University of Oklahoma, Norman, OK, USA

Kerry M. Green, PhD
Assistant Professor, Department of Behavioral and Community Health, University of Maryland School of Public Health, College Park, MD, USA

Ralph Hingson, ScD MPH
Director, Division of Epidemiology and Prevention Research, National Institute on Alcohol Abuse and Alcoholism, Bethesda, MD, USA

Steve Iliffe, FRCGP
Professor of Primary Care for Older People, Department of Primary Care & Population Health, University College London, London, UK

Stephen Jackson, MD FRCP
Professor of Clinical Gerontology, King's College Hospital, London, UK

Jonathan C. Lee, MD
Associate Medical Director, The Farley Center at Williamsburg Place, Williamsburg, VA, USA
Assistant Professor, Department of Psychiatric Medicine, Brody School of Medicine, East Carolina University, NC, UK

Sonne Lemke, PhD
Health Science Specialist, Program Evaluation and Resource Center, Department of Veteran Affairs, Menlo Park, CA, USA

Ting-Kai Li, MD
Professor, Department of Psychiatry
and Behavioral Sciences,
School of Medicine,
Duke University Medical Center,
Durham, NC, USA

**Susanne MacGregor, MA PhD
FRSA FAcSS**
Professor of Social Policy,
Department of Social and
Environmental Health Research,
Faculty of Public Health and Policy,
London School of Hygiene and
Tropical Medicine,
University of London,
London, UK

Paolo Mannelli, MD
Associate Professor,
Department of Psychiatry and
Behavioral Sciences,
School of Medicine,
Duke University Medical Center,
Durham, NC, USA

Jill Manthorpe, MA
Professor of Social Work,
Director of the Social Care
Workforce Research Unit,
King's College London,
London, UK

**Finbarr C. Martin, MD MSc FRCP
FCST**
Consultant Geriatrician at
Guys & St Thomas' NHS
Foundation Trust, London, UK
Honorary Professor of Medical
Gerontology, King's College London,
London, UK

Jane Carlisle Maxwell, PhD
Senior Research Scientist,
Addiction Research Institute,
Center for Social Work Research,
The University of Texas at Austin,
Austin, TX, USA

Maitreyee Mohanty, PhD
Pharmacotherapy and
Outcomes Science,
Virginia Commonwealth
University, Richmond, VA, USA

Rudolf H. Moos, PhD
Professor Emeritus,
Stanford University; Center for
Health Care Evaluation,
Veterans Affairs Palo Alto Health
Care System,
Menlo Park, CA, USA

Denis O'Mahony, MD FRCPI FRCP
Department of Medicine (Geriatrics),
University College Cork,
Cork, Ireland

**Andrew O'Neill, MB BaO
BCh MRCP**
Specialist Registrar in Geriatric
Medicine, University Hospital of
North Staffordshire,
Stoke-on-Trent, UK

Ashwin A. Patkar, MD MRC Psych
Professor, Department of Psychiatry
and Behavioral Sciences, Department
of Community and Family Medicine,
Medical Director,
Duke Addiction Programs &
Center for Addictive Behavior
and Change, School of
Medicine, Duke University
Medical Center,
Durham, NC, USA

Daniel J. Pilowsky, MD MPH
Assistant Professor of Clinical
Epidemiology and Psychiatry,
Department of Epidemiology,
Mailman School of Public Health;
and Department of Psychiatry,
Columbia College of Physicians
and Surgeons, Columbia University,
New York, NY, USA

Vijay A. Ramchandani, PhD
Investigator and Chief,
Section on Human
Psychopharmacology,
Laboratory of Clinical and
Translational Studies,
National Institute on Alcohol Abuse
and Alcoholism,
National Institutes of Health,
Bethesda, MD, USA

**Rahul (Tony) Rao, MD MSc
FRCPsych**
Visiting Researcher,
Department of Old Age Psychiatry,
Institute of Psychiatry,
London, UK and Lead for Dual
Diagnosis, Mental Health of Older
Adults and Dementia Clinical
Academic Group, South London and
Maudsley NHS Foundation Trust, UK

Kritika Samsi, MSc PhD
Research Fellow, Social Care
Workforce Research Unit,
King's College London, UK

Abdi Sanati, MD MSc MRCPsych
Consultant psychiatrist,
North East London NHS
Foundation Trust,
London, UK

Susan K. Schultz, MD
Professor, University of Iowa College
of Medicine,
Iowa City, IA, USA

Kathleen Schutte, PhD
Research Health Science Specialist,
Center for Health Care Evaluation,
Veterans Affairs Palo Alto Health Care
System, Menlo Park CA, USA

M. Shafi Siddiqui, MD
Linden Oaks Medical Group,
Naperville, IL, USA

Patricia W. Slattum, PharmD PhD
Director, Geriatric Pharmacotherapy
Program,
Professor of Pharmacotherapy and
Outcomes Science,
Virginia Commonwealth University,
Richmond, VA, USA

Carla L. Storr, MPH ScD
Professor, Department of Family &
Community Health,
University of Maryland School of
Nursing, Baltimore, MD, USA

Peter J. Taylor, DO MA
Consulting Geropsychiatrist
New Mexico Veterans Affairs Health
Care System,
Albuquerque, New Mexico, USA

**Derrett Watts, MBBCh DRCOG
MRCPsych MPhil**
Consultant Psychiatrist – Substance
Misuse, North Staffordshire
Combined Healthcare NHS Trust,
Stoke-on-Trent, UK

Dan Wilson, MB BChir MRCP
Department of Clinical Gerontology,
King's College Hospital NHS
Foundation Trust, London, UK

Li-Tzy Wu, ScD MA
Professor of Psychiatry,
Department of Psychiatry and
Behavioral Sciences,
School of Medicine,
Duke University Medical Center,
Durham, NC, USA

FOREWORD

This edited volume by Drs. Crome, Wu, Rao and Crome, *Substance Use and Older People,* arrives at just the right moment. To my knowledge this is the first book devoted to substance use disorders in older adults. And the substances include alcohol, illicit drugs and tobacco use, all challenges to the well-being of the elderly. Focus upon substance misuse has become increasingly timely, for the numbers of older adults will increase dramatically with the aging of the baby boomer generation (what some have called the grey tsunami). In addition, the relatively heavier burden of substance misuse in middle aged cohorts compared to older cohorts suggests that the burden will be even greater than simply projected by the increased number of elders. Not only is this volume timely, the chapters are comprehensive, in depth and they cover a range of critical topics, from psychopharmacology to the legal and ethical issues associated with substance misuse in this population. The multinational focus is also welcomed as concentration on one country, even one continent, will underestimate the valuable data which is emerging worldwide and which can inform clinical practice.

I recently chaired an Institute of Medicine (IOM) committee that produced the report, *The Mental Health and Substance Use Workforce for Older Adults: In Whose Hands?* (National Academies Press, Washington, DC, 2012). Our original charge was to explore the workforce needs for mental health problems in the elderly, yet within one hour of our first meeting the committee identified substance use disorders of enough importance that it received equal billing in our report. The demographic and epidemiological data presented in this volume clearly document the presence of problems, such as binge drinking of alcohol, that are already of public health significance among older adults. In addition, middle-aged cohorts carry a much higher burden than elders of substance misuse that cuts cross a variety of problems, from nonprescription use of prescription medications to use of illegal substances such as heroin and cocaine. We have not accumulated data to date that documents that this burden will persist as the middle aged enter late life. Nevertheless, past history and common sense suggests that we will face a higher burden clinically in the future among the elderly than we face today. And according to the IOM report, we do not have a workforce, both professional and volunteer, to meet the needs of these elders. To prepare investigators and practitioners to fill the emerging workforce need, this volume will be especially valuable as a basic text and ready reference for this workforce.

Substance use disorders and their functional as well as social limitations are complex and typically occur with other health problems. They often go unnoticed in large part because they are not viewed by health-care professionals and family as important enough to explore in clinical or even personal family communications. We do not wish to consider that our parents and grandparents, who we may have revered during our earlier lives, may suffer from an embarrassing problem that we typically identify with adolescents or young adults. If we are guilty of this oversight, we either consciously or inadvertently cover over substance misuse and, subsequently, the problems worsen and the older adult suffers. The chapter on elder abuse highlights that abuse may take the form of neglect of obvious problems and discouragement in seeking proper care.

Recent analyses of extant data focusing on the elderly, especially the National Survey of Drug Use and Health (NSDUH), has documented over the past ten years the burden in the elderly, a burden that was not well studied in past epidemiological studies. To put this another way, if we need solid numbers to back up our claim that substance use is a major public health problem among the elderly, the numbers are there! Chapters on epidemiology and demography within this text provide easy access for readers, especially valuable if readers are in a position to influence policy at local, state and federal levels.

The next section of the book focuses upon multidisciplinary approaches to substance misuse in the elderly. Treating substance use disorders at all ages, but especially in the elderly, requires a team. And that team may consist of members not usually associated with treatment at earlier ages, namely practitioners from clinical medicine. Older persons are vulnerable to a 'cascade effect' if they suffer from significant and ongoing problems in one area of health. For example, an older adult may have abused alcohol for many years and now encounters medical complications, such as liver disease. Yet another older person may suffer from low back pain and then begin to abuse opioid analgesics. Rarely can one specialist adequately treat substance misuse in isolation. This volume provides a framework for multidisciplinary as well as interdisciplinary approaches to care. I would propose that professionals treating older adults with substance use disorders may actually need transdisciplinary care, namely care from professionals who have skills which cross disciplines, such as substance use counselling, medical care of co-morbid problems and the effective use of psychotropic medications. That is, care of this population may benefit from a new type of professional in the future.

Treatment of substance use disorders across the life cycle is difficult, with few approaches leading to consistently dramatic improvements which persist through time. The authors of chapters on treatment and the system of health care focused on late life substance misuse recognize these challenges and provide useful guides for better treatment today and into the future. I would propose, however, that our knowledge base for effective treatment is incredibly limited for the elderly and we need much more research to inform our treatments. This volume provides a useful catalogue and description of current evidence-based as well as traditional treatments from which future treatments can evolve.

In conclusion, the authors appropriately consider policy. I refer back to the IOM volume, for the main purpose of that report was to shape policy. The response? Despite these tough economic times and the divisions in Washington, people are listening. So policy makers must speak up. The material in this volume will be welcomed by those who both set and advocate for policy. The time is right, the material is current, and the need is great. Congratulations to the authors and editors for their excellent work.

Dan G. Blazer MD, MPH, PhD
JP Gibbons Professor of Psychiatry and Behavioral Sciences
Duke University Medical Center
Durham, NC, USA

INTRODUCTION

Ilana B. Crome, Li-Tzy Wu, Rahul (Tony) Rao and Peter Crome

There are indications that the number of older people who use substances is increasing, and is likely to continue to do so over the next two decades [1, 2]. Projections suggest that the number of older illicit substance misusers will double from 2006 to 2020 [3]. Inappropriate prescribing, drug interactions and the use of over-the-counter medicines as well as those purchased on the Internet are further cause for concern, as they are likely to result in premature mortality and morbidity, as well as damage to social functioning. Experience in clinical practice (e.g. addiction, old age psychiatry, geriatric medicine, emergency medicine and trauma) suggests that this vulnerable group is a growing but neglected. Further investigation of this cohort is gaining momentum in research activities related to epidemiological trends, clinical treatment outcomes and professional education, and in health and social policy (e.g. models of service delivery). In 2011, the United Kingdom the Royal College of Psychiatrists produced a comprehensive report on older substance misusers, 'Our Invisible Addicts' – it generated enormous interest and reaction [4].

In this book we explore substance use and misuse (including smoking, drinking, illicit drug use, nonmedical prescription drug use, and dependence) in older people. We have covered thorny issues such as differences in the description and diagnosis of substance use, misuse and dependence in older people as compared with younger ages. By examination of recent trends, projections and predictors, we have charted the risk and resilience features, such as inequalities, culture and ethnicity, drawn from the longitudinal studies of ageing. We take the life course approach, which advances the understanding of older substance users from the social, biological, psychological and medical perspectives. We examine the effects and adverse acute and chronic impact of substances on the physical, psychological, psychiatric and social function. We have outlined what the core features of comprehensive geriatric assessment should encompass. We have paid special attention to the clinical consequences and complications – physical and psychiatric – including falls, trauma, pain, cancer, cardiovascular, respiratory, neuropsychiatric, dementia, confusion, depression, anxiety and paranoid disorders. This is because of the poorer outcomes associated and the greater likelihood that older people with substance problems might suffer from combined disorder.

Treatment interventions and outcomes in older people, in concert with the development of service delivery models, are a major focus. The spotlight has been on treatment options – being sensitive to the special needs of older people (sensory, mobility, cognitive); cultural context of treatment; the range of options (i.e. one-to-one, group, family); pharmacological (alcohol, opiate, nicotine and co-morbid disorders);

psychological/psychosocial approaches (e.g. general counselling), specific techniques (e.g. motivational enhancement and cognitive behavioural therapy); self-help/mutual aid, the role of social networks and creative programmes. Social factors in recovery and rehabilitation (including statutory services such as home care) and the impact of housing (e.g. sheltered accommodation) have been emphasized. Where available we have presented information on service models and service designs. Paramount is the identification of gaps that can stimulate future research. Recommendations for policy directives, in relation to current and future practice, build on the synthesis of knowledge acquired during the evolution of the book.

We have pointed to the diverse treatment settings at which older substance misusers might present or need emergency or continuing care. These include intensive care, trauma, pain management, cardiovascular and respiratory units, gastroenterology, oncology, neurology, ophthalmology, primary care, geriatric medicine, old age psychiatry wards, nursing homes, renal and urological units, and even prison. We have embraced ethics and philosophies of care of older people, such as the role of users, carers and communities.

We hope that the book will be of interest to old age psychiatrists, addiction psychiatrists, geriatricians, gerontologists, educators, epidemiologists, psychologists, clinical social workers, case managers, sociologists, policy makers, researchers, general health-care providers, commissioners, and politicians. Undergraduate and postgraduate students across the range of clinical, research and policy arenas as well as related specialist areas such as epidemiology, clinical medicine, psychology, economics, sociology, social and health policy should also find it engaging and stimulating.

Our aim has been to review, reflect upon and draw together the most up-to-date information available on a fast growing topic. We hope this will be a resource for practitioners (be it in geriatric medicine, old age psychiatry as well as other professional groups), policy makers and educators who are involved in the prevention of ill health of older people and who provide interventions. That the public, as well as professionals, become increasingly concerned is a key aspiration.

We have been so privileged to work with distinguished colleagues around the world who have enriched the process and have come together to produce something that we believe does take the field forward. We would like to acknowledge their passion, goodwill, enthusiasm, patience, humour and rigour.

References

1. Wu, L.T. and Blazer, D.G. (2011) Illicit and nonmedical drug use among older adults: A review. *Journal of Aging and Health*, **23**, 481–504.
2. Wu, L.T. and Blazer, D.G. (2014) Substance use disorders and psychiatric comorbidity in mid and later life: a review. *International Journal of Epidemiology*, 43(2), 304–317.
3. Han, B., Gfroerer, J.C., Colliver, J.D. and Penne, M.A. (2009) Substance use disorder among older adults in the United States in 2020. *Addiction*, **104**, 88–96.
4. Crome, I.B., Rao, T., Tarbuck, A. *et al.* (2011) Our Invisible Addicts. Royal College of Psychiatrists Council Report 165. Royal College of Psychiatrists, London.

LIST OF ABBREVIATIONS

AA	Alcoholics Anonymous
AADL	Advanced Activities of Daily Living
ACE-R	Addenbrooke's Cognitive Assessment – Revised
ADE	Adverse Drug Event
ADL	Activities of Daily Living
ADR	Adverse Drug Reaction
AIDS	Acquired Immune Deficiency Syndrome
ALN	Alcohol Liaison Nurse
ARPS	Alcohol-Related Problem Survey
ASAM	American Society of Addiction Medicine
AUD	Alcohol Use Disorder
AUDIT	Alcohol Use Disorders Identification Test
AUDIT C	Alcohol Use Disorders Identification Test Consumption
BAC	Blood Alcohol Concentration
BAL	Blood Alcohol Level
BI	Brief Intervention
BRFSS	Behavioural Risk Factor Surveillance System
BRITE	Brief Intervention and Treatment for Elders
CAGE	Cut down, Annoyed by criticism, Guilty about drinking, Eye-opener drinks
CARET	Co-morbidity Alcohol Risk Evaluation Tool
CBC	Complete Blood Count
CBT	Cognitive Behavioural Therapy
CDC	Centers for Disease Control and Prevention
CDT	Carbohydrate Deficient Transferase
CGA	Comprehensive Geriatric Assessment
CI	Confidence Interval
CIDI	Composite International Diagnostic Interview
CMHT	Community Mental Health Team
CNS	Central Nervous System
COPD	Chronic Obstructive Pulmonary Disease
CSAT	Center For Substance Abuse Treatment
CT	Computed Tomography
DA	Dopamine
DAST	Drug Abuse Screening Test
DAWN	Drug Abuse Warning Network
DHHS	Department of Health And Human Services

DSM	Diagnostic and Statistical Manual of Mental Disorders
DSM-IV	Diagnostic and Statistical Manual of Mental Disorders, Fourth Edition
DSM-5	Diagnostic and Statistical Manual of Mental Disorders, Fifth Edition
E-CBT	Extended Cognitive Behavioural Therapy
ECHR	European Convention of Human Rights
e-combined	Extended combined treatment
ED	Emergency Department
EEG	Electroencephalogram
EMCDDA	European Monitoring Centre for Drugs and Drug Addiction
E-NRT	Extended Nicotine Replacement Therapy
ENSPM	English National Survey of Psychiatric Morbidity
EtG	Ethyl Glucuronide
EtS	Ethyl Sulfate
FDA	Food and Drug Administration
FRAMES	Feedback, Responsibility, Advice, Menu of options, Empathy, Self-efficacy
GABA	Gamma-Aminobutyric acid
GATS	Global Adult Tobacco Survey
GFR	Glomerular Filtration Rate
GGT	Gamma-Glutamyl Transferase
GP	General Practitioner
HCV	Hepatitis C Virus
HIPAA	Health Insurance Portability Rehabilitation Act
HIV	Human Immunodeficiency Virus
IADL	Instrumental Activities of Daily Living
ICD-10	International Classification of Diseases, Tenth Revision
IDUs	Injection Drug Users
IP	Inappropriate Prescribing
IT	Information Technology
LCA	Latent Class Analysis
LSD	Lysergic Acid Diethylamide
LTCs	Long-Term Conditions
MAOI	Monoamine Oxidase Inhibitor
MAST	Michigan Alcoholism Screening Test
MAST-G	Michigan Alcoholism Screening Test – Geriatric version
MATCH	Matching Alcoholism Treatments to Client Heterogeneity
MCA	Mental Capacity Act
MCV	Mean Corpuscular Volume
MET	Motivational Enhancement Therapy
MH/SU	Mental Health/Substance Use
MI	Motivational Interviewing
MM	Moderation Management
MMAST-G	Mini-Michigan Alcoholism Screening Test – Geriatric
MMSE	Mini-Mental State Examination
mPFC	Medial Prefrontal Cortex
MRI	Magnetic Resonance Imaging

NCHS	National Center for Health Statistics
NCPIE	National Council on Patient Information and Education
NDTMS	National Drug Treatment Monitoring System
NESARC	National Epidemiologic Survey on Alcohol and Related Conditions
NGO	Non-Governmental Organization
NHIS	National Health Interview Survey
NHS	National Health Service
NHSDA	National Household Survey on Drug Abuse
NIAAA	National Institute on Alcohol Abuse and Alcoholism
NICE	National Institute for Health and Clinical Excellence
NIDA	National Institute of Drug Abuse
NLAES	National Longitudinal Epidemiologic Survey
NMDA	N-methyl-D-aspartate
NRT	Nicotine Replacement Therapy
NSAID	Non-Steroid Anti-Inflammatory Drug
NSAL	National Survey of American Life
NSDUH	National Survey on Drug Use and Health
OR	Odds Ratio
OTC	Over-The-Counter
PCMH	Patient-Centered Medical Home
PET	Phosphatidyl Ethanol
PIM	Potentially Inappropriate Medication
PPO	Potential Prescribing Omission
PTSD	Post-Traumatic Stress Disorder
QF	Quantity/Frequency
RPT	Relapse Prevention Therapy
SAMHSA	Substance Abuse and Mental Health Services Administration
SBIRT	Screening of substance misuse, Brief Intervention, and Referral to Treatment
SDDCARE	Senior Drug Dependents and Care Structure Project
shARPS	Short Alcohol-Related Problem Survey
SLCHS	Southeast London Community Health Survey
SMAST	Short Michigan Alcoholism Screening Test
SMAST-G	Short Michigan Alcoholism Screening Test – Geriatric Version
SMCD	Substance Misuse and Co-morbid Mental Disorders
STOPP	Screening Tool of Older Persons' Prescriptions
SUD	Substance Use Disorder
TEDS	Treatment Episode Data Set
THC	$\Delta 9$-tetrahydrocannabinol
TIP	Treatment Improvement Protocol
TSF	Twelve-Step Facilitation
UC	Usual Care
VTA	Ventral Tegmental Area
WHO	World Health Organization

LEGAL AND ETHICAL ASPECTS OF CARE FOR OLDER PEOPLE WITH SUBSTANCE MISUSE

Chapter 1

NEGOTIATING CAPACITY AND CONSENT IN SUBSTANCE MISUSE

Kritika Samsi

Social Care Workforce Research Unit, King's College London, UK

Introduction

Mental capacity is an individual's ability to make autonomous decisions for themselves, the significance of which has increased with greater recognition of the involvement of the individual as a 'self-governing welfare subject' [1] with greater emphasis on personal choice and self-determination of his or her own health and social care decisions [2].

The complexity of problems associated with substance use in older people means that there are particular risks around capacity or 'competency', through impairment in cognition, judgement and function [3]. There could be co-morbid mental health problems that may further contribute to their impairment [4]. Decision making capacity is vital not only for individuals to be able to express their preferences for long-term care but also in the case of immediate in-patient care, when practitioners may face complex decision making issues. Some of these issues include: (i) timing of capacity assessment; (ii) conflict between presence of capacity, alongside evidence of self-neglect and need for medical care; and (iii) the role of the practitioner in encouraging the older person to give up addictions that are harmful to them [3].

Substance abuse and capacity

There had been diagnostic limitations in the Diagnostic and Statistical Manual of Mental Disorders iv (DSM-iv) in how substance abuse and dependence were classified, resulting in what some believed were deceptively low rates of identification of older individuals with substance abuse and dependencies [5]. Some of the criteria used – such as giving up activities and the inability to fulfil major role obligation at work – were also criticized for being irrelevant to an older population [5].

The physiological impact of acute alcohol intoxication is more severe in the elderly, with an increase in the risk of delirium [5]. In the brain, alongside an acute confusional state, cerebral atrophy can result in global cognitive impairment [5].

Substance Use and Older People, First Edition.
Edited by Ilana B. Crome, Li-Tzy Wu, Rahul (Tony) Rao and Peter Crome.
© 2015 John Wiley & Sons, Ltd. Published 2015 by John Wiley & Sons, Ltd.

Mental capacity, judgment and ability to consent can also be affected. Most types of dementia are more prevalent in older people with alcoholism [6].

Impaired decision making capacity characterizes substance misuse. The diagnostic criteria according to the Diagnostic and Statistical Manual of Mental Disorders 5 (DSM-5) acknowledge this, as substance dependence is described as persistent use despite knowing the negative physical and psychological effects of the substance [7]. The self-destructive choices and decisions made by substance abusers have been termed 'myopia', which are deficits in emotional signalling that produce poor short-term decisions for immediate gains despite potential for higher losses in the future [8].

Mental capacity legislation

Several western countries have existing legislation that addresses and protects autonomy, capacity, dignity and decision making for vulnerable people. None of this legislation codifies 'age' as a specific vulnerability in itself, and safeguarding incapacity or deteriorating capacity more wholistically is prioritized instead. By handing over decision making powers to a trusted relative or nominated consultee, an individual can choose who makes decisions on their behalf and, thereby, assert their choices and preferences through them.

The Guardianship and Administration Act was introduced in 1993 in South Australia and in 2000 in Queensland, two of Australia's largest states. The Substitute Decisions Act and the Health Care Consent Act were introduced in Ontario, Canada, in 1992 and 1996, respectively. Most of these Acts incorporate the same principles, with variations in the way capacity assessments are carried out, and how care priorities are determined. Presuming an individual has capacity, unless proven otherwise, is the guiding principle in all of these Acts.

Scotland, England and Wales introduced legislation around capacity more recently. Scotland introduced the Adults with Incapacity Act in 2000, and the Mental Capacity Act 2005 was introduced in 2007 in England and Wales; both are applicable to those over the age of 16 years.

Using the Mental Capacity Act 2005 as a case example in England and Wales, the rest of this chapter illustrates some of the principles embedded in current legislation in the area of capacity and consent, focusing specifically on its applicability to those with a history of substance abuse.

Mental Capacity Act 2005

The Mental Capacity Act 2005 (MCA), implemented in England and Wales in 2007, introduced a variety of provisions to safeguard and enhance the rights of vulnerable people with compromised capacity [9]. Prior to the Act, it was sometimes challenging to ascertain 'mental capacity' to make decisions and different approaches were described under mental capacity legislation and mental health legislation [1].

A central principle of the MCA is the presumption that all adults have the capacity to make decisions for themselves, unless proven otherwise. Provisions for surrogate decision making should only be resorted to after it has been proved that an individual lacks capacity. The other four central principles of the Act include:

- A person must be given all practicable help before anyone treats them as not being able to make their own decisions.
- A person is not to be treated as unable to make a decision merely because he makes an unwise decision.
- Anything done or any decision made under this Act for or on behalf of a person who lacks capacity must be done, or made, in his/her best interests.
- Anything done or decided for or on behalf of a person who lacks capacity should be the least restrictive of their basic rights and freedoms.

Capacity assessment

There are a number of capacity and decision making assessment tools currently available [4]. In the MCA, a four-stage assessment of decision making ability is required to prove that an individual is unable to make a specific decision at that specific time. These include asking the following four questions:

1. Does the person have a general understanding of what decision they need to make and why they need to make it?
2. Does the person have a general understanding of the likely consequences of making, or not making, this decision?
3. Is the person able to understand, retain, use and weigh up the information relevant to this decision?
4. Can the person communicate their decision (by talking, using sign language or any other means)? Would the services of a professional (such as a speech and language therapist) be helpful?

Inherent to this assessment is the recognition that capacity is not an absolute state but varies over time and with the decision that is required to be made. For substance misusers, this becomes an even more crucial issue, as their states of incapacity may fluctuate according to the level of intoxication or delirium. Capacity should, therefore, be seen as decision specific, rather than all encompassing. If a person is deemed to be 'lacking capacity', it means that they lack capacity to make a particular decision or take a particular action for themselves at the time the decision or action needs to be taken. The MCA applies to anyone who has 'an impairment of or disturbance in the functioning of the mind or brain' and was warmly welcomed for not using the phrase 'mental disorder', which may not be appropriate to a person with substance abuse problems. Similarly, an 'incapable' adult is defined in the Scottish and the Canadian legislation as someone unable to act, make, communicate, understand or retain the memory of decisions.

Legal frameworks such as the MCA 2005, codifying complex phenomena that can threaten the autonomy of vulnerable individuals, have wide applicability: from types of decisions, such as day-to-day support [10], advance decision making about personal health and welfare [11], end of life care [12]; to different settings [13], such as medical encounters [14] and long-term care facilities [15]; and to a wide range of professionals [16–19].

Capacity and unwise decisions

A central feature of the Mental Capacity Act is the acknowledgement that individuals who have the capacity to make their own decisions are in a position to make what may be deemed 'unwise' decisions. In many cases, this applies to risk taking, such as gambling, forming relationships and choosing a certain type of lifestyle. In the case of substance misuse, individuals may choose to continue to use a substance in spite of being aware of its harmful effects. If that individual is deemed as having the capacity to make a decision for themselves – that is if that individual is shown as being able to weigh up the consequences of their decision and still choose to use a particular substance – the MCA safeguards that individual's decision making capacity by suggesting that decisions otherwise deemed 'unwise' are legally acceptable.

Consent, barriers to decision making and substituted decision making

If capacity is an individual's ability to make decisions, 'consent' can be seen as granting permission or agreeing to the decisions themselves. In relation to consenting, the relevance of the MCA covers three relevant areas: substituted decision making powers, best interest principles and independent decision makers.

The MCA facilitates substituted decision making through the uptake of Advance Care Planning (ACP) in three forms:

1. Statements of wishes and preferences for future care that an individual would want, that was made before they lost capacity. These can include requests for specific medical treatments, such as artificial nutrition and hydration. Although these written statements are not binding, a practitioner must consider them before making a proxy decision on an individual's behalf, and any reason they are choosing to go against the written statement of wishes should be clearly recorded.
2. Advance decisions to refuse certain treatment where an individual stipulates that they do not want a particular intervention, such as artificial nutrition or hydration, or withdrawal of life support system. These are more binding on practitioners. (Box 1.1 shows provisions outlined in the MCA).
3. Granting a trusted friend or relative Lasting Power of Attorney (LPA) to cover health and welfare decisions. Granting LPA is a powerful principle since the MCA was introduced, as it enables individuals to have their wishes and preferences included at a time when they may be unable to contribute themselves.

Box 1.1 Provisions for Advance decisions outlined in the MCA

24.1 'Advance decision' means a decision made by a person ('P'), after he has reached 18 and when he has capacity to do so, that if:

(a) at a later time and in such circumstances as he may specify, a specified treatment is proposed to be carried out or continued by a person providing health care for him, and

(b) at that time he lacks capacity to consent to the carrying out or continuation of the treatment, the specified treatment is not to be carried out or continued.

Box 1.2 Provisions for Lasting Power of Attorney outlined in the MCA

9.1 A lasting power of attorney is a power of attorney under which the donor ('P') confers on the donee (or donees) authority to make decisions about all or any of the following:

(a) P's personal welfare or specified matters concerning P's personal welfare, and

(b) P's property and affairs or specified matters concerning P's property and affairs, and which includes authority to make such decisions in circumstances where P no longer has capacity.

A health and welfare LPA can run in conjunction with a financial LPA, which sets out a decision maker for property and financial affairs. Surrogate decision makers may also be granted the power to make decisions about life-sustaining treatment. (Provisions relating to an LPA outlined in the MCA are outlined in Box 1.2.)

There are some pre-conditions that govern the behaviour of an LPA, such as any substitute decision must be made in the individual's best interest [20]. Moreover, there are a number of decisions that are outside the remit of substitute decision making, where it is deemed impossible to be able to gauge another's likelihood of consent (section 27 of the MCA). For instance, nothing in the Act permits a substituted decision to be made regarding any of the following:

- consenting to marriage or a civil partnership;
- consenting to have sexual relations;
- consenting to a decree of divorce on the basis of two years' separation;
- consenting to the dissolution of a civil partnership;
- consenting to a child being placed for adoption or the making of an adoption order;
- discharging parental responsibility for a child in matters not relating to the child's property; or
- giving consent under the Human Fertilisation and Embryology Act 1990.

> **Box 1.3 Best interest checklist in the MCA**
>
> - Can the decision be delayed to when the individual may have capacity?
> - No decision should be based on the person's appearance, age, medical condition, or behaviour.
> - All relevant information should be considered, and every attempt to involve the person in the decision should be made.
> - Any written or verbal statement expressing the individual's wishes, values, choices, preferences, beliefs and feelings should be considered.
> - Views of family members, partners or other supporters who may know the person better should be incorporated.
> - If the decision is about treatment, the decision maker should not be motivated by a desire to bring about their death, nor by assumptions of their quality of life.

Best interest decisions

An individual's best interest is always protected under capacity legislation. The MCA 2005 deems that all surrogate decisions should be in an individual's best interest. However, research has indicated prevalent discrepancies about how this may be rolled out in practice [21], especially in relation to challenges with resolving conflicts [22]. Best interest decision making includes a checklist, which takes into account key indicators of an individual's well-being. In complex cases, such as working with older people with substance misuse problems, assessing impaired capacity may not be straightforward and there may be additional criteria to take into account. Hazelton *et al.* [3] suggest delaying significant decisions for as long as possible, or at least until acute effects have passed, as well as differentiating between alcohol-related cognitive deficits and addiction-related denial. Using the least restrictive option is also always recommended. (Box 1.3 shows a best interest checklist outlined in the MCA.)

Independent decision makers

Family networks of older people with a history of substance misuse may be absent, chaotic and challenging to engage. A relationship between the older person and their family relative may not be based on trust or prior knowledge of preferences of the individual.

Legislation has provided for these cases through the establishment of new roles; for example, in England and Wales, that of an Independent Mental Capacity Advocate (IMCA), or someone who can step in to the role of substitute decision maker, to make major decisions regarding treatment or accommodation for a person with impaired capacity [23]. Definition of roles and remits in all of the legislation largely overlap, with their main remit being to consider the best interests of the vulnerable person in order to make the decision that contributes most to their well-being (Box 1.4).

Box 1.4   Stipulations covering an Independent Mental Capacity Advocate

36.2 The regulations may, in particular, make provision requiring an advocate to take such steps as may be prescribed for the purpose of:

(a) providing support to the person whom he has been instructed to represent ('P') so that P may participate as fully as possible in any relevant decision;
(b) obtaining and evaluating relevant information;
(c) ascertaining what P's wishes and feelings would be likely to be, and the beliefs and values that would be likely to influence P, if he had capacity;
(d) ascertaining what alternative courses of action are available in relation to P;
(e) obtaining a further medical opinion where treatment is proposed and the advocate thinks that one should be obtained.

Conclusion

The relevance of capacity and consent to older people with a history of substance misuse is significant, given that capacity to consent for this vulnerable group may be impaired, may fluctuate and many of them may have absent or chaotic social networks. This then leaves professionals working with this group with greater responsibilities to assess capacity, safeguard the interests of this group, uphold the dignity and enhance the autonomy of their patients. While there is availability of and access to training in these legal matters in some countries, and much of current legislation has been welcomed as being easy-to-read and apply, there needs to be greater emphasis on the availability of these resources in order that all professionals prioritize this in their daily work. Ultimately, creating a safer environment where patients are self-determining individuals making their own choices about their well-being is the goal of any health and social care system.

References

1. Newman, J. (2007) The double dynamics of activation. *International Journal of Sociology and Social Policy*, **27**, 364–375.
2. Okai, D., Owen, G., McGuire, H., *et al.* (2007) Mental capacity in psychiatric patients: systematic review. *British Journal of Psychiatry*, **191**(4), 291–297.
3. Hazelton, L., Sterns, G.L. and Chisholm, T. (2003) Decision-making capacity and alcohol abuse: clinical and ethical considerations in personal care choices. *General Hospital Psychiatry*, **25**(2), 130–135.
4. Jeste, D.V. and Saks, E. (2006) Decisional capacity in mental illness and substance use disorders: empirical database and policy implications. *Behavioural Science and Law*, **24**, 607–628.
5. Menninger, J.A. (2001) Assessment and treatment of alcoholism and substance-related disorders in the elderly. *Bulletin of the Menninger Clinic*, **66**(2), 166–183.
6. Thomas, V.S. and Rockwood, K.J. (2001) Alcohol abuse, cognitive impairment, and mortality among older people. *Journal of the American Geriatrics Society*, **49**(4), 415–420.

7. American Psychiatric Association (2013) *Diagnostic and Statistical Manual of Mental Disorders*, 5th edn. American Psychiatric Publishing, Arlington, VA.
8. Bechara, A., Dolan, S. and Hindes, A. (2002) Decision-making and addiction (Part II): myopia for the future or hypersensitivity to reward? *Neuropsychologia*, 40, 1690–1705.
9. Office of Public Sector Information (2005) The Mental Capacity Act 2005. http://www.legislation.gov.uk/ukpga/2005/9/contents (last accessed 27 March 2014).
10. Stanley, N. and Manthorpe, J. (2008) Small acts of care: exploring the potential impact of the Mental Capacity Act 2005 on day-to-day support. *Social Policy and Society*, 8(1), 37–48.
11. Dunn, M.C., Clare, I.C.H. and Holland, A.J. (2010) Living a life like ours: support workers' accounts of substitute decision-making in residential care homes for adults with intellectual disabilities. *Journal of Intellectual Disability Research*, 54(2), 144–160.
12. Schiff, R., Sacares, P., Snook, J., *et al.* (2006) Living wills and the Mental Capacity Act: a postal questionnaire survey of UK geriatricians. *Age and Ageing*, 35(2), 116–121.
13. Weiner, M.F., Davis, B., Martin-Cook, K., *et al.* (2007) A direct functional measure to help ascertain optimal level of residential care. *American Journal of Alzheimer's Disease and Other Dementias*, 22(5), 355–359.
14. Shah, A., Banner, N., Heginbotham, C. and Fulford, B. (2009) The application of the Mental Capacity Act 2005 among geriatric psychiatry patients: a pilot study. *International Psychogeriatrics*, 21(5), 922.
15. Manthorpe, J., Samsi, K., Heath, H. and Charles, N. (2011) 'Early days': knowledge and use of the Mental Capacity Act 2005 by care home managers and staff. *Dementia*, 10(3), 283–298.
16. Johnstone, C. and Liddle, J. (2007) The Mental Capacity Act 2005: a new framework for healthcare decision making. *Journal of Medical Ethics*, 33, 94–97.
17. Lyons, C., Brotherton, A., Stanley, N., *et al.* (2007) The Mental Capacity Act 2005: implications for dietetic practice. *Journal of Human Nutrition and Dietetics*, 20(4), 302–310.
18. Tullet, J. (2008) Legal and Ethical Frameworks for Mental Health Nursing. In: *Older People and Mental Health Nursing: A Handbook of Care* (eds R. Neno, B. Aveyard and H. Heath), Blackwell Publishing Ltd, Oxford, UK. doi: 10.1002/9780470692240.ch6.
19. Manthorpe, J. and Samsi, K. (2009) Implementing the Mental Capacity Act 2005: challenges for Commissioners. *Journal of Integrated Care*, 17(3), 39–47.
20. Brown, R. and Barber, P. (2008) *The Social Worker's Guide to the Mental Capacity Act 2005*. Learning Matters, Exeter.
21. Myron, R., Gillespie, S., Swift, P. and Williamson, T. (2007) Whose Decision? Preparation for and Implementation of the Mental Capacity Act in statutory and non-statutory services in England and Wales. The Mental Health Foundation, London.
22. Joyce, T. (2010) *Best Interests Guidance on Determining theBest Interests of Adults who Lack the Capacity to Make a Decision (or Decisions) for Themselves [England and Wales]*. The British Psychological Society, Leicester.
23. Ministry of Justice (2007) Mental Capacity Act 2005 Code of Practice. TSO (The Stationery Office), Norwich. http://webarchive.nationalarchives.gov.uk/+/http://www.dca.gov.uk/legal-policy/mental-capacity/mca-cp.pdf (last accessed 27 March 2014).

Chapter 2
ELDER ABUSE

Jill Manthorpe
Social Care Workforce Research Unit, King's College London, UK

Introduction

This chapter considers the complex relationships between substance misuse and the abuse, mistreatment and neglect of older people. While it is often suggested that the risks of elder abuse from a care giver, paid or unpaid, or a family member or social contact, are enhanced by substance misuse or dependency on behalf of the perpetrator, this chapter notes that older people who are being victimized may turn to alcohol or other substances to cope with their situations. Moreover, as this chapter outlines, there is some evidence that older people who are themselves substance misusers may be at particular risk of abuse because they are not able to adequately defend themselves or seek help. It is also possible that the stigma and shame of being victimized are reinforced by the known stigma and shame for older people of being judged as a substance misuser [1]. These risks may be compounded by ageism and ageist practices among professionals [2].

One further complication of this subject is that of the terms 'abuse' and 'abuser'. In the area of elder abuse research and services that have a focus on adult protection or safeguarding, the term abuse is often used broadly, covering financial abuse, physical abuse, psychological abuse and so on. The term 'abuser' or 'perpetrator' is often used to describe the individual who is responsible for this. In contrast, in other settings the terms 'abuser' and 'abuse' may be used to mean 'user' and 'misuse' of substances such as alcohol and illicit drugs. The rest of this chapter seeks to use these terms in their context but in practice this is an area ripe for misunderstanding and confusion.

Defining elder abuse

Defining elder abuse is not easy [3] and there is no universally accepted definition. In its absence the following definition is often referred to:

> 'A single or repeated act or lack of appropriate action occurring within any relationship where there is an expectation of trust, which causes harm or distress to an older person or violates their human and civil rights' [4].

Substance Use and Older People, First Edition.
Edited by Ilana B. Crome, Li-Tzy Wu, Rahul (Tony) Rao and Peter Crome.
© 2015 John Wiley & Sons, Ltd. Published 2015 by John Wiley & Sons, Ltd.

Types of elder abuse are generally categorized as physical, psychological (or emotional), financial, sexual and neglect. One or several of these abusive acts or omisions may be experienced in a person's own home, in community settings or in settings such as long-term care facilities and hospitals. As many of the studies mentioned in this chapter illustrate, the populations studied vary by age group, location and the form of abuse investigated, including incidence [5].

However, the subject of elder abuse is relatively isolated from other research and practice debates. Until recently, it has been relatively distant from debates about domestic violence (intimate partner violence) and 'hate' crimes.

Generally, elder abuse is a term used to refer to the ill treatment of an older person (usually defined as over age 65 years) by commission (abuse) or omission (neglect).

There is general agreement that most studies underestimate the prevalence of elder abuse [5] and, while general estimates of around 5% of the older population may be a reasonable conclusion, this may be much higher among people who are not able to express their fears or who are overlooked or disbelieved, which may include people who are misusing substances or drinking heavily. Evidence from the United States is that one in 10 older people experiences some form of elder abuse, but only one in 25 cases is reported to social services agencies [6], despite mandatory reporting in many parts of this country.

In most developed states, policies and procedures outline the expected response of national and local government to incidents and allegations of elder abuse [7]. In England, the term safeguarding is used to describe multiagency arrangements to prevent and respond to the abuse of 'vulnerable' (generally meaning frail or disabled) adults. Use of this term marks a shift in emphasis from reaction and rescue to prevention and harm minimization, in the hope that outcomes for the older person might be better and of their own choosing [8]. In other parts of the world the terminology referring to the organization of professionals working to investigate and respond to elder abuse may include adult protective services.

Main reviews

Alcohol and substance misuse risk factors

Early studies, mainly from the United States, drew attention to the need to examine the characteristics of perpetrators of elder abuse, rather than victims, and highlighted that substance dependence among perpetrators was a salient risk factor [9]. Risk of physical and verbal abuse appears to depend more on problematic characteristics associated with the perpetrator, particularly their physical and mental health (including dementia) but notably, in many studies, their consumption of and reliance on alcohol. For example, in a national study of referrals to protective services in Ireland [10], of those alleged perpetrators (n = 586) among whom a health problem ('issue') was identified, alcohol issues were noted among 31% and drug issues among 4% [10, Table 2]. Among the 1086 clients for whom there was cause for concern (alleged victims), drug issues featured among very few (0.3%) but alcohol problems featured among 8%. However, the first systematic review of risk factors for abuse in people aged 55 years and over [11, p.296] pointed out that while many of the studies reviewed highlighted risk factors among perpetrators of drug abuse, alcohol misuse and gambling, these were 'lower quality' studies.

There are few accounts of this from older people directly. In one of the few studies where older people who have been abusers provided an account of their actions, the following illustrates a husband's account of his assault of his wife when he was drunk:

> 'I got violent with it ... I got so violent that the police were called ... I had actually hit my wife and I couldn't remember it. The minute that I triggered off, I knew there was something desperately wrong, when you can't remember.
>
> All I remember was sitting down, watching the telly (TV) and everything else was a blank until the police came' (quoted in [12, p.12]).

There is little evidence that the stress of caring for an older person is, on its own, a cause of abuse. Risk appears to depend more on problematic characteristics associated with the abuser – notably, in many studies, their heavy consumption of alcohol or drug substances [13, 14, p.95]. As Lachs and Pillemer [15, p.1265] have also observed:

> '... people who commit elder abuse tend to be heavily dependent on the person they are mistreating. Abuse results in some cases from attempts by the relatives (and especially adult offspring) to obtain resources from the victim. Moreover, situations have been identified in which a tense and hostile family relationship is maintained because a financially dependent son or daughter is unwilling to leave and thus lose parental support.'

Much research has focused on domestic contexts but there is also some evidence that people working in services for older people, in care or health-related settings, may abuse older people as a consequence of their own substance misuse. For example, theft in nursing homes may be in the context of the staff member's own substance misuse or dependencies (or those of their social networks). Such theft and fraud may be of residents' medications or their property [16]. The practice of undertaking background checks or 'screening' job applicants or current staff working in jobs caring for older people for substance misuse and criminal histories is one way that employers seek to minimize the risks that these people may present [17].

Risk factors among older people

It is important not to over emphasize the role of substance misuse in heightening the risks of elder abuse in the context of the limitations of current knowledge. The most consistent correlates of mistreatment across abuse types among community-dwelling older people (aged 60 years and over) in a major US study recently revealed these to be low social support and previous traumatic event exposure [18].

While there are some indications that older people may turn to alcohol to cope with abuse – the idea of alcohol as an escape or coping mechanism is a powerful explanation – there are some accounts of how alcohol and substance misuse among older people makes them potentially vulnerable to abuse. Friedman *et al.* [19] tracked 41 cases of severe trauma among older people admitted to hospital in the United States and found that the victims of severe traumatic elder abuse were more likely to be female, to have a neurological or mental disorder, and to abuse drugs or alcohol than other case controls. One account from practice in a specialist agency working with older people with alcohol problems in London [12, p.9] described a case example where a family member sought control over their older relative by 'enabling them to drink'. This seemed to be a form of abuse in that the provision of alcohol was becoming a form of restraint or control. From Scotland, another practitioner, working in an addiction unit for people aged over 50 years old, reported:

> 'There is one (case) at the moment we have been working with from when the project started. It has been a long process, he has alcohol-related brain damage. He has a friend who helps him with his finances, and there is an issue whether he (the friend) is taking advantage or not' [12, p.11].

The effects of elder abuse

The World Health Organization (WHO) review of Elder Abuse and Alcohol [20] outlined how the impacts of elder abuse and harmful alcohol use could lead to similarly harmful consequences, covering three main areas:

1. Physical injury, financial problems, social withdrawal, malnourishment and emotional and psychological problems, including depression and cognitive and memory impairments. As older people are often physically weaker, physical violence may result in greater injury or their convalescence may take longer.
2. Since older people often have lower incomes and less opportunity to replace money, the economic consequences of financial abuse may be severe (although largely unmeasured).
3. Reduced life expectancy or depression may occur. In some cases harmful alcohol use becomes a coping strategy but lead to other life limiting health problems, such as cardiovascular diseases, cancers and unintentional injuries. Wider impacts of alcohol use in older people are substantial, including self-neglect, suicidal ideation/behaviour.

However, it is important for practitioners to be vigilant about elder abuse even where there are no strong indications of harm. For example, in a very large postal survey (N = 91 749) of postmenopausal women (aged 50–79 years) in the United States, Mouton *et al.* [21] found that some lifestyle factors were associated with exposure to abuse (those reporting 'Any Abuse'; n = 10 199).

Relevant to this chapter, alcohol use was less likely among those women surveyed who had been exposed to abuse – particularly verbal abuse – a finding the researchers reported to be surprising because, they commented, abuse victims (of intimate partner violence and elder abuse) generally have a higher rate of alcohol and substance use. The researchers suggested that the respondents to their survey '*did not perceive a need to "escape" an abusive relationship through alcohol use*' (p.609). Another possibility raised by the researchers was that '*these women perceived alcohol use as increasing their vulnerability and thus escalating their potential of being victimized by greater violence*' (p.609).

Discussion

This chapter has pointed to the potential for alcohol and substance misuse to be risk factors for elder abuse among older people and those providing them with care and support. Elder abuse takes many forms and health and care professionals working with older people need to be aware of their own roles and responsibilities in reducing the risks of this harm and ensuring that older people have their rights to live safely and without great fear of being mistreated or neglected. This requires professionals to be vigilant, have a high index of suspicion and to provide sufficient professional 'space' to older people to build up trust, and for them to confide when things are going wrong. As Wadd *et al.* [12, p.11] have also illustrated from practice accounts, there may be 'false positives' where things are not what they first seem, and 'jumping to conclusions' may be less likely if a multidisciplinary approach is adopted.

Practitioners and their managers also need to be aware of their own local or agency policies and procedures about reporting concerns, taking part in investigations, making decisions and monitoring. Practitioners with experience of substance misuse services have much to offer other professionals working with older people from their knowledge of about treatment options, including brief interventions, counselling, group or peer support, family interventions, risk assessment, monitoring and case management. They could also offer training (as recommended to family caregivers and care workers by Plant *et al.* [22]), participate in shared training among domestic violence practitioners and those working in elder protection services [23], and case consultation.

Conclusions and next steps

While there is growing evidence that the problem of elder abuse affects older people in all settings [5], there is far less evidence of what interventions work in prevention or what promotes resilience and survival among victims [24]. This chapter has explored three main issues: (i) the increased vulnerability of individual older people to elder abuse if they are misusing alcohol; (ii) increased risks to older people from people who are misusing alcohol or substances; (iii) the possibility that older people misusing alcohol may be doing so in the context of abusive experiences. As noted, there is limited but growing evidence, meaning that practitioners need vigilance and time to consider if an older person is at risk and should record their observations.

Awareness among professionals is increasing and there are substantial opportunities for multiagency and multidisciplinary practice to ensure that the rights of older people not to be abused or neglected are upheld. Practice in this area has been surprisingly underresearched. As this chapter has shown, the risk factors of alcohol and, to a lesser extent, substance abuse among the perpetrators of elder abuse have been identified for many years. This means that the knowledge and expertise of practitioners working in alcohol and substance misuse services could make a major impact in elder abuse prevention, and provide skilled care and support for victims and survivors.

References

1. Alcohol Concern Cymru (2011) Hidden Harm. Alcohol Concern Cymru, Cardiff.
2. Centre for Policy on Ageing (2009) Ageism and Age Discrimination in Primary and Community Health Care in the United Kingdom: A Review from the Literature. Centre for Policy on Ageing, London.
3. Dixon, J., Biggs, S., Tinker, A. *et al.* (2009) Abuse, Neglect and Loss of Dignity in the Institutional Care of Older People. King's College London.
4. World Health Organization (2002) A Global Response to Elder Abuse and Neglect: Building Primary Health Care Capacity to Deal with the Problem Worldwide: Main Report. World Health Organization, Geneva, Switzerland.
5. Cooper, C., Selwood, A. and Livingston, G. (2008) The prevalence of elder abuse and neglect: a systematic review. *Age and Ageing*, 37, 151–160.
6. Dong, X. (2012) Advancing the field of elder abuse: future directions and policy implications. *Journal of American Geriatrics Society*, 60, 2151–2156.
7. Sethi, D., Wood, S., Mitis, F. *et al.* (eds) (2011) European Report on Preventing Elder Maltreatment. World Health Organization, Geneva.
8. Manthorpe, J. (2013) Elder Abuse. In: *The Oxford Textbook of Old Age Psychiatry* (eds T. Dening and A. Thomas). Oxford University Press, Oxford.
9. Anetzberger, A. (2005) The reality of elder abuse. *Clinical Gerontologist*, 28, 1–25.
10. Clancy, M., McDaid, B., O'Neill, D. and O'Brien, J.G. (2011) National profiling of elder abuse referrals. *Age and Ageing*, 40, 346–352.
11. Johannesen, M. and LoGuidice, D. (2013) Elder abuse: a systematic review of risk factors in community-dwelling elders. *Age and Ageing*, 42, 292–298.
12. Wadd, S., Lapworth, K., Sullivan, M. *et al.* (2011) *Working with Older People*. University of Bedfordshire, Bedford.
13. O'Keefe, M., Hills, A., Doyle, M. *et al.* (2007) UK Study of Abuse and Neglect of Older People: Prevalence Survey Report. National Centre for Social Research, London.
14. Bonnie, R.J. and Wallace, R.B. (2003) Elder Mistreatment: Abuse, Neglect and Exploitation in an Aging America. National Research Council, Washington, DC.
15. Lachs, M. and Pillemer, K. (2004) Elder abuse. *The Lancet*, 364, 1263–1272.
16. Griffore, R.J., Barboza, G.E., Mastin, T. *et al.* (2009) Family members' reports of abuse in Michigan nursing homes. *Journal of Elder Abuse and Neglect*, 21(2), 105–114.

17. Galantowicz, S., Crisp, S., Karp, N. and Accius, J. (2010) Safe at Home? Developing Effective Criminal Background Checks and Other Screening Policies for Home Care Workers. AARP Public Policy Institute, Washington, DC.
18. Acierno, R., Hernandez, M.A., Amstadter, A. *et al.* (2010) Prevalence and correlates of emotional, physical, sexual, and financial abuse and potential neglect in the United States: The National Elder Mistreatment Study. *American Journal of Public Health,* **100**(2), 292–297.
19. Friedman, L., Avila, S., Tanouye, K. and Joseph, K. (2011) A case control study of severe physical abuse of older adults. *Journal of the American Geriatrics Society,* **59**(3), 417–422.
20. World Health Organization (2005) Elder abuse and alcohol. http://www.who.int/violence_injury_prevention/violence/world_report/factsheets/fs_elder.pdf (last accessed 27 March 2014).
21. Mouton, C.P., Rodabough, R.J., Rovi, S. *et al.* (2004) Prevalence and 3-year incidence of abuse among postmenopausal women. *American Journal of Public Health,* **94**(4), 605–612.
22. Plant, M., Curran, J. and Brooks, R. (2009) Alcohol and Ageing: the views of older women and carers. Gender Issues Network on Alcohol, Alcohol Focus Scotland, Glasgow, UK.
23. Payne, B. (2008) Training adult protective services workers about domestic violence: training needs and strategies. *Violence Against Women,* **14**(10), 1199–1213.
24. Ploeg, J., Fear, J., Hutchison, B. *et al.* (2009) A systematic review of interventions for elder abuse. *Journal of Elder Abuse and Neglect,* **21**(3), 187–210.

Chapter 3
THE UNITED STATES PERSPECTIVE

Cynthia M.A. Geppert[1] and Peter J. Taylor[2]

[1]New Mexico Veterans Affairs Health Care System/University of New Mexico School of Medicine, USA
[2]Haven Behavioral Hospital, USA

The ageing of the baby boomers and its impact on substance abuse

'Baby boomers' is an epithet for the generation born in the United States from 1946 to 1964. The term denotes the demographic cohort born after World War II but connotes a cultural group known historically for their championing of civil rights, emphasis on individual freedoms and increased use of substances of abuse. The baby boomers are the largest living generation, approximately 78 million, with the leading edge turning 65 in 2011, are changing the epidemiology of American substance misuse in an unprecedented way.

The Substance Abuse and Mental Health Services Administration (SAMSHA) Treatment Episode Data Set (TEDS) records demographic characteristics of admissions for substance abuse treatment, particularly facilities receiving public funding. While alcohol remained the most common substance of abuse among older adults, primary admissions for drugs other than alcohol rose 106% for elderly men and 119% for elderly women between the years 1999 and 2002 [1]. In the decade from 1995 to 2005, primary admissions for opioid misuse increased from 6.6 to 10.5% in persons 65 and older, as did admissions for cocaine and sedatives. The TEDS estimates that the number of adults over 50 with substance abuse problems will increase from 2.5 million in 1999 to 5.0 million by 2020 [2].

The social expectation is that substance misuse, especially of illicit drugs, decreases as individuals' progress through the life cycle. However, the baby boomers are the exception. Averaged data from the 2007–2009 National Survey on Drug Use and Health show that 4.8 million adults over the age of 50, about 5.2%, had used an illicit drug in the year prior to the survey. Marijuana use is predicted to triple from 2001 to 2020 in this generation and is the most frequently misused drug for men from 50 to 58 years old, with prescription drugs being more common in those over 60 [3]. Not only the prevalence but also the complexity and co-morbidity of elder substance misuse are increasing. In 2009, the proportion of older adults entering substance use treatment who were using alcohol in combination with

Substance Use and Older People, First Edition.
Edited by Ilana B. Crome, Li-Tzy Wu, Rahul (Tony) Rao and Peter Crome.
© 2015 John Wiley & Sons, Ltd. Published 2015 by John Wiley & Sons, Ltd.

other drugs more than tripled from 12.4 to 42%, as did the rate of elders with co-occurring substance and psychiatric problems (10.5 to 31.4%) [4].

Ethical and legal aspects of substance misuse in older adults

Several authors have commented upon how little attention substance misuse in elders has received in the professional literature [5]. The ethical and legal aspects of drug and alcohol use in older adults have been even more neglected [6]. Given the paucity of research, the information presented in this chapter is adapted from the small body of work on the legal and ethical aspects of substance abuse [7] and the more extensive scholarship on ethics and law relevant to the clinical care of elders [8]. Four dovetailing concepts – confidentiality, informed consent, decisional capacity and coercion – are most frequently involved in the ethical and legal dilemmas encountered in the treatment of older adults with substance misuse. These '4 Cs' will, accordingly, form the organizing and conceptual structure for the chapter.

Confidentiality

Confidentiality refers to the health care professional's obligation to not disclose a patients' health information without permission or as required by law, while *privacy* designates the patient's right to determine, within this regulatory framework, the conditions and circumstances under which they will permit their health information to be disclosed [9]. The stigmatization historically attached to misuse of substances in the United States has both religious and cultural roots in perceptions of addiction as a character flaw, sin or moral failing [10] rather than as a medical disease with social determinants [11]. Social stigma coupled with the illegality of much substance misuse in the United States has been a major obstacle to treatment seeking. In an effort to overcome this obstacle, the federal government passed stringent confidentiality regulations that designate data on substance use diagnosis and treatment as the most highly protected class of health information. These regulations supersede state statutes unless the latter are even more restrictive. There are two key regulations that govern the release of all substance use information: The Drug Abuse Prevention, Treatment and Rehabilitation Act (42 U.S.C; 42 C.F.R. Part 2) and the Health Insurance Portability and Accountability Act (HIPAA) of 1996 (45 C.F.R, part 160 and Subparts A and E of Part 164) [9]. The regulations apply to any programme that receives federal assistance, any health care entity that transmits health information electronically and to any individual who has either sought or been provided treatment. There are nine exceptions to these confidentiality rules; these are listed in Box 3.1.

The rigour of these regulations may generate ethical dilemmas for practitioners, particularly when state law is less strict. A dilemma that is frequently encountered in American practice is the older adult with alcohol dependence and early dementia who may be an impaired driver. Acting on nonmaleficence and the duty to safeguard

> **Box 3.1 Nine exceptions to privacy regulations**
>
> 1. Written informed consent utilizing the required form.
> 2. State mandated reporting of child or incapable elder abuse.
> 3. Medical emergencies.
> 4. Patient information that is not identifiable as related to substance misuse.
> 5. Disclosure under a special court order.
> 6. Interprofessional communications within a programme.
> 7. Authorized research, programme auditing for compliance or quality evaluation.
> 8. Disclosure to a qualified service organization.
> 9. Crime committed against programme staff on program premises.

the health of the public, the addiction professional will report the elder to the motor vehicle department, yet such reporting does not respect the patient's autonomy and could be a breach of confidentiality. The skilled clinician will work within the therapeutic alliance to try and persuade the older adult to voluntarily relinquish their keys. With the permission of the elder, the practitioner may involve friends or family to arrange alternative modes of transport to minimize the adverse effects of the loss of independence driving represents, especially in the United States. The difficulty of this all too common case underscores the need for clinicians to have familiarity with federal privacy regulations, state laws, professional guidance and institutional policies, and to have ready access to expert legal and ethical consultation.

Some experts question whether 42 C.F.R. Part 2 actually applies to the primary care settings where older adults usually receive care for substance misuse; yet, there is no doubt that HIPAA is in force in general medical settings. Practitioners often struggle with how to balance the duty to document the diagnosis and treatment of substance misuse accurately to ensure appropriate medical care, especially in an emergency, while also protecting the confidentiality of the information. Discrimination may result from even inadvertent release of this information to insurance companies, social service agencies or families, with the potential for refusal of coverage, denial of benefits or interpersonal conflict, all of which represent threats to the elders' economic and legal self-determination [12]. This is a form of social injustice that particularly burdens older adults and deters them from seeking treatment for substance misuse.

Informed consent

In the area of substance misuse, older adults are most often asked to provide informed consent for disclosure of substance use information and for treatment both for the primary substance use disorder and for associated medical and psychiatric conditions. The practice of informed consent for clinical treatment is foundational in Anglo-American ethics and law and operationalizes the principles of respect for persons and autonomy. There is consensus in the bioethics and legal communities that an adequate informed consent process must include discussion of diagnosis, prognosis with and without intervention (detoxification, outpatient therapy, residential or inpatient treatment, medications etc.) and the biopsychosocial risks and benefits of the various options.

Practitioners have an ethical, and indeed legal, obligation to take reasonable steps to enable an older adults' ability to provide informed consent, which practically means employing efforts to enhance decisional capacity. Empirical ethics work has found that the use of audiovisual aids, involvement of friends and family (with patient permission), repetition of information, educational materials congruent with the older adults' educational level, cultural background and intellectual ability can all improve the ability of even older adults with mild-to-moderate dementia to provide informed consent [13]. An older patient with acute alcohol intoxication or opioid withdrawal may be unable to provide informed consent for extended substance use treatment during the index episode but to conclude they totally lack decision making capacity is not ethically justifiable. Even when an older adult is unable to provide consent for complex treatment decisions, the same elders are often able to choose a surrogate decision maker, thereby maximizing remaining autonomy.

Capacity

Intact decisional capacity along with appropriately delivered information and reasonable voluntarism are the three requisite components for authentic informed consent. In the United States, the clinical judgment of decision making capacity is differentiated from the legal concept of competence. Capacity may be partial or fluctuating depending on medical and psychiatric conditions, and thus can be judged on a continuum, while competency is a legal determination of a court and is much more comprehensive [14]. The clinical capacity evaluation generally informs the legal competency adjudication but the two can also diverge, generating ethical conflicts for patients, families and professionals. A capacity evaluation could include assessment of an individual's ability to both perform specific tasks (finances, driving etc.) and/or to make specific decisions (i.e. choosing a power of attorney for health care and financial affairs). Appelbaum and colleagues have posited core abilities of decisional capacity that are now widely adopted in American health care and legal settings [15]. Clinical examples of these faculties relevant to older adults with substance misuse are summarized in Table 3.1.

The higher order faculties of reasoning and appreciation, as the table vignette's illustrate, present more shades of grey and result in a less clear-cut assessment of capacity than the simpler faculties of communication and understanding. Clinician's will often encounter an older adult with alcohol-related dementia who appears to lack insight into the harm resulting from the substance misuse. The awareness of harm and potential benefit of help are critical elements of the diagnosis of substance dependence and of authentic informed consent for treatment. In such a situation the clinician will need to implement a harm reduction programme based on a best interest model. The primacy of patient autonomy in the United States

Table 3.1 Elements of decisional capacity with clinical examples

Ability	Definition	Clinical example
• Communication	• Express a clear and consistent choice about proposed treatment	• Mr C, a 67-year-old admitted for a series of seizures secondary to methamphetamine use, is asked if he is willing to speak to a substance abuse counsellor. The patient responds with paranoid ideation and tangential thoughts but never answers the question.
• Understanding	• Comprehend the medical problem, the proposed treatment, any alternatives and the outcome of the various options	• Mrs R, a 75-year-old woman, is able to repeat back in her own words the risks of overtaking her prescription opioids. She is able to review and sign an opioid agreement.
• Reasoning	• Weigh the respective benefits and burdens of proposed treatments	• Mr J, a 69-year-old with cocaine and marijuana misuse, agrees to enter a residential programme. Mr J will have to take time off from work for the treatment and fears his boss may learn of his substance problem. But knows he has failed outpatient treatment multiple times because his wife uses. Mr J thinks he has more chance of being fired if he continues to use.
• Appreciation	• Link discussions about pros and cons of choices to a concrete situation facing the patient, specific to their priorities and needs	• Mrs B, an 80-year-old woman with alcohol-related dementia, is repeatedly in the emergency department after falling at home when intoxicated. She insists she does not have a drinking problem and is just clumsy and tripped over things. She refuses inpatient substance use treatment because she wants to remain home with her little dog. A social worker involves the patient's adult children who intervene to have their mother admitted for detoxification.

often leaves practitioners with few legal or social mechanisms for acting with even beneficent paternalism.

There are tools that clinicians and the courts can use to assess capacity but these have been criticized for their lack of clinical usefulness, being too theoretical and not evaluating the patient's ability to actually navigate a decision and implement it in the real world. Clinical guidelines around capacity assessment have also been developed based on formal neuropsychological testing of abilities, such as attention, executive function and visual-spatial reasoning, all of which chronic and heavy substance use may impair [16]. Although specific instruments and procedures are likely to miss much of the nuance of capacity assessment, there is evidence that relying on clinical acumen alone is also problematic. In a study by Kim *et al.*, five experts were asked to watch the same videos of patients and decide if they had the capacity to perform various tasks. The variation between experts is notable. One expert thought 43% of the patients had capacity to identify a surrogate, another thought 83% had this capacity [17].

A major ethical challenge of capacity assessment is often one of omission: lack of capacity and/or misuse of substances are frequently not detected in health care settings where the focus is on the diagnosis and treatment of medical disorders [18]. Identifying substance misuse or incapacity in an older adult can often complicate discharge planning, generating provider and system incentives to ignore the problems.

While dementia is a common source of impaired capacity in older adults, denial also diminishes capacity in persons who misuse substances. Individuals with substance use problems frequently deny or lack insight into the social, interpersonal and health-related risks of their drinking and drug use [19]. Denial is especially common when the substance of abuse is legal, such as alcohol, tobacco or prescription opioids. The cultural history of baby boomer substance misuse may render this generation less likely to recognize and admit problematic behaviour.

Alcohol-related dementia has been less studied than other types of dementia. However, some research suggests that up to 10% of patients with alcohol-related problems have or will progress to alcohol-induced persisting dementia [20]. Retrograde amnesia, confabulation, executive function deficits, problems with new learning and visual-spatial and constructional deficits characterize Wernicke–Korsakoff syndrome [21]. Alcohol-induced dementia differs from other dementias clinically and ethically. Firstly, the intermittent nature of alcohol-related cognitive problems has led some experts in the field to question whether the threshold for capacity for disposition should be raised to account for a predictable relapse and loss of ability to care for oneself once out of a supervised setting. However, other experts have disagreed and argue that such prognostication is neither clinically or ethically justifiable [22].

Secondly, alcohol-induced dementia is one of the few forms of cognitive impairment that is at least partially reversible with sobriety, good nutrition and medical care. A paradoxical situation thus ensues: an older adult admitted to hospital when intoxicated or withdrawing is initially incapable of participating in discharge planning. Just as social workers are making disposition plans that could include the appointment of a surrogate decision maker or even a guardian of person and placement in a skilled nursing facility, the elder makes a recovery sufficient to refuse the discharge plan or convinces a judge they can make their own decisions, even though they may not be in their best interest [22]. Court rulings in the United States have upheld the doctrine of the least restrictive alternative, allowing an older adult with substance misuse, and even marginal capacity, to function independently in spite of repeatedly making poor choices regarding both continued substance misuse and unsafe living conditions [23].

Coercion

The baby boomer's well-known rejection of authority may change the research finding that older adults are often more deferential than younger individuals to physicians or family in regards to health care decisions. Currently, older adults are less likely to be referred to substance misuse treatment by the criminal justice system or an employer. Data from the Drug and Alcohol Information System found that, in 2002, 42% of older adults were self-referred compared to 7% of younger patients. Healthcare providers referred 35% of older patients but only 11% of younger patients [24]. While these data seem to support the presumptive voluntariness of older adults' engagement in substance misuse treatment, they may also conceal undue influence from relatives or practitioners. Emotional or financial dependence on partners or adult children, lack of access to other health care resources or fears of abandonment by providers if they do not comply with recommendations for treatment represent potentials for hidden coercion [25].

More obvious forms of coercion arise when family members, or other care takers, provide the older adult with the chosen substance of misuse as a means of exerting personal or economic control; in most jurisdictions this constitutes elder abuse. However, if the elder does not meet the legal standard of incapacity, the courts and adult protective services may not become involved, leaving the clinician with the moral distress of knowing that the elder is being taken advantage of but lacking the legal standing to intervene.

Unlike some European countries, most American states do not consider substance misuse or substance-induced dementia *per se* as a mental illness subject to commitment laws and mental health codes (without a co-morbid psychiatric diagnosis). Thus, an elder who is a chronic alcoholic presenting severely depressed with suicidal tendencies can be admitted to a mental health facility for treatment on grounds of a danger to self and receive care for both disorders. Yet, another older adult who is seriously misusing prescription opioids, but has not threatened self or others and lacks criteria for grave passive neglect, may not be involuntarily admitted to a psychiatric or a medical facility [26].

For elders with legally adjudicated incompetence, the courts can appoint an independent guardian of person, fiduciary or conservator for finances. However, older adults without the financial or familial wherewithal to hire private attorneys may wait months or years to obtain such protections in states with few legal and public health resources. In these situations, the clinician should use all the powers of persuasion at their disposal, as well as the assistance of social workers, community advocacy groups and less self-interested relatives or friends, to protect the elder.

Conclusion

The baby boomer generation of elders will continue to alter the landscape of substance use disorder and its treatment for the next 30 years, just as it has changed youth and middle-age culture in the last 60 years. Health care providers expect that their clinical, legal and ethical responsibilities to these patients will need to respond to this new geography of old age. This chapter has summarized the current mental health, legal and ethical literature mapping this field in the United States.

References

1. SAMHSA (2005) Older Adults in Substance Abuse Treatment: Update. The DASIS Report, Office of Applied Studies, Substance Abuse and Mental Health Services Administration (SAMHSA), Rockville, MD.
2. SAMHSA (2007) Adults Aged 65 or Older in Substance Abuse Treatment: 2005. The DASIS Report, Office of Applied Studies, Substance Abuse and Mental Health Services Administration (SAMHSA), Rockville, MD.
3. SAMHSA (2011) Illicit Drug Use among Older Adults. The NSDUH Report, Center for Behavioral Statistics and Quality, Substance Abuse and Mental Health Services Administration (SAMHSA), Rockville, MD.
4. SAMHSA (2011) Older Adult Admissions Reporting Alcohol as a Substance of Abuse: 1992 and 2009. The TEDS Report, Center for Behavioral Statistics and Quality, Substance Abuse and Mental Health Services Administration (SAMHSA), Rockville, MD.
5. Patterson, T.L. and Jeste, D.V. (1999) The potential impact of the baby-boom generation on substance abuse among elderly persons. *Psychiatric Services*, **50**(9), 1184–1188.
6. Koenig, T.L. and Crisp, C. (2008) Ethical issues in practice with older women who misuse substances. *Substance Use & Misuse*, **43**(8–9), 1045–1061.
7. Geppert, C.M.A. and Robers, L.W. (2008) *The Book of Ethics: Expert Guidance for Professionals Who Treat Addiction*. Hazelden, Center City, MN.
8. Blank, K. (2004) Legal and Ethical Issues. In: *Comprehensive Textbook of Geriatric Psychiatry* (eds J. Sadavoy, L.F. Jarvik, G.T. Grossberg and, B.S. Meyers), 3rd edn. Norton, New York, NY.
9. Washington, D.B. and Demask, M. (2008) *Legal and Ethical Isssues For Addiction Professionals*. Hazelden, Center City, MN.
10. Morse, S.J. (2004) Medicine and morals, craving and compulsion. *Substance Use & Misuse*, **39**(3), 437–460.
11. Room, R. (2005) Stigma, social inequality and alcohol and drug use. *Drug and Alcohol Review*, **24**(2), 143–155.
12. Brooks, M.K. (1998) Appendix A - Legal and Ethical Issues. In: *Substance Abuse Among Older Adults*. Treatment Improvement Protocol (TIP) Series 26, Center for Substance Abuse Treatment.Substance Abuse and Mental Health Services Administration (SAMHSA), Rockville, MD.
13. Dunn, L.B. and Jeste, D.V. (2001) Enhancing informed consent for research and treatment. *Neuropsychopharmacology*, **24**(6), 595–607.
14. Jonsen, A.R., Seigler, M. and Winslade, W.J. (2010) *Clinical Ethics: A Practical Approach to Ethical Decisions in Clinical Medicine*, 7th edn. McGraw-Hill, Inc., New York.
15. Appelbaum, P.S. (2007) Clinical practice. Assessment of patients' competence to consent to treatment. *The New England Journal of Medicine*, **357**(18), 1834–1840.

16. Lai, J.M. and Karlawish, J. (2007) Assessing the capacity to make everyday decisions: a guide for clinicians and an agenda for future research. *American Journal of Geriatric Psychiatry*, 15(2), 101–111.
17. Kim, S.Y., Appelbaum, P.S., Kim, H.M. *et al.* (2011) Variability of judgments of capacity: experience of capacity evaluators in a study of research consent capacity. *Psychosomatics*, 52(4), 346–353.
18. Weintraub, E., Weintraub, D., Dixon, L. *et al.* (2002) Geriatric patients on a substance abuse consultation service. *American Journal of Geriatric Psychiatry*, 10(3), 337–342.
19. Duffy, J.D. (1995) The neurology of alcoholic denial: implications for assessment and treatment. *Canadian Journal of Psychiatry*, 40(5), 257–263.
20. Parsons, O.A. (1994) Determinants of cognitive deficits in alcoholics: the search continues. *The Clinical Neuropsychologist*, 8(1), 39–58.
21. Ridley, N.J., Draper, B. and Withall, A. (2013) Alcohol-related dementia: an update of the evidence. *Alzheimer's Research & Therapy*, 5(1), 3.
22. Hazelton, L.D., Sterns, G.L., and Chisholm, T. (2003) Decision-making capacity and alcohol abuse: clinical and ethical considerations in personal care choices. *General Hospital Psychiatry*, 25(2), 130–135.
23. Appelbaum, P.S. and Gutheil, T.G. (2007) *Clinical Handbook of Psychiatry and the Law*, 2nd edn. Lippincott, Williams & Wilkins, Philadelphia, PA.
24. SAMHSA (2005) Older Adults in Substance Abuse Treatment: Update. The DIAS Report, Office of Applied Studies, Substance Abuse and Mental Health Services Administration (SAMHSA), Rockville, MD.
25. Wild, T.C., Newton-Taylor, B. and Alletto, R. (1998) Perceived coercion among clients entering substance abuse treatment: structural and psychological determinants. *Addictive Behaviors*, 23(1):81–95.
26. Layde, J.B. (2008) Forensic issues in the treatment of addictions. In: *The Book of Ethics: Expert Guidance for Professionals who Treat Addiction* (eds C.M. Geppert and L.W. Roberts). Hazelden, Center City, MN.

Chapter 4

THE EUROPEAN PERSPECTIVE

Abdi Sanati[1] and Mohammed Abou-Saleh[2]

[1] North East London NHS Foundation Trust, UK
[2] St George's, University of London, UK

Introduction

In this chapter, the focus on the European Perspective of the ethical and legal status of substance misuse in people age over 65 year of age. To address this issue, there are few considerations that need to be clarified.

Firstly, the majority of studies in substance misuse have been carried out in adults of working age. Whilst there are issues specifically concerning the elderly, there is the potential for some extrapolation from studies concerning younger adults to the elderly population. Also, the legal and ethical aspects that apply to adults of working age apply to the elderly, too, which includes legal issues concerning drug misuse. Here emphasis is on matters that are specifically pertinent to the elderly population.

Secondly, any discussion on substance misuse pre-supposes the status of this condition as a mental disorder. Debates over this matter will undoubtedly affect the ethical and legal foundations of practice. The acknowledgement of the status of substance misuse as a mental disorder entails all the ethical and legal issues concerning doctor–patient/ service user–provider relationship. It also puts a responsibility on the service providers to provide appropriate and evidence-based treatments and services to improve outcomes for this group of patients.

With regards to the legal issues, there are different laws in different countries in Europe covering substance misuse. Here the focus is mainly, but not exclusively, on the United Kingdom. Since people above the age of 18 are considered as adults, there are no differences in law with regard to the elderly population compared with younger adults.

This chapter aims to address some of the relevant ethical and legal issues. After a summary of the approach in Europe to use, possession and associated crime, the influence of the European Convention of Human Rights is discussed. Then, the discussion moves on to the ethical issues concerning providing service and care for the elderly population with substance misuse.

Substance Use and Older People, First Edition.
Edited by Ilana B. Crome, Li-Tzy Wu, Rahul (Tony) Rao and Peter Crome.
© 2015 John Wiley & Sons, Ltd. Published 2015 by John Wiley & Sons, Ltd.

Use and possession

Under UK law, illegal substances are referred to as 'controlled drugs' [1]. They are divided into three categories, carrying different penalties for possession or dealing: *Class A* includes ecstasy, LSD, heroin, cocaine, crack, magic mushrooms and amphetamines (if prepared for injection); *Class B* includes amphetamines, cannabis, methylphenidate (Ritalin), pholcodine; and *Class C* includes tranquilizers, some painkillers, gamma hydroxybutyrate (GHB) and ketamine.

By and large, Europe has a more liberal approach to the illicit substances compared to the USA [2]. While misuse of illicit substances is not considered a crime in all European countries, the possession of substances is considered a crime. According to European Monitoring for Drugs and Drug Addictions, 'It is often considered that the difference between penalising use of drugs, and penalising possession of drugs for personal use, is an academic one – it is impossible to use drugs without possessing them' [3]. There are notable exceptions when it comes to actual use of the drug. For example, in The Netherlands, the sale of cannabis in certain coffee shops is allowed. In Portugal, possession and use of cannabis is no longer an offence punishable by criminal imprisonment.

Crime

There is clear evidence that use of illicit substances and crime are intricately related. According to the National Treatment Agency for Substance Misuse in the United Kingdom, 'All the evidence indicates that problem drug users are responsible for a large percentage of acquisitive crime, such as shoplifting and burglary' [4]. There has been a convergence between the criminal justice system and health agencies in tackling crime, as it is clear that effective treatment of the substance misuse has a definite impact in reducing crime.

There is an important issue specifically pertaining to the elderly. There is an increase in the population of elderly and they are one of the most vulnerable groups when it comes to prison sentences [5].

It is, therefore, extremely important to address the problem of substance misuse in this age group to avoid involvement of the criminal justice system.

European Convention of Human Rights

The European Convention of Human Rights (ECHR) is the overarching legal framework with which all the European signatories have to comply. It was developed in Europe post World War II in order to protect the human rights and freedom of European citizens. Its signatories include all 47 members of the European Council. There are several articles that are relevant to the topic under study here [6].

Article 5 specifies the right of liberty. It states that, 'Everyone has the right to liberty and security of person. No one shall be deprived of his liberty save in the following cases and in accordance with a procedure prescribed by law'. Interestingly, Section 1 (e) describes one of the exceptions as 'the lawful detention of persons for the prevention of the spreading of infectious diseases, of persons of unsound mind, alcoholics or drug addicts or vagrants'. It is clear that the act allows for the detention of people with substance misuse problems, but the conditions for this need to be specified.

In Article 8, 'Right to respect for private and family life', it is stated that, 'There shall be no interference by a public authority with the exercise of this right except such as is in accordance with the law and is necessary in a democratic society in the interests of national security, public safety or the economic well-being of the country, for the prevention of disorder or crime, for the protection of health or morals, or for the protection of the rights and freedoms of others.' Drug addiction can be inquired and reported on the basis of this exception. On the other hand, in Article 10 there is emphasis on 'preventing the disclosure of information received in confidence', which can be used to protect the information provided by substance users for the clinicians. The way the ECHR is interpreted here depends on the context.

While there can be discrimination against substance users, Article 14, 'Prohibition of Discrimination', can be used to challenge any discrimination suffered by these people. The important factor is that these problems should be considered as medical problems, so any discrimination can be defined in the disability framework. If it is decided that these problems are not medical but moral, then it would be difficult to use this Article as a legal leverage against the discrimination.

Delivering services for the elderly with substance misuse – ethical aspects

In the United Kingdom, the Royal College of Psychiatrists highlighted the problems in substance misuse in the elderly in the document 'Our Invisible Addicts' [7]. Whilst the focus of this document is mainly on the United Kingdom, the conclusions are applicable in other countries of the European Union, as the legal and ethical framework used is the same.

There are several ethical issues that are touched on in this report. It confirms that the ethical–legal issues cannot separated from the practice. It is noted that, 'Between 2001 and 2031, there is projected to be a 50% increase in the number of older people in the United Kingdom. The percentage of men and women drinking more than the weekly recommended limits has also risen, by 60% in men and 100% in women between 1990 and 2006' [7]. This fact puts ethical and legal obligations to ensure that appropriate services are provided for this population. Failure to do so can be construed as a breach of their human rights and discrimination under Article 14 of the European Convention of Human Rights. The ethical argument has more weight when considering the increase in the rate of substance misuse in the elderly, the complexities of care given the increase in physical and mental health problems, and the increase in the mortality rate in this population when complicated by substance misuse.

The high rate of prescribing hypnotics and sedatives [8] in the ageing population puts an ethical obligation on the services to:

- Tackle the problem of overprescribing.
- Provide treatment for patients with addiction to the prescribed medications.

The issue of overprescribing (e.g. benzodiazepines) for the elderly needs special attention. There is evidence that misuse of prescription drugs is a significant problem in the elderly population [8]. It should be considered an ethical obligation that the misuse of these substances is investigated and the risk of misuse of these substances is acknowledged.

In line with universal best practice, providing treatment in the primary care setting is recommended: screening for substance misuse, brief interventions and referral of more complex substance use disorders to specialized services [9]. Moreover, there is a need for building capacity (training) and capability (staff) in medical and other health professionals in all health care settings to enable them to undertake effective assessments and interventions in elderly people with substance misuse.

Research and development

There is need for research and development for better and integrated care for elderly people with substance misuse. Currently, there is a paucity of research and evidence for treatment interventions and services for the management of substance use disorders in older adults. It is clear that research and development in this area is an ethical imperative. The majority of the research in this area is generated in the USA. It can be questioned whether the results can equally be applied to Europe. There are differences in the accessibility and organization of health care systems between Europe and the USA.

The social milieu in Europe is different from the USA and needs different approaches. It is important that European countries develop their own epidemiological databases and services that fit the local population best. It is crucial to produce good quality research locally.

In the United Kingdom, the Royal College of Psychiatrists recommends:

'Examination of trends in the extent, nature and predictors of substance use problems in older people is required; standardized age-appropriate assessment and outcome measures that encourage comparability should be developed; Effective interventions for adults should be evaluated and innovative treatments for older people developed;

Service models with a particular focus on long-term outcome should be developed and evaluated.' [7]

Policy making

At the policy level, the health organizations have a duty to develop policies to ensure easier access to the services, eliminating any discrimination on the basis of age, jointly working with the patients and developing services. There is an ethical obligation to promote inclusion of this group in making policies and addressing its complex needs. The needs of elderly substance misuse patients should be reflected at different levels, including, public health, service delivery, education and treatment.

In the United Kingdom, the Royal College of Psychiatrists recommends that, 'At the ethical level, developing, implementing and promoting service delivery based on need, but targeted in an age-appropriate way through multi-agency partnership is the way forward.' [7]

Some differences between Europe and the USA

One of the differences between Europe and the USA is the use of different classificatory systems for mental disorders. Unfortunately, substance misuse in the elderly is not acknowledged in either diagnostic classification. Given the differences in the demographics and presentation of substance misuse in the elderly, there is a need for this category to be acknowledged in the future editions of the International Classification of the Diseases (ICD). Also, in the ever moving, multicultural Europe, it is an ethical imperative to achieve cross-cultural validity in diagnosing substance misuse in elderly.

'A very different picture has emerged in the USA, with a specific Treatment Improvement Protocol (TIP) guide for the implementation of substance misuse services for older people, to which we should aspire.' [7] In terms of policies they have moved forward in acknowledging this patient group and its needs. The lack of substance misuse services in the elderly in the United Kingdom gives the wrong impression of discrimination against this age group.

Substance misuse in elderly Treatment Improvement Protocol 26 highlights problems faced in the USA. Two of the main problems identified are (i) the relationship between patient autonomy and the services' obligation to inform and (ii) accurate communication and documentation without disclosing information [10]. Both problems can be construed as problems concerning confidentiality and ownership of information. Since the late 1990s the legal provisions for notifying the authorities of people with substance misuse has been suspended in the United Kingdom [11].

One big difference between the USA and Europe is that while in the USA, 'in most settings where older adults receive care or services, Federal confidentiality laws and regulations do not apply' [9], in Europe in countries that have signed the European Convention of Human Rights, this legislation trumps all local laws. And the right of privacy has been clarified in Article 8 of the ECHR.

While in the USA some states require elderly substance misuse to be reported [7], in the United Kingdom the disclosure of information is strictly guided by the General Medical Council's confidentiality guidelines [12].

In communication with other professionals the practice is guided, again, by the General Medical Council's guidelines and is on a need to know basis [12]. Patient's consent is essential in the communications.

Ethical issues regarding treatment

When it comes to treatment, some of the interventions, such as detention in hospital, can potentially infringe on patients' human rights. For example, it was stated in the Royal College of Psychiatrists' document, 'Often the problem has to be approached by environmental manipulation, for example working with the family to reduce the amount of alcohol they purchase or supply to the individual concerned. Sometimes the only way forward may be to "take control of the money supply" (e.g. by activating a financial lasting power of attorney or referral to the Court of Protection), on the basis that this is in the older person's best interests, or by moving the person into more supervised accommodation such as residential care.' [7] Cases like this require the need to involve the courts to ensure compliance with the ECHR.

The fact that substance misuse increases the risk of suicide among elderly [7] (who are already at higher risk of suicide) makes it an ethical imperative to address this problem as a means to reduce premature death because of suicide in the society.

Stigma

One aspect of substance misuse in elderly that has ethical implication is the associated stigma. The stigma leads to further marginalization within the community and also within the other substance misusers who are younger. It also interferes in appropriate detection of these problems.

In the United Kingdom, there has been an initiative by the Royal College of Psychiatrists to live up to this ethical task and ensure the stigma associated with drug misuse in elderly is addressed.

Underprescribing controlled drugs

While the main focus in discussions over substance misuse is on abusing illegal substances or overprescribing addictive medications, there is an important area which has serious ethical implications. This area concerns underprescribing the controlled drugs, which can have a crucial role in management of different illnesses. This issue has been addressed in detail by the World Health Organization [13].

The international treaties for drug control rightly target the abuse of illicit substances and ways of tackling it [14]. However, there needs to be an equal emphasis on ensuring that controlled substances are available for medical and scientific purposes. This is especially relevant in our discussion, as the elderly are more likely to need the controlled substances.

As opioid analgesics are an important part of management of different symptoms, especially pain, lack of their availability can be interpreted as degrading treatment which is prohibited under ECHR. The fact that these drugs are of relatively low cost adds to the moral dimension of the argument. The WHO also emphasizes the potential to discriminate against groups such as the elderly which is prohibited under ECHR [6].

Given the fact that only a very small minority of the patients with no history of substance abuse who receive opioids for pain develop dependence syndrome there is a moral argument for their judicious use [13].

There is an emphasis on availability, accessibility, affordability and control of these drugs. The WHO endorses the principle of balance, which puts dual responsibility on governments to ensure availability of these substances for medical use while preventing their abuse. Unfortunately, preference is mostly given to the obligation to prevent abuse.

In some countries, laws and regulations intended to prevent the misuse of controlled substances are overly restrictive and impede patient access to medical treatment with such substances [13]. Policy makers should devise and implement enabling policies that promote widespread understanding about the therapeutic usefulness of controlled substances and their rational use. On the other hand, it is necessary to be aware of the risks of overprescribing drugs, such as benzodiazepines, as they have a propensity to cause addiction. The issue is relevant in the elderly as it is shown that a large group of elderly patients who are prescribed benzodiazepines continue to use them for the long term and suffer from dependence. The dependence on benzodiazepines is associated with co-morbid illnesses such as anxiety disorder, sleep disorder and affective disorders [8]. There is an ethical implication as the duty of the doctor is to first do no harm. In the United Kingdom, specific guidelines limit prescribing this group of drugs [8].

Summary

This chapter has reported on and critically discussed some of the important ethical and legal aspects of substance misuse in the elderly from a European perspective. As it is hard to define a unified European perspective, the focus has mostly been on the United Kingdom. It is important to reiterate that the ethical and legal framework largely depends on the status of substance misuse as a mental disorder. As things stand, there are serious ethical and legal issues to be considered in this population. It is clear that while there are general outlines in the law, it will take time for case law to develop, as law does evolve in time. The ethics of practice to a great extent concern the poor service these patients receive currently and the imperative to develop services, treatments and policies to support them through a population specific research and development programme.

References

1. Drug penalties. The Home Office, UK. http://www.homeoffice.gov.uk/drugs/drug-law/ (last accessed 28 March 2014).
2. National Organization for the Reform of Marijuana Laws (2003) European Drug Policy: 2002 Legislative Update. http://norml.org/component/zoo/category/european-drug-laws (last accessed 28 March 2014).
3. European Monitoring Centre for Drug and Drug Addiction (2010) Illegal Consumption of Drugs. http://www.emcdda.europa.eu/html.cfm/index5747EN.html (last accessed 28 March 2014).
4. National Treatment Agency for Substance Misuse (2009) Breaking the link: The role of drug treatment in tackling the crime. http://www.nta.nhs.uk/uploads/nta_criminaljustice_0809.pdf (last accessed 28 March 2014).
5. Howse, K. (2003) Growing Old in Prison. Prison Reform Trust, UK. http://www.prisonreformtrust.org.uk/Portals/0/Documents/Growing%20Old%20in%20Prison%20-%20a%20scoping%20study.pdf (last accessed 28 March 2014).
6. European Court of Human Rights. European Convention of Human Rights. Council of Europe, Strasbourg, France (available online).
7. Royal College of Psychiatrists (2011) Our invisible addicts: First Report of the Older Persons' Substance Misuse Working Group of the Royal College of Psychiatrists. College Report CR165, Royal College of Psychiatrists, London, UK.
8. Sanati, A. and Abou-Saleh, M.T. (2012) The use and abuse of prescribed medicines. In: *Pathy's Principles and Practice of Geriatric Medicine* (eds A.J. Sinclair, J.E. Morley and B. Vellas), 5th edn. John Wiley & Sons Ltd, Chichester, pp. 1495–1501.
9. Abou-Saleh, M.T., Nuzhat, A. and Camacho, P. (2012) Substance use disorder in primary care mental health. In: *Companion to Primary Care Mental Health* (ed. G. Ivbijaro). Radcliff Publishing, London, Part VI. http://www.radcliffehealth.com/shop/companion-primary-care-mental-health (last accessed 28 March 2014).
10. SAMHSA (1998) Substance Abuse Among Older Adults. Treatment Improvement Protocol (TIP) Series, No. 26, Substance Abuse and Mental Health Services Administration (SAMHSA), Rockville, MD.
11. UK Government (1997) The Misuse of Drugs (Supply to Addicts) Regulations 1997. http://www.legislation.gov.uk/uksi/1997/1001/made (last accessed 28 March 2014).
12. GMC (2007) Confidentiality. The General Medical Council, UK. http://www.gmc-uk.org/static/documents/content/Confidentiality_0910.pdf (last accessed 28 March 2014).
13. WHO (2011) Ensuring balance in national policies on controlled substances: Guidance for availability and accessibility of controlled medicines. World Health Organization (WHO), Geneva, Switzerland. http://www.who.int/medicines/areas/quality_safety/GLs_Ens_Balance_NOCP_Col_EN_sanend.pdf (last accessed 28 March 2014).
14. Room, R. and Reuter, P. (2012) How well do international drug conventions protect public health? *The Lancet*; **379**, 84–91.

Chapter 5

CLINICAL MEDICINE AND SUBSTANCE MISUSE: RESEARCH, ASSESSMENTS AND TREATMENT

Amit Arora[1], Andrew O'Neill[2], Peter Crome[3] and Finbarr C. Martin[4]

[1] University Hospital of North Staffordshire/Keele University, UK
[2] University Hospital of North Staffordshire, UK
[3] Institute for Social Sciences and Medical School, Keele University/Department of Primary Care and Population Health, University College London, UK
[4] Guys & St Thomas' NHS Foundation Trust/King's College London, UK

Introduction

With the increase in population numbers of older people over recent decades, the demands of caring for this diverse and complex group have become a firmly established health priority. In the United Kingdom alone, the number of people aged 65 and older increased by 20% to 10.3 million during the period 1985–2010. Current estimates suggest that this growth will continue for at least the next few decades, with those aged 65 and over accounting for 23% of the total population in 2035 and one quarter by 2050. Over a similar period, those aged over 80 will increase from a current population of three million to around eight million by 2050 [1].

An ability to live longer lives has led to a greater emphasis on making those lives healthier, not just for the benefit of the individual but also to reduce the medical, social and economic burdens placed on societies by the frailty and ill health that can accompany ageing.

Despite historically receiving little attention, issues surrounding substance misuse and dependence in older adults are coming to the fore. A growing realization that the elderly can struggle with addiction is driving attempts to improve professional awareness and service provision, along with social policy recognition of the baggage of drug and alcohol abuse brought with the 'baby boomer' generation as it ages.

Data from England indicates that 20% of men and 10% of women aged over 65 are exceeding recommended alcohol intake guidelines [2], with older men as likely to exceed the guidelines as those aged 16–24. Studies into medication misuse suggest a prevalence of between 1 and 26%, depending on the definitions used [3, 4]. In Blazer and Wu's national United States study, 60% of those over 50 had used

Substance Use and Older People, First Edition.
Edited by Ilana B. Crome, Li-Tzy Wu, Rahul (Tony) Rao and Peter Crome.

alcohol during the past year, 2.6% marijuana and 0.41% cocaine [5]. These figures are predicted to rise, with Colliver *et al.* suggesting a 60% increase in illicit drug use among American over 50 years old and a doubling of those who use psychotherapeutic drugs for nonmedical reasons [6].

Reflecting this increase, hospital admissions in England involving drug-related mental health or behavioural disorders have doubled over the period 2000–2010 [7]. Gfroerer *et al.* suggest that around 4.4 million US adults aged over 50 will require treatment for substance abuse problems by 2020 – a 70% increase on current treatment rates [8].

In contrast to younger cohorts, where substance misuse often presents to healthcare professionals with psychiatric sequelae, older patients frequently present with physical complications caused by substance abuse [9] rather than seeking assistance and treatment for addiction in itself [10]. Healthcare interactions with older patients who have had falls, confusion, mood disturbance or evidence of self-neglect may have the potential to reveal underlying substance misuse.

Despite increasing prevalence rates, it is also known that older people are less likely to complain about health problems [11, 12] and have a lower propensity to seek out specialist care, especially psychiatric care [13]. As a consequence, the majority of physical symptoms will be assessed and treated by nonaddiction specialists, and it is in this scenario that clinical medicine has an important role to play. Those involved in the delivery of geriatric medicine are highly likely to be involved in this process of both identification and treatment.

This chapter covers three main areas. Firstly, it summarizes the potential for identification of those affected and the pitfalls and difficulties for clinicians in this process. Secondly, it clarifies some of the physical effects experienced by those affected, concentrating on the so-called 'geriatric giants'. Finally, it identifies some of the potential avenues through which the identification and care of those at risk can be improved.

Why is clinical medicine important?

The majority of healthcare professionals working today can expect to have some contact with an older patient in the course of their everyday work. Considering that the average over 75 year old in the United States has at least three medical conditions and uses five prescribed drugs, it comes as no surprise that those over 65 visit their doctor an average of eight times a year as opposed to the five of their younger counterparts [14]. Usage of secondary care resources is similarly significant, with around two-thirds of all United Kingdom National Health Service (NHS) beds occupied by adults over the age of 65 [15]. Financially, a cohort of only 5% of US patients manages to consume 50% of the total healthcare budget; over half this group is aged over 65 [16].

Despite high levels of service use, substance abuse issues amongst older people are not routinely volunteered by those affected. Various combinations of social isolation, poor access to services, low expectations, limited information and a degree of resignation all appear to contribute to an inability to seek help [17]. Even when seeking assistance, an older person may well not be aware that their problems are related to their use of alcohol or other substances.

For the clinician, the typical situations, symptoms and outcomes of substance abuse witnessed in younger patients may not be present. Symptoms such as confusion, falls and incontinence, which would be immediately identified as abnormal in younger adults may be wrongly considered to be normal in an older person, or there may be multiple potential causes which obscure the main underlying reasons. It is this complex combination of factors which can result in patients presenting initially to general or geriatric medicine.

So why is clinical medicine important when addressing the issue of substance abuse in older adults? There are two main areas; these are covered here.

Identification

Many older substance abusers may not recognize their use as problematic and it may only be through presentation with physical or occasionally psychiatric complications that a link with use can be identified. As a consequence, most problems are currently identified through surrogate issues picked up during interactions with primary care practitioners or through assessment in secondary care by frontline medical, surgical and psychiatric services [17, 18]. It is within this scenario that healthcare professionals need to be proactive in raising issues around substance abuse and is where clinical medicine can play an essential role.

Unfortunately, research suggests that it is currently struggling to fulfil its potential. Despite high levels of interaction, studies consistently show poor identification skills in doctors presented with potential substance misuse [4]. Researchers looking at acute medical admissions to The Johns Hopkins Hospital found that only 37% of older alcoholic patients were identified by junior doctors through the use of CAGE (Cut down, Annoyed by criticism, Guilt about drinking, needing Eye-opener) and SMAST (Short Michigan Alcohol Screening Test) questionnaires compared with 60% of the younger alcoholic patients [19]. McInnes and Powell reported that junior doctors looking after medical inpatients were only able to identify one-third of hazardous or harmful drinkers, with similar problems identifying benzodiazepine users (only 3 out of 88 of those using harmful amounts identified) and smokers (29 out of 77 identified) [20]. In a cross-sectional prevalence study using interviews and screening questionnaires, Adams et al. noted that only 20% of older alcohol abusers were identified by clinical staff [21].

This research suggests a significant level of diagnostic uncertainty and potential for misdiagnosis amongst health professionals. As a consequence, clinicians may unwittingly apply inappropriate investigations and interventions which may exacerbate underlying issues and ultimately fail to resolve potentially treatable substance use problems [19].

There are multiple factors that can contribute to this uncertainty. Firstly, patients may present in an acute, unannounced and atypical fashion; secondly, they may have a significant number of co-morbid conditions that can obfuscate underlying causes; thirdly, a high degree of suspicion is required as standard diagnostic and screening criteria are often insensitive or inappropriate; fourthly, the same social conditioning that prevents elders from presenting may also limit practitioner insight and result in misinterpreted clinical triggers; finally, the finite amount of time imposed by modern day healthcare demands may mean that clinicians are tempted to pay more attention to immediate physical ailments at the expense of more routine screening questions [22].

A common theme when caring for older people is the atypical or subtle fashion in which complaints can present. While older adults can suffer from virtually every disease affecting younger people, they often present with a fairly limited range of symptoms which are often nonspecific in themselves. Issues such as lethargy, confusion, poor oral intake and reduced mobility may represent a spectrum of disease from the benign to the sinister.

As a consequence, clinicians may have a wide range of differential diagnoses when a patient becomes ill or simply when concerns arise. Symptoms such as confusion or memory loss, anxiety, depression, tremor, incontinence, poor sleep pattern, falls, self-neglect or unusual responses to medication may represent the effects of numerous conditions. A significant temptation is to attribute these to 'normal' ageing when the underlying reason may be alcohol or drugs. In 1998, researchers from the National Center on Addiction and Substance Abuse in the United States identified significant shortcomings in the diagnoses physicians consider when confronted with nonspecific symptoms. Using theoretical case scenarios detailing patient histories which included symptoms such as low energy levels, weight loss, irritability, chronic heartburn and trouble sleeping, they identified that a diagnosis of substance abuse in an older woman was only considered by 1% of physicians, despite physical signs of alcohol and prescription drug abuse [22].

In addition to this nonspecificity, overlying co-morbid conditions can complicate the diagnostic process by diverting the clinician's attention from substance use issues when presented with physical ill health or functional decline. Conditions such as the confusion of alcohol withdrawal syndrome may be misinterpreted as the delirium of infection. The tremor associated with alcohol withdrawal may be incorrectly assumed to be a sign of Parkinson's disease [23]. Indirect effects on general well-being, such as poor nutrition, neglect of hygiene, financial difficulties or functional decline, may be seen as primary issues rather than triggers for further enquiry.

The assumed (or real) physical limitations associated with ill health (e.g. reduced mobility resulting in transport problems) may also discourage professionals from referring older patients to effective treatment programmes. However if they are identified and referred, empirical evidence clearly shows that older people, and in particular those who commence substance misuse later in life, respond favourably to treatment programmes. In comparison to young and middle aged patients, they are more likely to engage with treatment programmes which, in turn, results in better long-term outcomes [24, 25]. Those older adults who manage to complete treatment programmes report significant improvements in their mental health, cognitive functioning, energy levels and use of medication [26].

Ultimately, issues around substance misuse can be difficult for a health professional to address satisfactorily in the course of their work. A combination of insufficient knowledge and awareness, limited research, societal programming and the technical limitations of hurried visits which have to address multiple co-morbidities will continue to result in healthcare providers missing substance abuse and dependency in older adults [9, 19, 20].

The health effects of substance abuse

The second area of interest concerns the marked effects on health that can accompany substance abuse. These are largely encountered and addressed within the remit of clinical medicine and can carry both significant mortality and morbidity. The chronic effects of alcohol, cigarettes and prescription medication on the adult population are well established, and dealing with their health consequences is part of daily medical work. The impact of associated cardiovascular disease, cancer and alcoholic liver disease are recognized as public health priorities and become increasingly significant as individuals age.

In addition to the direct effects of intoxication, overdose and withdrawal, the physical complications of substances of abuse are numerous and manifest in almost all organs. Serious medical disorders among elderly people who misuse alcohol are much more common than among the overall population of a similar age, with prevalent impairments in physical, psychological, social and cognitive health.

Within geriatric medicine, attempts have been made to shift attention away from diagnostic labels and instead concentrate on those physical issues which impact most on an older person's life. Five main areas – the 'Geriatric Giants' – are widely recognized as the targets of this approach. These include impaired memory, instability, immobility, incontinence and sensory impairment. Substance abuse can have implications in all these areas. A sixth 'I' – iatrogenesis – refers to the heightened sensitivity of older patients to the primary effects of drugs, drug–drug interactions as well as withdrawal.

Cognitive impairment

The spectre of cognitive impairment and its resultant mental, physical and functional consequences are well known and feared. A recent survey of over 50 year olds found that 80% rated dementia as the disease they most feared developing – joint first with cancer [27]. Worldwide, 35.6 million people have dementia and there are 7.7 million new cases every year [28]. A recent study identified objective evidence of cognitive impairment in 25% of nondemented adults aged over 65 [29]. Between 65 and 80% of those affected will progress to dementia within five years of diagnosis [30].

The effect of medication on cognition is well recognized, with studies reporting medication as the main factor behind delirium in between 11 and 30% of elderly medical inpatients [31, 32]. In those with more chronic cognitive impairment, and in particular those with suspected dementia, medication toxicity is suggested to play a role in between 2 and 12% of patients affected [33, 34]. This prevalence presents significant challenges for the physician trying to screen for potentially reversible causes, with at least 10% of patients referred to memory clinics displaying cognitive impairments directly contributable to the effects of medication [35].

Commonly prescribed medications associated with cognitive impairment include those with anticholinergic effects (such as antihistamines and drugs used for incontinence), hypnotics, antidepressants, analgesics, anticonvulsants, corticosteroids and cardiac drugs such as beta blockers and digoxin [36]. Benzodiazepines and opioid analgesics – the two most commonly misused medications in older populations – sit squarely within this group.

Multiple studies identify a strong link between benzodiazepine use and cognitive decline [37–39] and even dementia [40]. In those using benzodiazepines, symptoms such as daytime sleepiness, unsteadiness and forgetfulness may lead families and carers to suspect dementia. Clinical evaluation may reveal deficits in attention and memory, along with impaired psychomotor abilities, which may result in a drug related delirium or pseudo-dementia being wrongly labelled as Alzheimer's disease.

Even among those with age-related cognitive decline, the additional effects of sedatives can have significant repercussions for the preservation of cognition and maintenance of daily functioning. Several longitudinal studies have demonstrated a more rapid decline in markers of cognition and attention in long term users of benzodiazepines when compared to nonusers [38, 39].

Similar to benzodiazepines, opiate analgesics have marked effects on cognition, even at low doses [41]. Experimental studies in younger people demonstrate that opiates impair balance, coordination, vision and judgement [42, 43]. Extrapolation would suggest that older people are at least, if not more, susceptible to their effects. With longer term use, their cumulative effects on cognition may result in a drug induced pseudo-dementia being missed, resulting in the introduction of unnecessary medication, functional decline and subsequent loss of independence.

Alcohol is widely used in most societies for a variety of purposes and is consumed by adults of all ages. Culberson reports 50% of community-dwelling persons aged 65 and older regularly consume alcohol [44]. This trend of continued use through life may have significant consequences in later years, particularly if levels of consumption are sustained. Empirical neuropsychological studies consistently show that older adults suffer detrimental effects on their cognition and spatial-motor abilities at much lower levels of alcohol consumption than younger adults [45]. Consumption of more than 14 units of alcohol per week by older adults has been associated with significant impairment of IADLs (Instrumental Activities of Daily Living) and to a lesser extent AADLs (Advanced Activities of Daily Living) [46].

The relationship between alcohol consumption and cognitive impact is well documented [47], with the chronic toxic effects of alcohol producing cerebral degeneration and eventual dementia. Where memory is preserved, isolated and irreversible cerebellar damage and dysfunction is not uncommon, resulting in instability and incoordination [48]. Even older adults with levels of intake well within recommended guidelines [49] may suffer cognitive effects which mimic dementia or other organic brain diseases.

Chronic cognitive impairment may also be precipitated by nutritional deficiencies related to chronic alcohol misuse, in particular thiamine deficiency. Classically described as a triad of ocular disturbance, ataxia and global confusion, Wernicke's encephalopathy refers to the effects of acute thiamine deficiency, most common in alcoholic patients [50]. In the chronic phase, symptoms may progress to Korsakoff's psychosis, which is characterized by a lack of insight, apathy and anterograde amnesia with confabulaton. Early identification and treatment is essential, and those patients presenting with a history of chronic alcohol abuse should be treated with parenteral thiamine as a priority. By the time amnesia and psychosis are evident, complete recovery is highly unlikely, with half of patients only experiencing partial improvement in symptoms [51].

While an association between cigarette smoking, small vessel disease and cognitive decline may seem logical, data to support a direct correlation are currently lacking. Multiple methodological incompatibilities have prevented effective meta-analysis but most studies appear to suggest that there is a trend toward faster decline in global cognition and executive function as smokers age, particularly in middle aged men [52, 53].

Instability, falls and immobility

Falls in the elderly are a major cause for concern, with unintentional injury currently the fifth leading cause of death in older adults. Falls account for two thirds of these injury-related deaths [54]. Decreased attention, altered motor coordination and cognitive dysfunction with impaired judgement all combine in older adults to increase risk of falling. In the United Kingdom, just over one in three adults aged over 65 will fall each year – approximately 3.4 million. One-half of those aged over 80 will fall each year. This brings a daily cost of 4.6 million pounds [55].

Over one-quarter of those aged over 80 who fall will suffer a significant injury, with reports recently of an increasing incidence of traumatic spinal cord injury among older adults [56]. Aside from the impact on a person's health, falls reduce confidence and instil a fear of further falls in previously mobile adults. This results in constriction of activities and socialization, precipitating family concern and may eventually end in institutionalization. Several risk factors for falls have been identified but none is as potentially preventable or reversible as medication use [57].

With current estimates suggesting that alcohol is responsible for between 6 and 45% of all injury-related adult Emergency Department attendances, its role in increasing risk of injury is well established. Around 5.2 million people die each year from alcohol-related injuries [58]. Alcohol interferes with balance and coordination, predisposing to unsteadiness and falls. It also impairs judgement and increases risk taking and impulsivity, which may result in a variety of injuries, ranging from simple falls to drink-driving related fatalities and extending to acts of domestic violence [59].

Physically, alcohol affects multiple parts of the neuromuscular system, which can result in impairment of mobility and falls. Alcohol-related muscle atrophy affects 40–60% of those with chronic alcohol dependence, producing progressive weakness and neuralgia [60]. There may be a reduction in sensory awareness and peripheral neuropathy may result in foot drop, which along with cerebellar degeneration causes a classically described wide-based ataxic gait [60].

In addition to this increased risk of trauma, reduced bone mass and osteoporosis can follow, resulting in a higher incidence of low impact fractures [61]. Concurrent poor nutrition and associated smoking habits can also contribute to this heightened risk of fracture.

While alcohol is a well described risk factor for fracture, its relationship with falls in the elderly is less well characterized in the literature. Consumption of more than 14 units of alcohol per week was found to increase risk of falls by 25% in a study by Mukamal *et al.* [62]. However, Cawthon *et al.* identified that it was those with a history of heavy alcohol use, rather than those with high current levels of use, who were at higher risk of falls [63]. This suggests that it is the chronic physical changes associated with alcohol which are most pertinent, rather than acute intoxication.

Amongst community dwellers, benzodiazepines are a significant risk factor for falls [64]. Despite a reduction in use over recent decades [65] as evidence of side effects has accumulated, they remain widely prescribed [66]. Estimates suggest that between 16 and 33% of adults over the age of 65 in North America, Australia and Europe use sedative hypnotics on a regular basis – a significantly higher number than in younger cohorts [67]. In the United Kingdom, older adults receive around 80% of all benzodiazepine prescriptions [68], with the main reasons for use being anxiety, agitation or insomnias.

While this sedative intent is the primary effect of benzodiazepines, even when used in therapeutic doses, the chronic use of sedatives by older adults is associated with a variety of other adverse nervous system effects [69]. These may include diminished psychomotor performance, impaired reaction time, loss of coordination, ataxia, falls, excessive daytime drowsiness and confusion – all of which contribute to falling. Over 80 year olds who use benzodiazepines are twice as likely to fall in comparison to those who do not. Those under 80 years old are 1.5 times more likely to fall. Almost 10% of those falls will be fatal [64]. For those who remain independent, use of benzodiazepines while driving produces an increased risk of involvement in motor vehicle accidents [70, 71].

The effect of opioids on balance cannot be underestimated. While there is a lack of robust data to suggest a direct link between use and falls, it is known that both cognitive impairment and psychomotor retardation are risk factors for falls [72]. Additionally, older adults are more likely to be seriously injured when they fall and have an increased rate of mortality from common fall-related injuries, such as hip fracture. Several studies have demonstrated a definite link between opioid use and fracture [73], with one study in 2011 by Miller *et al.* suggesting a fourfold increase in fracture rates amongst users in comparison to those using nonsteroidals [74].

Of increasing significance, cannabis use has been demonstrated to affect judgement, slow reaction times and impair perceptual-motor coordination and motor performance [75]. General population studies display a link between use and an increased risk of motor vehicle accidents [76]. With extrapolation, it seems reasonable to assume that any level of increased psychomotor retardation would lead to an increased risk of falls.

Incontinence

Urinary incontinence is a prevalent condition among frail older people. Large population surveys reveal a prevalence in women of 23% in those aged 60–79 and 32% in those over 80 [77]. Around 16% of men aged over 75 are affected by incontinence [78]. In comparison to community dwellers, those who live in nursing homes appear to have significantly higher rates of incontinence, ranging from 43 to 77% [79]. Incontinence significantly impacts on the quality of life of older adults, primarily through detrimental effects on physical function and social interaction. It has a significant financial impact on patients, families and healthcare systems, being one of the most common reasons for older people to be admitted to institutional care [80, 81].

The chain of interlinked physiological factors that allows for normal urinary continence is vulnerable to adverse drug effects at a number of levels. Alcohol has well recognized diuretic effects. In addition to an increase volume of fluid, alcohol suppresses the thirst sensation and vasopressin production, resulting in a period of significant diuresis post-ingestion. Through its effect on mobility, alcohol may affect an individual's ability to get to a toilet in time, increasing the risk of a fall [82]. The loss of a significant volume of fluid may well also precipitate orthostatic hypotension, again affecting risks of falling [83].

Both urinary retention and incontinence are recognized as results of benzodiazepine use [78, 84]. Physiologically, benzodiazepines cause relaxation of striated muscle, resulting in decreased urethral pressure and subsequent stress incontinence. Additionally, there may be reduced awareness of the need to void, along with impairments in dexterity and mobility. A 2003 study of nursing home residents by Landi *et al.* found that benzodiazepine use was associated with a 45% increase in risk of urinary incontinence [85].

Opioids can cause faecal and urinary incontinence by a number of mechanisms. They act as a potent constipating agent, and with chronic use can result in faecal impaction and overflow. The faecal mass effect can cause urinary tract compression and precipitate urinary retention and overflow. Additionally, opioids can act directly upon the bladder itself, inhibiting innervation and causing a reduced sensation of bladder fullness along with bladder muscle relaxation. Their anticholinergic effects may also promote urinary retention with resultant overflow incontinence.

Iatrogenesis

Drug–drug interactions
Older people generally have the largest burden of illness and consume many categories of medications. The use of medication among the elderly population has increased tremendously over recent decades. Almost five out of six older US citizens

are on at least one medication, with around half of these on three or more medications [86]. Over half of the UK NHS drug budget is used in providing medication to over 60 year olds [87].

Older people are also significant self-medicators. Around 40% of all over-the-counter medication purchases are made by over 65 s [88]. Commonly bought medications include analgesics, laxatives, cough and cold products, which may interact with prescribed medication or have side effects of their own.

While these medications may have significant benefits, their administration is always accompanied by the potential for harm, even when prescribed at recommended doses based on appropriate guidelines. Those who have dementia are particularly vulnerable, where patients may not be able to recognize the effects of the drugs themselves and their carers may fail to distinguish between the effects of medication and the symptoms of the disease itself.

The World Health Organization reports that drug interactions are a leading cause of morbidity and mortality [89]; this relates as much to illicit substances as those prescribed [90]. This prevalence places two responsibilities on clinicians – firstly, to diagnose and treat the side effects of drug reactions and, secondly, to be aware of the consequences of their own prescribing patterns. An inability to distinguish drug-related symptoms from those of primary medical conditions often results in the addition of medication to treat the symptoms. This, in turn, leads to an increased risk of further adverse effects – the so-called 'prescribing cascade'.

It is estimated that the rate of adverse drug reaction (ADR) related hospital admissions is 16.6% in the elderly, as opposed to 4% in younger patients [91]. As many as 88% of these episodes are considered preventable [92]. In addition, poisoning is now one of the leading causes of accidental death, with the United States seeing a 145% increase in poisoning deaths between 1999 and 2007. Drug–drug interactions have been identified as a major factor in this growth [86].

Chronic alcohol misuse can alter the effect of a wide range of medication. Sedative drugs such as tricyclic antidepressants, antihistamines and hypnotic sedatives (e.g. benzodiazepines, barbiturates and 'Z' drugs) will have their effects enhanced, resulting in CNS depression and impaired psychomotor performance. Analgesic use may also be affected through alteration of the pharmacokinetics of extended release morphine preparations, resulting in unpredictable absorption rates. Gastric mucosal damage as a consequence of excess alcohol may potentiate the ability of nonsteroidal drugs to cause irritation and haemorrhage. Chronic use also increases the risk of paracetamol overdose, even if recommended levels are adhered to. Several cases of fulminant hepatic failure have been reported in unwitting users [93].

Those using antibiotics may see their effect impaired or enhanced, or may have an increased sensitivity to the effects of alcohol. In diabetics, use of alcohol and hypoglycaemic agents increases the incidence of severe hypoglycaemic episodes and their associated risks of injury [94]. Use with antihypertensives may precipitate hypotension, resulting in falls, whereas mixing monoamine-oxidase inhibitor (MAOI) antidepressants and tyramine-rich alcohol can result in severe hypertension [95, 96].

In patients with epilepsy who abuse alcohol, acute intoxication may precipitate seizures [97] by reducing their seizure threshold in the context of poor concordance with anticonvulsant therapy. The primary interaction between alcohol and anticonvulsants appears to be an enhanced sedative effect, with increased sensitivity to the intoxicating effects of alcohol.

In those using benzodiazepines and opioids, combination with other drugs with inherent sedative effects can result in the potentiation of CNS depressant effects, resulting in greater functional impairment. As a consequence of impaired reaction times and coordination, there is an increased chance of injury, particularly given the heightened risk of the subject being unaware of being affected. It is estimated that around one in four deaths involving opioids also involves alcohol [98].

Use of anti-ageing drugs
In the United Kingdom the use of anti-ageing vitamins, other nutrients and herbal medicines is becoming more common despite lack of effectiveness in clinical trials. More worryingly, ready access to online pharmacies and aggressive marketing strategies have seen an increase in the use of more potent anti-ageing remedies, such as recombinant growth hormone, androgenic steroids and testosterone, despite evidence that they are largely unneeded [99] and may have significant potential for harm [100].

Many of the more benign preparations are available freely as over-the-counter drugs and have the potential to have 'drug–drug interactions'. Though not strictly 'substance misuse', this could manifest itself in variable ways in clinical practice.

Withdrawal
Older adults are particularly susceptible to the effects of drug withdrawal, due to a combination of lower physiological reserve, a larger number of co-existing premorbid diseases and a greater sensitivity to medications commonly used to treat withdrawal symptoms.

Alcohol withdrawal syndrome refers to the variety of symptoms suffered by an individual when they stop or dramatically reduce their alcohol intake after a period of excessive consumption. Withdrawal may present with a spectrum of symptoms ranging from mild anxiety, through tremor and delirium and ending in convulsions and death. As a consequence, it can be classified as mild, moderate and severe. Withdrawal may be planned in advance and addressed in a controlled manner, or precipitated acutely by crises such as a lack of funds, acute illness or injury, or an inability to ingest alcohol through nausea or vomiting.

Symptoms normally start between six and forty eight hours after the last alcoholic drink. Clinical examination may reveal signs such as tremor, diaphoresis, agitation, tachycardia or hypertension. Serious symptoms and events such as hallucinations, seizures and delirium tremens normally occur in later phases of withdrawal. Delirium tremens has a mortality rate of about 5% with severity generally being related to a previous history of delirium tremens, heavy alcohol consumption and the presence of physical illness, with those over the age of 45 most at risk from fatal withdrawal reactions [101]. Seizures can occur with any degree of severity of withdrawal [102].

The effect of advanced age is drawing attention as a factor that enhances the potential severity of withdrawal [103]. Alcohol withdrawal syndrome is more common in elderly individuals who stop or reduce an intensive alcohol intake and may be evident following relatively infrequent or low volume intake in comparison with younger adults [104]. The effects of withdrawal on elderly subjects have also been shown to be of a greater magnitude and more prolonged than those of younger people [105] and require more prolonged periods of hospitalization [9, 102]. With their increased burden of co-morbidity, heightened sensitivity to the adverse effects of drug treatment, susceptibility to kindling and overall limited physiological reserve, older people are at a significantly higher risk of complicated alcohol withdrawal [103].

Similar to alcohol, benzodiazepine withdrawal syndrome is well documented and can have serious consequences, with the elderly being particularly susceptible. In general, those who have longer treatment periods, higher doses or undergo sudden discontinuation are more likely to suffer side effects [106]. While specific research into the elderly is lacking, general population studies into benzodiazepine withdrawal indicates that while those who are on short-term (<2–3 months), low dose regimes may experience mild symptoms of withdrawal [107]. In those who are on long-term (>1 year), low dose regimes, moderate to severe withdrawal symptoms occur in 20–100% of patients [108]. Regardless, there is significant variability in patient sensitivity to discontinuation and administration for anything more than a few weeks should trigger the use of tapering doses [109].

After the abrupt discontinuation of therapeutic doses of benzodiazepines a characteristic abstinence syndrome may develop. The milder form may manifest in headache, insomnia, increased anxiety, low mood, tremor and myoclonic jerks. In those who are withdrawing from prolonged treatment, significantly more dramatic symptoms may be experienced, with nausea, vomiting, delirium, hallucinations, depersonalization and generalized seizures potentially ensuing.

Opiate withdrawal can be an unpleasant experience, but is not life-threatening or particularly dangerous in comparison to untreated withdrawal from benzodiazepines [107, 110]. It is usually accompanied by agitation and insomnia, dysphoria, gastrointestinal upset, myalgia and difficulties with thermoregulation resulting in fever. Supportive therapy is usually required to prevent the combination of craving and uncomfortable symptomatology precipitating a relapse to drug use.

Challenges for the future

As outlined above, clinical medicine is well placed to play a significant role in the identification and management of substance abuse issues in the elderly. An increasingly aged population with multiple co-morbidities, polypharmacy and functional issues will continue to place significant demands on those delivering frontline medicine, with geriatric medicine particularly affected. In addition, changing attitudes and patterns of use amongst middle aged adults are likely to influence consumption over further decades, which will require not only changes in current service provision but also modification of clinician skills and attitudes.

Obviously, these challenges will demand significant developments in the delivery of clinical medicine. These developments fall into three main categories: research trends, identification tools and clinician training.

Research

The role of further research into multiple aspects of elder substance abuse cannot be overemphasized. It is clear that three significant areas of research need to be addressed. Firstly, there is little clear data on the epidemiology of all forms of substance use and abuse among older populations and their prevalence in geriatric medical and other old age specialist services. Secondly, the atypical nature of presentation has been largely unexplored and the relationship often seen between functional difficulties and substance abuse is objectively untested. Thirdly, there is little or no supportive evidence for the management regimes used in the withdrawal syndromes experienced by older adults. The sensitivity of older patients to iatrogenesis warrants that any pharmaceutical intervention should have a sound evidence base. This currently does not exist.

However this is not going to be achieved easily and indicators of progress are not positive. Evidence suggests that representation of older people in clinical trials has not been in keeping with the prevalence and incidence amongst them. Although age as such has been removed as an exclusion criteria from many recent trials, there seem to be other criteria in place that have enabled the systematic exclusion of older people from clinical trials. Many barriers to recruiting older people in such trials have been described [111].

The UK Clinical Research Network Study Portfolio (2014) includes no current studies relevant to the identification or management of alcohol or substance abuse in general adult or older peoples' health services. Only two papers undertaking original research into the area are readily identifiable on PubMed for 2013–2014 [112, 113].

Identification tools

A large gap in knowledge also exists on how those affected are screened and identified. When tasked with creating diagnostic definitions and criteria for substance abuse, committees usually envisage an average patient who is a socially active young or middle-aged adult of normal physiology. The medical, psychological and social frailties of an older adult are rarely considered. The Diagnostic and Statistical Manual of Mental Disorders, 5th Edition (DSM-5), describes substance use disorders as '…*a cluster of cognitive, behavioural, and physiological symptoms indicating that the individual continues using the substance despite significant substance-related problems*' (p. 481). Criteria for diagnosis include impaired control, social impairment, risky use and pharmacological responses such as tolerance and withdrawal [114].

However, for those who may not be employed, do not drive and who have limited and rather insular social networks, these criteria are often inapplicable. Levels of intake below those suggested by guidelines designed and advertised for younger adults may not be seen as harmful by either patient or clinician. The symptoms associated with intoxication, craving and withdrawal may be atypical.

As a consequence, while in relatively healthy older adults approaches to the identification of substance misuse, assessment and treatment are largely similar to those employed in younger cohorts, for those who are frailer and less healthy the use of standard methods may be inappropriate or even misleading.

Commonly used office-based screening tools such as the CAGE questionnaire are notoriously insensitive when applied to older people [115]. Less well known among nonspecialists, tools such as the MAST-G (Michigan Alcoholism Screening Test – Geriatric version) screen may prove more appropriate [116]. It may also be that moving away from concentrating on individual issues to take an overall assessment of an older patient's health may provide more useful results.

With this in mind 'Comprehensive Geriatric Assessment (CGA)' could prove a useful framework. Developed as a means of ascertaining a frail older person's medical co-morbidities, mental health status, day-to-day functioning and continuing social circumstances, professionals involved in care can anticipate and treat complications, identify potential for rehabilitation, offer social care support and determine follow up plans. While a single trained physician can provide a basic assessment, a multidisciplinary team involving a physician, nurse and social worker is most effective. However, it can also draw upon an extended team of physical and occupational therapists, nutritionists, pharmacists, psychiatrists, psychologists, dentists, audiologists, podiatrists and opticians.

It has been repeatedly validated as a sensitive approach to identifying and addressing the physical, pharmacological and functional limitations that may impact on a frail person's well-being [117, 118]. Given that substance misuse affects all three of the above factors in older people, its deployment may reveal hidden physical and social effects. In addition, for those who suffer ill effects as a consequence of self-medication or substance misuse, the identification and elimination of reversible conditions may remove important triggers, such as self-medication for depression or chronic pain.

While the time and resource demands of CGA mean that it is currently unfeasible for it to be deployed as a general measure, specific triggers for its use might include: an acute illness accompanied by functional deterioration; the presence of one or more of the 'geriatric giants' (immobility, instability, impaired memory/intellect, incontinence and sensory impairment); or a proposed change in care environment. In this manner, the true impact of ill health shifts to a much more practical footing, rather than concentrating on the correction of basic physiological parameters.

Training and support

While current research may be lacking, there is a strong body of evidence to support the assertion that substance abuse is a growing problem among older people. This changing situation will be reflected among those users of older hospital and specialist health services. Despite early governmental and public health initiatives, there has been little response by medical services to address the implications of these changes. While assessing and treating substance abuse is identified as a core competency in UK general medicine training, the current syllabus for specialist geriatric training makes only limited reference to substance misuse within the context of health promotion rather than specific patient care. None of the core geriatric textbooks devote significant attention to the issue. Neither the British nor American Geriatrics Societies offer any form of guidance or best practice guidance for the identification or management of substance abuse in older patients. Unless the training and experience provided to clinicians change, it seems unlikely that clinical practice and service provision will improve.

Conclusions

Substance misuse in older people is a growing but underrecognized problem. The current generation of younger and middle aged people may be more exposed to substance misuse, partly because of easier availability or due to wider societal acceptance. As they enter older age, substance misuse could become more prevalent.

The varied presentation of diseases in older people could make identification and assessment of substance misuse difficult unless there is sufficient awareness and training of health and social care staff and organizations concerned. This will pose challenges, such as evidence gathering and further research, developing best practice guidelines, development of curriculums and training of healthcare professionals.

Ultimately, with improved health promotion amongst older adults and concurrent advances in understanding, training and education of healthcare professionals about the unique challenges and frailties of older people, it is hoped that there will be a subsequent improvement in both identification and management of substance misuse.

References

1. Office for National Statistics (2011) *National Population Projections, 2010-Based Statistical Bulletin*. Office for National Statistics. http://www.ons.gov.uk/ons/dcp171778_235886.pdf (last accessed 22 April 2014).
2. Robinson, S. and Harris, H. (2011) *Smoking and Drinking Among Adults, 2009 Report*. Office for National Statistics, UK. http://www.ons.gov.uk/ons/rel/ghs/general-lifestyle-survey/2009-report/smoking-and-drinking-among-adults--2009.pdf (last accessed 29 March 2014).
3. Simoni-Wastila, L. and Yang, H.K. (2006) Psychoactive drug abuse in older adults. *Am J Geriatr Pharmacother*, **4**(4), 380–394.
4. Jinks, M.J. and Raschko, R.R. (1990) A profile of alcohol and prescription drug abuse in a high-risk community-based elderly population. *DICP*, **24**(10), 971–975.
5. Blazer, D.G. and Wu, L.-T. (2009) The epidemiology of substance use and disorders among middle aged and elderly community adults: National Survey on Drug Use and Health (NSDUH). *Am J Geriatr Psychiatry*, **17**(3), 237–245.
6. Colliver, J.D., Compton, W.M., Gfroerer, J.C. and Condon, T. (2006) Projecting drug use among aging baby boomers in 2020. *Ann Epidemiol*, **16**(4), 257–265.
7. NHS Information Centre (2012) *Statistics on Drug Misuse: England, 2012*. The Health and Social Care Information Centre. http://www.hscic.gov.uk/catalogue/PUB09140/drug-misu-eng-2012-rep.pdf (last accessed 29 March 2014).

8. Gfroerer, J., Penne, M., Pemberton, M. and Folsom, R. (2003) Substance abuse treatment need among older adults in 2020: the impact of the aging baby-boom cohort. *Drug Alcohol Depend*, **69**(2), 127–135.

9. Mulinga, J.D. (1999) Elderly people with alcohol-related problems: where do they go? *Int J Geriatr Psychiatry*, **14**(7), 564–566.

10. Crome, I.B. and Day E. (1999) Substance misuse and dependence: older people deserve better services. *Rev Clin Gerontol*, **9**(4), 327–342.

11. Gjørup, T., Hendriksen, C., Lund, E. and Strømgård, E. (1987) Is growing old a disease? A study of the attitudes of elderly people to physical symptoms. *J Chronic Dis*, **40**(12), 1095–1098.

12. Morgan, R., Pendleton, N., Clague, J.E. and Horan, M.A. (1997) Older people's perceptions about symptoms. *Br J Gen Pract*, **47**(420), 427–430.

13. Garrido, M.M., Kane, R.L., Kaas, M. and Kane, R.A. (2011) Use of mental health care by community-dwelling older adults. *J Am Geriatr Soc*, **59**(1), 50–56.

14. Robinson, T.E., 2nd, White, G.L., Jr and Houchins, J.C. (2006) Improving communication with older patients: tips from the literature. *Fam Pract Manag*, **13**(8), 73–78.

15. NAO (National Audit Office) (2000) *Inpatient Admissions and Bed Management in NHS Acute Hospitals*. http://www.nao.org.uk/wp-content/uploads/2000/02/9900254.pdf (last accessed 29 March 2014).

16. NIHCM (National Institute For Health Care Management) (2012) *The Concentration of Health Care Spending*. http://www.nihcm.org/pdf/DataBrief3%20Final.pdf (last accessed 29 March 2014).

17. Center for Substance Abuse Treatment (1998) *Substance Abuse Among Older Adults*. Treatment Improvement Protocol (TIP) Series, No. 26, Substance Abuse and Mental Health Services Administration (SAMHSA), Rockville, MD. Available from: http://www.ncbi.nlm.nih.gov/books/NBK64419/ (last accessed 29 March 2014).

18. Whelan, G. (2003) Alcohol: a much neglected risk factor in elderly mental disorders. *Curr Opin Psychiatry*, **16**(6), 609–614.

19. Curtis, J.R., Geller, G., Stokes, E.J. *et al.* (1989) Characteristics, diagnosis, and treatment of alcoholism in elderly patients. *J Am Geriatr Soc*, **37**(4), 310–316.

20. McInnes, E. and Powell, J. (1994) Drug and alcohol referrals: are elderly substance abuse diagnoses and referrals being missed? *BMJ*, **308**(6926), 444–446.

21. Adams, W.L., Magruder-Habib, K., Trued, S. and Broome, H.L. (1992) Alcohol abuse in elderly emergency department patients. *J Am Geriatr Soc*, 1992 **40**(12), 1236–1240.

22. The National Center on Addiction and Substance Abuse at Columbia University (1998) *Under the Rug: Substance Abuse and the Mature Woman*. http://www.casacolumbia.org/download/file/fid/650 (last accessed 22 April 2014).

23. Shen, W.W. (1984) Extrapyramidal symptoms associated with alcohol withdrawal. *Biol Psychiatry*, **19**(7), 1037–1043.

24. Lemke, S. and Moos, R.H. (2003) Treatment and outcomes of older patients with alcohol use disorders in community residential programs. *J Stud Alcohol*, 2003 **64**(2), 219–226.

25. Lemke, S. and Moos, R.H. (2003) Outcomes at 1 and 5 years for older patients with alcohol use disorders. *J Subst Abuse Treat*, **24**(1), 43–50.

26. Outlaw, F.H., Marquart, J.M., Roy, A. *et al.* (2012) Treatment outcomes for older adults who abuse substances. *J Appl Gerontol*, **31**(1), 78–100.

27. SAGA (2013) *Over 50s Fear Dementia More Than Cancer*. http://www.saga.co.uk/newsroom/press-releases/2013/february/over-50s-fear-dementia-more-than-cancer.aspx (last accessed 29 March 2014).

28. WHO (World Health Organization) (2012) *Dementia*.http://www.who.int/mediacentre/factsheets/fs362/en/index.html (last accessed 29 March 2014).

29. Caracciolo, B., Gatz, M., Xu, W. *et al.* (2012) Differential distribution of subjective and objective cognitive impairment in the population: a nation-wide twin-study. *J Alzheimers Dis*, **29**(2), 393–403.
30. Busse, A., Angermeyer, M.C. and Riedel-Heller, S.G. (2006) Progression of mild cognitive impairment to dementia: a challenge to current thinking. *BJP*, **189**(5), 399–404.
31. Francis, J., Martin, D. and Kapoor, W.N. (1990) A prospective study of delirium in hospitalized elderly. *JAMA*, **263**(8), 1097–101.
32. George, J., Bleasdale, S. and Singleton, S.J. (1997) Causes and prognosis of delirium in elderly patients admitted to a district general hospital. *Age Ageing*, **26**(6), 423–427.
33. Larson, E.B., Kukull, W.A., Buchner, D. and Reifler, B.V. (1987) Adverse drug reactions associated with global cognitive impairment in elderly persons. *Ann Intern Med*, **107**(2), 169–173.
34. Katz, I.R., Parmelee, P. and Brubaker, K. (1991) Toxic and metabolic encephalopathies in long-term care patients. *Int Psychogeriatr*, **3**(2), 337–347.
35. Starr, J.M. and Whalley, L.J. (1994) Drug-induced dementia. Incidence, management and prevention. *Drug Saf*, **11**(5), 310–317.
36. Flaherty, J.H. (1998) Psychotherapeutic agents in older adults. Commonly prescribed and over-the-counter remedies: causes of confusion. *Clin Geriatr Med*, **14**(1), 101–127.
37. Barker, M.J., Greenwood, K.M., Jackson, M. and Crowe, S.F. (2004) Cognitive effects of long-term benzodiazepine use: a meta-analysis. *CNS Drugs*, **18**(1), 37–48.
38. Verdoux, H., Lagnaoui, R. and Begaud, B. (2005) Is benzodiazepine use a risk factor for cognitive decline and dementia? A literature review of epidemiological studies. *Psychol Med*, **35**(3), 307–315.
39. Paterniti S., Dufouil, C. and Alpérovitch, A. (2002) Long-term benzodiazepine use and cognitive decline in the elderly: the Epidemiology of Vascular Aging Study. *J Clin Psychopharmacol*, **22**(3), 285–293.
40. Billioti de Gage S., Begaud B., Bazin F. *et al.* (2012) Benzodiazepine use and risk of dementia: prospective population based study. *BMJ*, **345**, e6231.
41. McMorn, S., Schoedel, K.A. and Sellers, E.M. (2011) Effects of low-dose opioids on cognitive dysfunction. *JCO*, **29**(32), 4342–4343.
42. Sjogren, P., Thomsen, A.B and Olsen, A.K. (2000) Impaired neuropsychological performance in chronic nonmalignant pain patients receiving long-term oral opioid therapy. *J Pain Symptom Manage*, **19**(2), 100–108.
43. Davis, P.E., Liddiard, H. and McMillan, T.M. (2002) Neuropsychological deficits and opiate abuse. *Drug Alcohol Depend*, **67**(1), 105–108.
44. Culberson, J.W. (2006) Alcohol use in the elderly: beyond the CAGE. Part 2: Screening instruments and treatment strategies. *Geriatrics*, **61**(11), 20–26.
45. Oscar-Berman, M. and Marinković, K. (2007) Alcohol: effects on neurobehavioral functions and the brain. *Neuropsychol Rev*, **17**(3), 239–257.
46. Moore, A.A., Endo, J.O. and Carter, M.K. (2003) Is there a relationship between excessive drinking and functional impairment in older persons? *J Am Geriatr Soc*, **51**(1), 44–49.
47. Zuccalà, G., Onder, G., Pedone, C. *et al.* (2001) Dose-related impact of alcohol consumption on cognitive function in advanced age: results of a multicenter survey. *Alcohol Clin Exp Res*, **25**(12), 1743–1748.
48. Ridley, N.J., Draper, B. and Withall, A. (2013) Alcohol-related dementia: an update of the evidence. *Alzheimers Res Ther*, **5**(1), 3.
49. ICAP (International Centre for Alcohol Studies) (2010) *International Drinking Guidelines*. http://www.icap.org/Table/InternationalDrinkingGuidelines (last accessed 29 March 2014).

50. Thomson, A.D. and Marshall, E.J. (2006) The natural history and pathophysiology of Wernicke's Encephalopathy and Korsakoff's Psychosis. *Alcohol Alcohol*, **41**(2), 151–158.

51. Sechi, G. and Serra, A. (2007) Wernicke's encephalopathy: new clinical settings and recent advances in diagnosis and management. *Lancet Neurol*, **6**(5), 442–455.

52. Dregan, A., Stewart, R. and Gulliford, M.C. (2013) Cardiovascular risk factors and cognitive decline in adults aged 50 and over: a population-based cohort study. *Age Ageing*, **42**(3), 338–345.

53. Sabia, S., Elbaz, A., Dugravot, A. *et al.* (2012) Impact of smoking on cognitive decline in early old age: The Whitehall II Cohort Study. *Arch Gen Psychiatry*, **69**(6), 627–635.

54. Stevens, J.A., Corso, P.S., Finkelstein, E.A. and Miller, T.R. (2006) The costs of fatal and non-fatal falls among older adults. *Inj Prev*, **12**(5), 290–295.

55. Age UK (2012) *Stop Falling: Start Saving Lives and Money*. http://www.ageuk.org.uk/documents/en-gb/falls/stop_falling_report_web.pdf (last accessed 29 March 2014).

56. Van den Berg, M.E.L., Castellote, J.M., Mahillo-Fernandez, I. and de Pedro-Cuesta, J. (2010) Incidence of spinal cord injury worldwide: a systematic review. *Neuroepidemiology*, **34**(3), 184–192.

57. Lord, S.R., Clark, R.D. and Webster, I.W. (1991) Physiological factors associated with falls in an elderly population. *J Am Geriatr Soc*, **39**(12), 1194–1200.

58. WHO (World Health Organization) (2007) *Alcohol and Injury In Emergency Departments*. http://www.who.int/substance_abuse/publications/alcohol_injury_summary.pdf (last accessed 29 March 2014).

59. Anderson, P. (1988) Excess mortality associated with alcohol consumption. *BMJ*, **297**(6652), 824–826.

60. Preedy, V.R., Adachi, J., Ueno, Y. *et al.* (2001) Alcoholic skeletal muscle myopathy: definitions, features, contribution of neuropathy, impact and diagnosis. *Eur J Neurol*, **8**(6), 677–687.

61. Berg, A.O. (2003) Screening for osteoporosis in postmenopausal women: recommendations and rationale. *Am J Nurs*, **103**(1), 73–81.

62. Mukamal, K.J., Mittleman, M.A., Longstreth, W.T., Jr *et al.* (2004) Self-reported alcohol consumption and falls in older adults: cross-sectional and longitudinal analyses of the cardiovascular health study. *J Am Geriatr Soc*, **52**(7), 1174–1179.

63. Cawthon, P.M., Harrison, S.L., Barrett-Connor, E. *et al.* (2006) Alcohol intake and its relationship with bone mineral density, falls, and fracture risk in older men. *J Am Geriatr Soc*, **54**(11), 1649–1657.

64. Pariente, A., Dartigues, J.-F., Benichou, J. *et al.* (2008) Benzodiazepines and injurious falls in community dwelling elders. *Drugs Aging*, **25**(1), 61–70.

65. Gorevski, E., Bian, B., Kelton, C.M.L. *et al.* (2012) Utilization, spending, and price trends for benzodiazepines in the US Medicaid program: 1991–2009. *Ann Pharmacother*, **46**(4), 503–512.

66. Reed, K., Bond, A., Witton, J. *et al.* (2011) The changing use of prescribed benzodiazepines and z-drugs and of over-the-counter codeine-containing products in England: a structured review of published English and international evidence and available data to inform consideration of the extent of dependence and harm. National Addiction Centre. http://www.appgita.com/wp-content/uploads/2011/05/Report-1-NAC-Benzos-and-z-drug-addiction.pdf (last accessed 29 March 2014).

67. Bogunovic, O.J. and Greenfield, S.F. (2004) Practical geriatrics: Use of benzodiazepines among elderly patients. *Psychiatr Serv*, **55**(3), 233–235.

68. Curran, H.V., Collins, R., Fletcher, S. *et al.* (2003) Older adults and withdrawal from benzodiazepine hypnotics in general practice: effects on cognitive function, sleep, mood and quality of life. *Psychol Med*, **33**(7), 1223–1237.

69. Leipzig, R.M., Cumming, R.G. and Tinetti, M.E. (1999) Drugs and falls in older people: a systematic review and meta-analysis: I. Psychotropic drugs. *J Am Geriatr Soc*, **47**(1), 30–39.
70. Rapoport, M.J., Lanctôt, K.L., Streiner, D.L. *et al.* (2009) Benzodiazepine use and driving: a meta-analysis. *J Clin Psychiatry*, **70**(5), 663–673.
71. Orriols, L., Delorme, B., Gadegbeku, B. *et al.* (2010) Prescription medicines and the risk of road traffic crashes: A French registry-based study. *PLoS Med*, **7**(11), e1000366.
72. Chen, T.Y., Peronto, C.L. and Edwards, J.D. (2012) Cognitive function as a prospective predictor of falls. *J Gerontol B Psychol Sci Soc Sci*, **67**(6), 720–728.
73. Vestergaard, P., Rejnmark, L. and Mosekilde, L. (2006) Fracture risk associated with the use of morphine and opiates. *J Intern Med*, **260**(1), 76–87.
74. Miller, M., Stürmer, T., Azrael, D. *et al.* (2011) Opioid analgesics and the risk of fractures in older adults with arthritis. *J Am Geriatr Soc*, **59**(3), 430–438.
75. Ramaekers, J.G., Kauert, G., van Ruitenbeek, P. *et al.* (2006) High-potency marijuana impairs executive function and inhibitory motor control. *Neuropsychopharmacology*, **31**(10), 2296–2303.
76. Asbridge, M., Hayden, J.A. and Cartwright, J.L. (2012) Acute cannabis consumption and motor vehicle collision risk: systematic review of observational studies and meta-analysis. *BMJ*, **344**, e536.
77. Nygaard, I., Barber, M.D., Burgio, K.L. *et al.* (2008) Prevalence of symptomatic pelvic floor disorders in US women. *JAMA*, **300**(11), 1311–1316.
78. Markland, A.D., Goode, P.S., Redden, D.T. *et al.* (2010) Prevalence of urinary incontinence in men: results from the national health and nutrition examination survey. *J Urol*, **184**(3), 1022–1027.
79. Offermans, M.P.W., Du Moulin, M.F.M.T., Hamers, J.P.H. *et al.* (2009) Prevalence of urinary incontinence and associated risk factors in nursing home residents: a systematic review. *Neurourol Urodyn*, **28**(4), 288–294.
80. Thom, D.H., Haan, M.N. and Van Den Eeden, S.K. (1997) Medically recognized urinary incontinence and risks of hospitalization, nursing home admission and mortality. *Age Ageing*, **26**(5), 367–374.
81. Morrison, A. and Levy, R. (2006) Fraction of nursing home admissions attributable to urinary incontinence. *Value Health*, **9**(4), 272–274.
82. Foley, A.L., Loharuka, S., Barrett, J.A. *et al.* (2012) Association between the Geriatric Giants of urinary incontinence and falls in older people using data from the Leicestershire MRC Incontinence Study. *Age Ageing*, **41**(1), 35–40.
83. Ooi, W.L., Hossain, M. and Lipsitz, L.A. (2000) The association between orthostatic hypotension and recurrent falls in nursing home residents. *Am J Med*, **108**(2), 106–111.
84. Benazzi, F. (1998) Urinary retention with sertraline, haloperidol, and clonazepam combination. *Can J Psychiatry*, **43**(10), 1051–1052.
85. Landi, F., Cesari, M., Russo, A. *et al.* (2003) Potentially reversible risk factors and urinary incontinence in frail older people living in community. *Age Ageing*, **32**(2), 194–199.
86. CDC (2011) Visits To Physician Offices, Hospital Outpatient Departments, and Hospital Emergency Departments, by Age, Sex, and Race: United States, Selected Years 1995–2009. http://www.cdc.gov/nchs/data/hus/hus11.pdf#083 (last accessed 29 March 2014).
87. Philp, I.A (2007) Recipe for Care – Not a Single Ingredient. UK Department of Health. http://webarchive.nationalarchives.gov.uk/20070402085944/http://dh.gov.uk/prod_consum_dh/idcplg?IdcService=GET_FILE&dID=85995&Rendition=Web (last accessed 22 April 2014).
88. Amoako, E.P., Richardson-Campbell, L. and Kennedy-Malone, L. (2003) Self-medication with over-the-counter drugs among elderly adults. *J Gerontol Nurs*, **29**(8), 10–15.

89. WHO (World Health Organization) (2002) Safety of Medicines: A guide to detecting and reporting adverse drug reactions. http://archives.who.int/tbs/safety/esd_safety.pdf (last accessed 22 April 2014).

90. Lindsey, W.T., Stewart, D. and Childress, D. (2012) Drug interactions between common illicit drugs and prescription therapies. *Am J Drug Alcohol Abuse*, 38(4), 334–343.

91. Lazarou, J., Pomeranz, B.H. and Corey, P.N. (1998) Incidence of adverse drug reactions in hospitalized patients: a meta-analysis of prospective studies. *JAMA*, 279(15), 1200–1205.

92. Beijer, H.J.M. and de Blaey, C.J. (2002) Hospitalisations caused by adverse drug reactions (ADR): a meta-analysis of observational studies. *Pharm World Sci*, 24(2), 46–54.

93. Schiødt, F.V., Rochling, F.A., Casey, D.L. and Lee, W.M. (1997) Acetaminophen toxicity in an urban county hospital. *N Engl J Med*, 337(16), 1112–1117.

94. Signorovitch, J.E., Macaulay, D., Diener, M. *et al.* (2013) Hypoglycaemia and accident risk in people with type 2 diabetes mellitus treated with non-insulin antidiabetes drugs. *Diabetes Obes Metab*, 15(4), 335–341.

95. Flockhart, D.A. (2012) Dietary restrictions and drug interactions with monoamine oxidase inhibitors: an update. *J Clin Psychiatry*, 73(Suppl 1), 17–24.

96. Shulman, K.I., Tailor, S.A., Walker, S.E. and Gardner, D.M. (1997) Tap (draft) beer and monoamine oxidase inhibitor dietary restrictions. *Can J Psychiatry*, 42(3), 310–312.

97. Hillbom, M.E. (1980) Occurrence of cerebral seizures provoked by alcohol abuse. *Epilepsia*, 21(5), 459–466.

98. Warner, M., Chen, L.H., Makuc, D.M. *et al.* Drug poisoning deaths in the United States, 1980–2008. *NCHS Data Brief*, 2011 81, 1–8.

99. Wu, F.C.W., Tajar, A., Beynon, J.M. *et al.* (2010) Identification of late-onset hypogonadism in middle-aged and elderly men. *N Engl J Med*, J363(2), 123–135.

100. Liu, H., Bravata, D.M., Olkin, I. *et al.* (2007) Systematic review: the safety and efficacy of growth hormone in the healthy elderly. *Ann Intern Med*, 146(2), 104–115.

101. DeBellis, R., Smith, B.S., Choi, S. and Malloy, M. (2005) Management of delirium tremens. *J Intensive Care Med*, 20(3), 164–173.

102. Schuckit, M.A., Tipp, J.E., Reich, T. *et al.* (1995) The histories of withdrawal convulsions and delirium tremens in 1648 alcohol dependent subjects. *Addiction*, 90(10), 1335–1347.

103. Wojnar, M., Wasilewski, D., Zmigrodzka, I. and Grobel, I. (2001) Age-related differences in the course of alcohol withdrawal in hospitalized patients. *Alcohol Alcohol*, 36(6), 577–583.

104. Kraemer, K.L., Conigliaro, J. and Saitz, R. (1999) Managing alcohol withdrawal in the elderly. *Drugs Aging*, 14(6), 409–425.

105. Liskow, B.I., Rinck, C., Campbell, J. and DeSouza, C. (1989) Alcohol withdrawal in the elderly. *J Stud Alcohol*, 50(5), 414–421.

106. Schweizer, E. and Rickels, K. (1998) Benzodiazepine dependence and withdrawal: a review of the syndrome and its clinical management. *Acta Psychiatr Scand*, 98, 95–101.

107. Vorma, H., Naukkarinen, H.H., Sarna, S.J. and Kuoppasalmi, K.I. (2005) Predictors of benzodiazepine discontinuation in subjects manifesting complicated dependence. *Subst Use Misuse*, 40(4), 499–510.

108. Schweizer, E., Rickels, K., Case, W.G. and Greenblatt, D.J. (1990) Long-term therapeutic use of benzodiazepines. II. Effects of gradual taper. *Arch Gen Psychiatry*, 47(10), 908–915.

109. Iyer, S., Naganathan, V., McLachlan, A.J., and Le Couteur, D.G. (2008) Medication withdrawal trials in people aged 65 years and older: a systematic review. *Drugs Aging*, 25(12), 1021–1031.

110. Pétursson, H. (1994) The benzodiazepine withdrawal syndrome. *Addiction*, **89**(11), 1455–1459.
111. Fernando, P., Arora, A. and Crome, P. (2014) Inclusion of older people in interventional clinical trials. *Clin Investig*, **4**(1), 87–99.
112. Nickel, C.H., Ruedinger, J.M., Messmer, A.S. *et al.* (2013) Drug-related emergency department visits by elderly patients presenting with non-specific complaints. *Scand J Trauma Resusc Emerg Med*, **21**(1), 15.
113. Ekeh, A.P., Parikh, P.P., Walusimbi, M. *et al.* (2014) The prevalence of positive drug and alcohol screens in elderly trauma patients. *Subst Abus*, **35**(1), 51–55.
114. American Psychiatric Association (2013) *Diagnostic and Statistical Manual of Mental Disorders: DSM-5*, 5th edn. American Psychiatric Association, Washington, DC.
115. Adams, W.L., Barry, K.L. and Fleming, M.F. (1996) Screening for problem drinking in older primary care patients. *JAMA*, **276**(24), 1964–1967.
116. Blow, F., Brower, K.J., Schulenberg, J. *et al.* (1992) The Michigan Alcoholism Screening Test-geriatric version (MAST-G): a new elderly-specific screening instrument. *Alcohol Clin Exp Res*, **16**, 372.
117. Stuck, A., Siu, A., Wieland, G. *et al.* (1993) Comprehensive geriatric assessment: a meta-analysis of controlled trials. *The Lancet*, **342**(8878), 1032–1036.
118. Ellis, G., Whitehead, M.A., Robinson, D. *et al.* (2011) Comprehensive geriatric assessment for older adults admitted to hospital: meta-analysis of randomised controlled trials. *BMJ*, **343**, d6553.

EPIDEMIOLOGY AND DEMOGRAPHY

Chapter 6

CIGARETTE SMOKING AMONG ADULTS AGED 45 AND OLDER IN THE UNITED STATES, 2002–2011*

Shanta R. Dube[1] and Li-Tzy Wu[2]

[1] Division of Epidemiology and Biostatistics, School of Public Health, Georgia State University, USA
[2] Department of Psychiatry and Behavioral Sciences, School of Medicine, Duke University Medical Center, USA

Introduction

Tobacco use continues to be the leading cause of preventable morbidity and mortality in the United States and worldwide [1, 2]. Recent data from 16 countries in the Global Adult Tobacco Survey (GATS) show that current cigarette smoking prevalence among persons aged ≥15 years ranges from 5.8% in India to 38.8% in Russia, including 17.7% in the USA, 14.2% in Bangladesh, 16.9% in Brazil, 27.7% in China, 16.3% in Egypt, 15.6% in Mexico, 27.9% in Philippines, 30.2% in Poland, 23.5% in Thailand, 31.1% in Turkey, 28.6% in Ukraine, 24.7% in Uruguay, 19.9% in Vietnam and 21.0% in the United Kingdom [3]. Annually, 443 000 deaths among adults in the United States can be attributed to cigarette smoking and second-hand smoke exposure [4]. Moreover, the annual health care and labour costs incurred as a result of smoking in the United States amount to approximately $193 billion annually [4].

While there have been significant reductions in the prevalence of smoking since the release of the 1964 Surgeon General's report on smoking and health, in more recent years the rates of decline for cigarette smoking in the overall US population have slowed [5]. In 2011, 19% of adults and 18.5% of high school students were current cigarette smokers [5]. Variations in adult smoking continue to be observed across demographic characteristics such as gender, race/ethnicity and socioeconomic status [5]. For example, in 2011, 21.6% of men and 16.5% of women were current cigarette smokers. By race/ethnicity, current smoking prevalence was lowest among non-Hispanic Asians (9.9%) and highest among non-Hispanic American Indians/Alaska Natives (31.5%). Prevalence was higher among adults living below

---

*The findings and conclusions in this report are those of the authors and do not necessarily represent the official position of the Georgia State University and of Duke University.

Substance Use and Older People, First Edition.
Edited by Ilana B. Crome, Li-Tzy Wu, Rahul (Tony) Rao and Peter Crome.
© 2015 John Wiley & Sons, Ltd. Published 2015 by John Wiley & Sons, Ltd.

the federal poverty level (29.0%) compared with those living at or above this level (17.9%). Across age groups, the highest current prevalence was noted among adults aged 25–44 years (22.1%) and middle-to-older-age adults 45–64 years (21.4%) [5].

Cigarette smoking is associated with multiple health conditions which include, but are not limited to, malignancies, cardiovascular disease, lung disease and exacerbation of other chronic disorders, such as diabetes [2] and the biological mechanisms of how cigarette smoking causes these diseases have been documented [2]. Due to the age-related risks associated with these chronic disorders, smoking has a particularly negative impact on the health of older adults. As the 45–64-year old group continues to age, the unavoidable rise in the burden of smoking-related illnesses, such as chronic obstructive pulmonary disease, cardiovascular diseases and cancer, is expected to increase over time [6]. Therefore, smoking prevalence rates of demographic subgroups of adults aged 45 and older need to be closely monitored.

It is without a doubt that the US population has experienced rapid changes in its demography, including changes in the age structure. Census data indicate that, between 2000 and 2010, there was a dramatic shift in the number of persons aged 45–64 years and ≥65 years [7], which is largely due to the ageing 'baby boom' population, including persons born between the years of 1946 to 1964. From 2000 to 2010, growth rates of 31.5% and 15.1% were observed for persons aged 45–64 years and ≥65 years, respectively [7], which illustrates the rising population size of the ageing baby boom generation.

As we continue to progress into the twenty-first century, the United States will experience one of the largest ageing populations in its history through the baby boom generation. The implications for public health and health services will be many given that the baby boomers contribute to a large population living longer and, potentially, with a high prevalence of chronic medical disorders. The *Epidemiologic Transition Theory* provides a framework that describes how changing demographic patterns in populations such as shifts in age structure may contribute to changes in observed disease patterns and, consequently, health care needs and use [8]. For example, over time the United States has experienced reduced birth rates and death rates, and increased life expectancy, which were largely due to medical advances in reproductive health and infectious disease control, resulting in improved health and longevity. As a result, the leading causes of death are now chronic and degenerative diseases [8, 9]. A similar pattern of rising population sizes of older adults – due to improved longevity – is observed globally [10].

Because of the observed shift in the number of ageing adults and the implications this may have for public health, chronic disease management and demands for health care, examining social and behavioural determinants of disease [9], including the epidemiology of preventable risk behaviours such as cigarette smoking is needed for older adults. This chapter presents the prevalence of current cigarette smoking among two age strata of US adults: 45–64 years and ≥65 years using the US National Health Interview Survey (NHIS) between 2000 and 2011. Sociodemographic characteristics of current smokers in these two strata are presented as well as trends over time. Implications for public health and tobacco control efforts are discussed.

Evaluation methodology

To examine the epidemiology of cigarette smoking among adults aged 45 years or older, data from the National Health Interview Survey (NHIS) were used. The NHIS is a large-scale household interview survey of a statistically representative sample of the US civilian noninstitutionalized population (http://www.cdc.gov/nchs/nhis.htm). The NHIS serves as a principal source of information on the health of the US population by providing data to track health status, health care access and progress toward achieving national health objectives [11, 12].

The NHIS adult core questionnaire collects national health information on illness and disability. The questionnaire was administered by in-person interview and included a random probability sample of civilian adults aged ≥18 years. To examine changes over a 10-year period, data from the independent surveys of 2002 and 2011 NHIS were used. The total number of persons aged 45 or older was 15 322 (45–64 years: n = 9462; ≥65 years: n = 5860) in 2002 and 17 980 in 2011 (45–64 years: n = 11 078; ≥65 years: n = 6908).

Cigarette smoking status was defined by using two questions, 'Have you smoked at least 100 cigarettes in your entire life?' and 'Do you now smoke cigarettes every day, some days, or not at all?' Survey respondents who had smoked at least 100 cigarettes during their lifetime and, at the time of interview, reported smoking every day or some days were classified as current smokers. Smoking status for 45–64 years and ≥65 years was examined by sex, race/ethnicity, education, poverty status, region and employment status. For this report, poverty status was defined using 2008 poverty thresholds published by the US Census Bureau in 2009; family income was reported by the family respondent, who might or might not have been the same as the sample adult respondent from whom smoking information was collected.

The NHIS data were adjusted for nonresponse and weighted to provide national estimates of cigarette smoking prevalence. Firstly, the socioeconomic profiles of adults aged 45 or older (i.e. sex, race/ethnicity, education, poverty status, geographic region of residence and employment stats) were examined by age strata and by calendar year to explore changes in the estimated population size for demographic groups over a period of 10 years. Secondly, the prevalences of current cigarette smoking as well as daily smoking and nondaily smoking were calculated for each calendar year to determine potential changes in national trends of smoking among adults aged 45–64 and those ≥65 years, respectively. Thirdly, the national prevalences of current smoking by socioeconomic variables were examined. Finally, the analysis sample was stratified by age group and conducted adjusted logistic regression procedures to determine the strength of associations between socioeconomic variables and current smoking. Adjusted odds ratio estimates of socioeconomic correlates of current smoking in 2002 and in 2011 are reported to explore similarities and differences in correlates of smoking. In all analyses, 95% confidence intervals (95% CI) were calculated for each estimate to account for the survey's multistage probability sample design. Estimates with relative standard error of ≥30% (low level of precision) are not reported.

Results

Sociodemographic characteristics of older adults: 2002 versus 2011

Adults aged 45–64 years: During 2002 and 2011, among adults ≥18 years, the proportion of persons aged 45–64 years increased from 31.4% (95% CI = 30.8–32.1%) to 34.9% (95% CI = 34.3–35.6%), a relative increase of about 11% (Figure 6.1). By race/ethnicity, the proportion of non-Hispanic White decreased, while the proportion of Hispanic and Asian populations increased (Table 6.1). By education, the proportion of adults aged 45–64 years without high school diploma decreased, as did the proportion of adults who graduated high school. An increase was observed for 45–64 year olds who had some undergraduate college or associate degree and for those who completed undergraduate college. In this age group, there was also an increase in the proportion of adults who were not employed and a decreased in the proportion of adults who were currently employed.

Adults aged ≥65 years: During 2002 and 2011, among adults ≥18 years, the proportion of older adults aged ≥65 years increased from 16.1% (95% CI = 15.5–16.6%) to 17.2% (95% CI = 16.6–17.7%), a relative increase of 7%. There was a significant decline in the proportion of non-Hispanic Whites, while there was an increase in the proportion of non-Hispanic Asians in this older age group. By education, there was a significant decline in the proportion of older adults who did not graduate high school and an increase in the proportion of older adults with some college or Associate degree and who completed graduate degree.

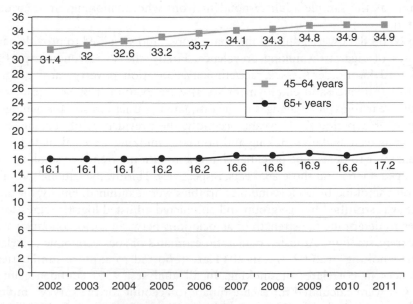

Figure 6.1 Ten-year trends in the proportion (%) of US adults aged 45–64 years and 65+ years (US National Health Interview Survey, 2002–2011).

Table 6.1 Overall characteristics of US adults aged 45 years or older (US National Health Interview Survey, 2002 and 2011)

| Characteristics | Adults 45–64 Years | | | | Adults 65+ Years | | | |
| | 2002 | | 2011 | | 2002 | | 2011 | |
	% (95% CI)		% (95% CI)		% (95% CI)		% (95% CI)	
Sex								
Male	48.4 (47.3–49.5)		48.6 (47.5–49.7)		42.8 (41.4–44.2)		44.0 (42.6–45.4)	
Female	51.6 (50.5–52.7)		51.4 (50.3–52.5)		57.2 (55.8–58.6)		56.0 (54.6–57.4)	
Race/Ethnicity								
White, non-Hispanic	**76.7 (75.5–77.8)**		**72.0 (70.9–73.2)**		**82.4 (81.1–83.7)**		**79.2 (77.9–80.5)**	
Black, non-Hispanic	10.3 (9.4–11.1)		11.2 (10.3–12.0)		8.2 (7.3–9.1)		8.4 (7.6–9.3)	
Hispanic	**8.5 (7.8–9.2)**		**10.8 (10.1–11.5)**		6.4 (5.6–7.2)		7.3 (6.6–8.0)	
American Indian/Alaska Native	0.5 (0.3–0.6)		0.5 (0.4–0.7)		—*		0.6 (0.3–1.0)	
Asian, non-Hispanic	**3.3 (2.8–3.7)**		**4.4 (3.9–4.8)**		**2.0 (1.4–2.5)**		**3.7 (3.2–4.2)**	
Multiple Race, non-Hispanic	0.8 (0.6–1.1)		1.1 (0.9–1.3)		0.8 (0.5–1.1)		0.7 (0.5–0.9)	
Education								
No diploma	**14.1 (13.3–14.9)**		**12.4 (11.6–13.2)**		**28.8 (27.3–30.3)**		**21.4 (20.1–22.7)**	
GED	3.2 (2.8–3.7)		3.0 (2.6–3.3)		2.7 (2.3–3.2)		2.3 (1.9–2.7)	
High School graduate	27.3 (26.1–28.4)		23.6 (22.6–24.7)		31.9 (30.5–33.3)		29.2 (28.0–30.5)	
Some college/Associate	**27.4 (26.3–28.4)**		**30.5 (29.5–31.5)**		**20.3 (19.0–21.5)**		**23.3 (22.1–24.4)**	

(continued)

Table 6.1 (continued)

| Characteristics | Adults 45–64 Years | | | | Adults 65+ Years | | | |
| | 2002 | | 2011 | | 2002 | | 2011 | |
	% (95% CI)		% (95% CI)		% (95% CI)		% (95% CI)	
Undergraduate degree	16.5 (15.5–17.4)		18.7 (17.7–19.7)		9.7 (8.6–10.7)		9.7 (8.6–10.7)	
Graduate degree	11.6 (10.8–12.4)		11.9 (11.0–12.7)		6.4 (5.7–7.1)		10.9 (9.9–11.9)	
Poverty Status								
At or above poverty level	70.0 (68.8–71.2)		79.4 (78.4–80.3)		56.7 (55.2–58.2)		72.0 (70.7–73.3)	
Below poverty level	5.9 (5.4–6.5)		9.9 (9.2–10.5)		7.6 (6.8–8.4)		8.4 (7.7–9.1)	
Unknown	24.1 (22.9–25.2)		10.8 (10.1–11.5)		35.7 (34.2–37.3)		19.6 (18.4–20.8)	
Region								
Northwest	20.4 (19.3–21.4)		19.1 (18.1–20.1)		20.2 (18.9–21.6)		19.6 (18.1–21.1)	
Midwest	24.3 (23.0–25.5)		23.3 (22.1–24.5)		24.1 (22.6–25.6)		22.1 (20.6–23.7)	
South	36.3 (34.9–37.8)		35.6 (34.3–36.8)		37.4 (35.3–39.4)		35.8 (34.1–37.5)	
West	19.0 (18.0–20.1)		22.0 (20.9–23.1)		18.3 (16.6–20.1)		22.5 (21.0–24.0)	
Employment status								
Currently employed	71.2 (70.1–72.4)		67.2 (66.0–68.4)		12.9 (11.9–13.9)		15.7 (14.7–16.7)	
Not currently employed	21.3 (20.2–22.3)		24.8 (23.7–25.9)		12.7 (11.7–13.7)		9.9 (9.0–10.7)	
Retired	7.5 (6.8–8.2)		8.0 (7.3–8.6)		74.4 (73.2–75.6)		74.4 (73.2–75.6)	

Boldface: The estimate in 2002 differs from the estimate in 2011 ($p < 0.05$).
*Estimates suppressed because of imprecise estimates due to small sample size.

In contrast with the 45–64-age group, there was an increase in the proportion of older adults who were currently employed but a decrease in the proportion of older adults who were not employed.

National trend in current smoking prevalence: 2002–2011

Current smoking (Figure 6.2): During the 10-year period (2002–2011), the prevalence of current smoking ranged from 21.0% (2007) to 22.7% (2002) among adults aged 45–64 years. Test for trends indicated no significant changes from 2002 (22.7%) and 2011 (21.4%) among adults 45–64 years. Among older adults aged ≥65 years, the prevalence of current smoking ranged from 7.9% (2011) to 10.2% (2006) during the 10-year period, and there was no significant changes in prevalence of smoking from 2002 (9.3%) and 2011 (7.9%).

Daily smoking (Figure 6.3): Between 2002 and 2011, the prevalence of current daily cigarette smoking ranged from 17.0% (2007) to 19.4% (2002) among adults aged 45–64 and from 6.6% (2011) to 8.5%(2002) among older adults aged ≥65 years. In both age groups, test for trends indicated that there were no significant changes in daily smoking prevalence during the period 2002 to 2011.

Nondaily smoking (Figure 6.3): During the span of 10 years, the prevalence of nondaily smoking ranged from 3.1% (2006) to 4.0% (2007) among adults aged 45–64 years and from 1.1% (2002) to 1.9% (2009) among older adults aged ≥65 years. During the period 2002–2011, among adults 45–64 years a statistically significant linear increase was observed for nondaily smoking ($p < 0.05$), but not for adults ≥65 years.

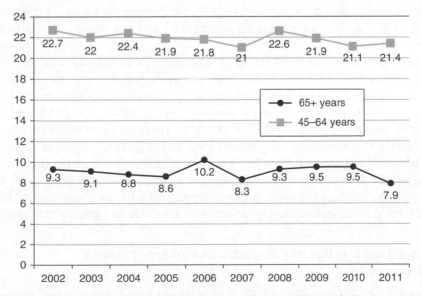

Figure 6.2   Ten-year trends in current cigarette smoking prevalence (%) among US adults aged 45–64 years and ≥65 years (US National Health Interview Survey, 2002–2011).

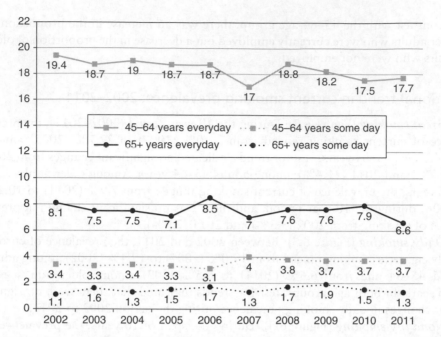

Figure 6.3 Ten-year trends in 'some day' and 'everyday' cigarette smoking prevalence (%) in the past month among US adults aged 45–64 years and 65+ years (US National Health Interview Survey, 2002–2011).

Current smoking prevalence by socioeconomic status: 2002 versus 2011

Table 6.2 summarizes smoking prevalence by socioeconomic status for the two age groups as well as changes in smoking prevalence by socioeconomic factors in 2002 versus 2011.

Adults aged 45–64 years (Table 6.2): Compared with the smoking prevalence among adults aged 45–64 in 2002 versus the corresponding prevalence in 2011, there were a significant declines in prevalence ($p < 0.05$) among women (21.1% vs. 18.5%), individuals at or above the poverty level (22.2% vs. 19.9%), and those who are currently employed (21.3% vs. 18.4%). There were no changes in smoking prevalence by race/ethnicity, educational level and geographic region of residence.

Adults aged ≥65 years (Table 6.2): Compared with the current smoking prevalence among adults aged ≥65 years in 2002 versus the corresponding prevalence in 2011, there were no significant changes in smoking prevalence by sex, race/ethnicity, educational level, poverty status, geographic region of residence and employment status.

Adjusted odds ratios of correlates of current smoking: 2002 versus 2011

Correlates of smoking among adults aged 45–64 years (Table 6.3): The overall patterns in associations of socioeconomic correlates with smoking were generally similar in 2002 and 2011.

Table 6.2 Current cigarette smoking among US adults aged 45 years or older by selected sociodemographic characteristics (US National Health Interview Survey, 2002 and 2011)

Characteristics	Adults 45–64 Years				Adults 65+ Years			
	2002		2011		2002		2011	
	% (95% CI)		% (95% CI)		% (95% CI)		% (95% CI)	
Total	22.7 (21.8–23.7)		21.4 (20.4–22.4)		9.3 (8.4–10.1)		7.9 (7.2–8.6)	
Sex								
Male	24.5 (23.0–25.9)		24.4 (22.9–25.9)		10.1 (8.7–11.5)		8.9 (7.7–10.1)	
Female	**21.1 (19.9–22.3)**		**18.5 (17.3–19.8)**		8.6 (7.6–9.7)		7.1 (6.2–8.0)	
Race/Ethnicity								
White, non-Hispanic	23.3 (22.2–24.4)		22.6 (21.3–23.8)		8.9 (8.0–9.9)		7.8 (7.0–8.6)	
Black, non-Hispanic	25.9 (23.2–28.5)		23.2 (20.9–25.6)		13.4 (10.6–16.2)		11.0 (8.8–13.2)	
Hispanic	17.2 (14.8–19.7)		13.5 (11.4–15.5)		7.4 (4.9–9.9)		7.2 (5.3–9.2)	
American Indian/Alaska Native	41.3 (25.5–57.1)		43.1 (28.7–57.4)		11.8 (−2.1–25.7)		6.7 (−1.9–15.3)	
Asian, non-Hispanic	10.4 (6.1–14.6)		11.3 (7.6–15.0)		6.6 (0.0–13.3)		3.6 (1.5–5.8)	
Multiple Race, non-Hispanic	24.8 (13.9–35.8)		32.3 (23.1–41.4)		21.9 (8.2–35.6)		13.1 (4.9–21.3)	
Education								
No diploma	32.8 (30.1–35.6)		33.8 (30.9–36.8)		11.9 (10.3–13.6)		10.4 (8.6–12.1)	
GED	41.6 (35.2–48.0)		52.4 (46.2–58.6)		8.8 (7.3–10.4)		16.4 (10.2–22.6)	
High School graduate	27.1 (25.0–29.1)		27.6 (25.5–29.8)		9.4 (4.5–14.3)		7.6 (6.4–8.8)	

(continued)

Table 6.2 (continued)

Characteristics	Adults 45–64 Years		Adults 65+ Years	
	2002	2011	2002	2011
	% (95% CI)	% (95% CI)	% (95% CI)	% (95% CI)
Some college/Associate	23.0 (21.2–24.9)	21.6 (19.8–23.3)	8.6 (7.0–10.2)	8.2 (6.6–9.8)
Undergraduate degree	12.9 (10.9–14.9)	9.9 (8.3–11.6)	6.9 (4.4–9.4)	6.0 (4.1–7.9)
Graduate degree	8.0 (6.3–9.6)	5.5 (4.0–7.0)	5.5 (2.9–8.1)	3.3 (1.7–4.8)
Poverty Status				
At or above poverty level	**22.2 (21.1–23.3)**	**19.9 (18.8–21.0)**	9.6 (8.4–10.8)	7.9 (7.0–8.7)
Below poverty level	38.6 (34.2–43.0)	36.0 (33.1–38.9)	14.5 (11.5–17.6)	14.3 (11.6–17.0)
Unknown	20.3 (18.4–22.1)	18.8 (16.1–21.5)	7.6 (6.3–8.9)	5.3 (3.9–6.7)
Region				
Northwest	21.0 (19.0–22.9)	19.3 (16.9–21.6)	10.1 (8.0–12.1)	7.8 (6.1–9.4)
Midwest	24.6 (22.6–26.7)	24.1 (21.9–26.4)	8.9 (7.5–10.3)	7.9 (6.5–9.4)
South	25.6 (24.1–27.1)	23.5 (21.8–25.3)	9.4 (8.0–10.8)	8.2 (7.0–9.4)
West	16.7 (14.8–18.6)	16.7 (15.0–18.5)	8.6 (6.6–10.6)	7.5 (5.9–9.0)
Employment status				
Currently employed	**21.3 (20.2–22.4)**	**18.4 (17.3–19.6)**	9.3 (7.2–11.5)	7.5 (5.7–9.3)
Not currently employed	29.5 (27.3–31.7)	31.2 (29.4–33.0)	12.3 (9.5–15.0)	13.3 (10.5–16.1)
Retired	16.9 (13.9–19.9)	15.8 (12.6–19.1)	8.7 (7.8–9.7)	7.3 (6.5–8.1)

Boldface: The estimate in 2002 differs from the estimate in 2011 (p < 0.05).

Table 6.3 Adjusted odds ratios (AOR) of correlates of current cigarette smoking among US adults aged 45 years or older by age strata and by year (US National Health Interview Survey, 2002 and 2011)

Adjusted logistic regression model*	Cigarette smoking among adults 45–64 years				Cigarette smoking among adults 65+ years			
	2002*		2011*		2002*		2011*	
	AOR	95% CI	AOR	95% CI	AOR	95% CI	AOR	95% CI
Sex								
Male	1.00		1.00		1.00		1.00	
Female	0.75	0.67–0.83	0.66	0.59–0.75	0.78	0.63–0.97	0.72	0.58–0.88
Race/Ethnicity								
White, non-Hispanic	1.00		1.00		1.00		1.00	
Black, non-Hispanic	0.87	0.74–1.03	0.73	0.62–0.85	1.27	0.95–1.70	1.19	0.91–1.57
Hispanic	0.52	0.43–0.65	0.34	0.27–0.43	0.60	0.39–0.91	0.66	0.47–0.92
American Indian/ Alaska Native	1.94	1.01–3.75	1.85	0.98–3.49	1.10	0.34–3.62	0.59	0.13–2.67
Asian, non-Hispanic	0.45	0.28–0.73	0.53	0.36–0.79	0.68	0.23–1.98	0.42	0.23–0.76
Multiple Race, non-Hispanic	0.90	0.49–1.63	1.54	0.97–2.46	2.78	1.24–6.23	1.56	0.73–3.32
Education								
No diploma	5.88	4.44–7.79	9.09	6.58–12.55	2.42	1.42–4.12	3.22	1.85–5.60
GED	7.90	5.43–11.49	16.15	10.96–23.80	1.84	0.85–3.96	5.51	2.70–11.26
High School graduate	4.26	3.29–5.50	6.08	4.47–8.27	1.86	1.09–3.17	2.58	1.52–4.36
Some college/ Associate	3.51	2.71–4.54	4.51	3.32–6.12	1.74	1.01–3.01	2.69	1.56–4.64

(continued)

Table 6.3 (continued)

Adjusted logistic regression model*	Cigarette smoking among adults 45–64 years				Cigarette smoking among adults 65+ years			
	2002*		2011*		2002*		2011*	
	AOR	95% CI	AOR	95% CI	AOR	95% CI	AOR	95% CI
Undergraduate degree	**1.77**	**1.31–2.41**	**1.84**	**1.30–2.62**	1.35	0.71–2.56	**1.96**	**1.06–3.62**
Graduate degree	1.00		1.00		1.00		1.00	
Poverty Status								
At or above poverty level	1.00		1.00		1.00		1.00	
Below poverty level	**1.54**	**1.24–1.90**	**1.45**	**1.23–1.71**	**1.46**	**1.06–1.99**	**1.73**	**1.30–2.29**
Unknown	**0.82**	**0.72–0.94**	0.90	0.74–1.09	**0.78**	**0.62–0.99**	**0.62**	**0.46–0.84**
Region								
Northwest	1.00		1.00		1.00		1.00	
Midwest	1.16	0.98–1.37	1.21	0.99–1.47	0.81	0.60–1.08	1.00	0.73–1.36
South	1.15	0.99–1.34	1.15	0.96–1.38	0.85	0.64–1.14	0.99	0.74–1.31
West	**0.79**	**0.65–0.96**	0.90	0.74–1.09	0.88	0.62–1.24	1.10	0.79–1.54
Employment Status								
Currently employed	1.00		1.00		1.00		1.00	
Not currently employed	**1.22**	**1.05–1.42**	**1.48**	**1.30–1.69**	1.16	0.79–1.69	**1.54**	**1.05–2.27**
Retired	**0.71**	**0.56–0.89**	**0.74**	**0.57–0.98**	0.86	0.63–1.16	0.87	0.64–1.19

Boldface: $p < 0.05$.
*Each adjusted logistic regression model included all covariates listed in the first column.

In 2011, male sex, being White (versus being Black, Hispanic, or Asian), less educated, below the poverty level and being unemployed (versus being employed) were associated with elevated odds of current smoking. In particular, there was a strong association between lower education levels and elevated odds of smoking.

Correlates of smoking among adults aged ≥65 years (Table 6.3): The overall patterns of results in this older group were similar to that of the 45–64-age group. In 2011, male sex, being White (versus being Hispanic or Asian), less educated, below the poverty level and being unemployed (versus being employed) were associated with elevated odds of current smoking.

Discussion

Results from the national samples in the NHIS confirm an increased population size of adults aged 45 or older. Between 2002 and 2011, there were also changes in the sociodemographic make-up, including an increase in the proportion of nonwhite groups (Hispanics, Asians) and adults with college education. The increase in the proportion of nonwhite groups is also noted in other data sources; this trend is expected to continue [5, 13]. Therefore, surveillance for tobacco use will need to monitor the trend in patterns of tobacco use and related morbidity among different subgroups of older nonwhites. In addition, the 45–64-age group represents a large proportion (34.9% in 2011) of the US adult population and has a much higher prevalence of current cigarette smoking (21.4%) than the older group (7.9%). Survey data from 13 low-to-middle income countries in the Global Adult Tobacco Survey have identified higher prevalences of current tobacco use among middle aged adults than among the younger group (15–24 years) [14]. These findings highlight a particular need for research and intervention efforts to increase smoking cessation rates in the middle-to-older-age population.

Another important finding is the lack of major changes in the overall current smoking prevalence over a 10-year period, and this pattern is observed in both age strata. Smoking initiation often occurs in adolescence or young adulthood and prevention efforts have rightly focused more on adolescents and young adults than older adults [15]. As noted from the national Monitoring the Future study, smoking prevalence rates have declined significantly among US adolescents in the 8th (aged 12–13) 10th (aged 15–16) and 12th (aged 17–19) grades during the past decade [16]. The present findings revealed that the majority of current cigarette smokers – 83% among smokers aged 45–64 years, 84% among smokers aged ≥65 years in 2011 – are daily smokers and that this pattern has remained stable during 2002–2011. In addition, among adults 45–46 years, there were significant increases in prevalence of nondaily cigarette use. Nondaily use may be an indication that smokers perceive occasional use as less harmful. Unless effective measures are implemented to decrease smoking prevalences substantially, the smoking-related burden and health care use are expected to rise over time as the baby boomer generation continues to grow older. These findings reiterate the need to identify and implement secondary or targeted prevention efforts to increase quitting and reduce smoking related morbidity among older adults.

The findings also identify several subgroups of middle aged and elderly adults who show elevated odds of current smoking, including men, non-Hispanic Whites, less educated people, adults living below the federal poverty level, and unemployed adults. Additionally, elderly adults who are Black, American Indian/Alaska Native or mixed race (multiple races] are as likely as Whites in odds of current smoking. Collectively, the pattern demonstrates that cigarette smoking disproportionally affects socioeconomically disadvantaged middle aged and elderly adults, and that there is little geographic variation in smoking prevalence. The overall pattern is in line with other research, suggesting that indicators of low socioeconomic status are robust correlates of cigarette smoking [17].

The data source of the NHIS has some limitations. The results should be interpreted within the context of its limitations. Causal inferences cannot be made because the data are cross-sectional. The results are based on survey respondents' self-reports, which may be influenced by reporting errors. The survey's sampling framework does not cover the homeless and institutionalized adults. These results from the NHIS should be considered conservative estimates of smoking prevalences among noninstitutionalized adults in the community. In addition, this study does not consider mental illness, a correlate of smoking [11, 18]. Other national survey data have estimated that approximately 20% of adults aged ≥18 years in the United States have a mental illness (defined as a mental, behavioural or emotional disorder, excluding developmental and substance use disorders) in the past 12 months [11]. Among adults with a mental illness, 36.1% are current cigarette smokers, compared with 21.4 % among adults without a mental illness [11]. Among adults with a mental illness, high prevalences of cigarette smoking are also noted among men and adults with a lower level of education or living below the poverty level [11].

Conclusion

More than one in five adults aged 45–64 is a current cigarette smoker, and one in 12 adults aged 65 or older is a current smoker. Most current users smoke cigarettes daily. The data suggest that adults with a lower socioeconomic status use more cigarettes than adults with a higher socioeconomic status. A similar pattern of associations between a lower socioeconomic status and greater prevalences of current tobacco use is also observed in survey data from 13 low-to-middle income countries in the Global Adult Tobacco Survey [14]. The smoking-related burden of illnesses is expected to have a particularly negative impact on adults with a lower socioeconomic status; they, unfortunately, also show disparities in the overall health status compared with individuals with a higher socioeconomic status [19].

The stability of smoking prevalence over a span of 10 years demonstrates a need for concerted research efforts to identify effective tobacco control programmes specifically targeting middle aged and older adults, especially men without a college degree. Additionally, increasing routine screening for cigarette smoking in the general medical settings and providing brief intervention and treatment (e.g. pharmacotherapy) as indicated is needed to promote smoking quitting and cessation [20, 21]. While healthcare providers have not offered older tobacco-using patients tobacco cessation information consistently [22, 23], research has demonstrated that offering nurses and other allied health professionals training on tobacco cessation intervention can improve practitioner attitudes toward helping older adults quit tobacco [24]. Quitting smoking improves health and can contribute to reduced healthcare costs and improved quality of life. The increasing populations of older adults in the United States and other countries require additional research efforts to inform tobacco control programmes and to promote effective use of smoking cessation treatment.

References

1. WHO (World Health Organization). WHO report on the global tobacco epidemic, 2011: Warning about the dangers of tobacco. World Health Organization, Geneva, Switzerland.
2. US Department of Health and Human Services (2010) 2010 Surgeon General's Report – How tobacco smoke causes disease: the biology and behavioral basis for smoking-attributable disease: a report of the Surgeon General. US Department of Health and Human Services, CDC, Atlanta, GA. http://www.cdc.gov/tobacco/data_statistics/sgr/2010/index.htm (last accessed 31 March 2014).
3. Giovino, G.A., Mirza, S.A., Samet, J.M. *et al.* (GATS Collaborative Group) (2012) Tobacco use in 3 billion individuals from 16 countries: an analysis of nationally representative cross-sectional household surveys. *Lancet*, 380(9842), 668–679.
4. Centers for Disease Control and Prevention (2008) Smoking-attributable mortality, years of potential life lost, and productivity losses – United States, 2000–2004. *MMWR Morb Mortal Wkly Rep*, 57(45);1226–1228.
5. Centers for Disease Control and Prevention (CDC) (2012) Current cigarette smoking among adults – United States, 2011. *MMWR Morb Mortal Wkly Rep*, 61(44): 889–894.
6. Feenstra, T.L., van Genugten, M.L. *et al.* (2001) The impact of aging and smoking on the future burden of chronic obstructive pulmonary disease: a model analysis in the Netherlands. *Am J Respir Crit Care Med*, 164(4), 590–6.
7. US Census Bureau (2011) Age and Sex Composition: 2010. Economics and Statistics Administration, US Department of Commerce. http://www.census.gov/prod/cen2010/briefs/c2010br-03.pdf (last accessed 31 March 2014).
8. Omran, A.R. (1971) The epidemiologic transition. A theory of the epidemiology of population change. *Milbank Mem Fund Q*, 49(4), 509–538.
9. McKeown, R.E. (2009) The epidemiologic transition: Changing patterns of mortality and population dynamics. *Am J Lifestyle Med*, 3(1 Suppl), 19S–26S.
10. Kinsella, K. and He, W. (2009) An Aging World: 2008. International Population Reports, P95/09-1, US Government Printing Office, Washington, DC.
11. Centers for Disease Control and Prevention (CDC) (2013) Vital signs: current cigarette smoking among adults aged ≥18 years with mental illness – United States, 2009–2011. *MMWR Morb Mortal Wkly Rep*, 62(5), 81–87.
12. Centers for Disease Control and Prevention (CDC). National Health Interview Survey: The principal source of informationon the health of the U.S. population. http://www.cdc.gov/nchs/data/nhis/brochure2010January.pdf (last accessed 31 March 2014).

13. Wu, L.T., Swartz, M.S., Burchett, B. *et al.* (2013) Tobacco use among Asian Americans, Native Hawaiians/Pacific Islanders, and mixed-race individuals: 2002–2010. *Drug Alcohol Depend*, **132**(1–2), 87–94

14. Palipudi, K.M., Gupta, P.C., Sinha, D.N. et al. (GATS Collaborative Group) (2012) Social determinants of health and tobacco use in thirteen low and middle income countries: evidence from Global Adult Tobacco Survey. *PLoS One*, 7(3), e33466.

15. Freedman, K.S., Nelson, N.M. and Feldman, L.L. (2012) Smoking initiation among young adults in the United States and Canada, 1998–2010: a systematic review. *Prev Chronic Dis*, **9**, E05.

16. Johnston, L.D., O'Malley, P.M., Bachman, J.G. and Schulenberg, J.E.(2013) Monitoring the future national results on drug use: 2012 overview, key findings on adolescent drug use. Institute for Social Research, University of Michigan, Ann Arbor, MI.

17. Blazer, D.G. and Wu, L.T. (2012) Patterns of tobacco use and tobacco-related psychiatric morbidity and substance use among middle-aged and older adults in the United States. *Aging Ment Health*, **16**(3), 296–304.

18. Dube, S.R., Caraballo, R.S., Dhingra, S.S. *et al.* (2009) The relationship between smoking status and serious psychological distress: findings from the 2007 Behavioral Risk Factor Surveillance System. *Int J Public Health*, **54**(Suppl 1), 68–74.

19. National Center for Health Statistics/Centers for Disease Control and Prevention (2012) Health, United States, 2011: With special feature on socioeconomic status and health. National Center for Health Statistics, Hyattsville, MD.

20. Lai, D.T., Cahill, K., Qin, Y. and Tang, J.L. (2010) Motivational interviewing for smoking cessation. *Cochrane Database of Systematic Reviews* **1** (Art. No.: CD006936). doi: 10.1002/14651858.CD006936.pub2 .

21. Stead, L.F., Perera, R., Bullen, C. *et al.* (2012) Nicotine replacement therapy for smoking cessation. *Cochrane Database of Systematic Reviews* **11** (Art. No.: CD000146). doi: 10.1002/14651858.CD000146.pub4 .

22. Steinberg, M.B., Akincigil, A., Delnevo, C.D. *et al.* (2006) Gender and age disparities for smoking-cessation treatment. *Am J Prev Med*, **30**(5), 405–412.

23. Watt, C.A., Carosella, A.M., Podgorski, C. and Ossip-Klein, D.J. (2004) Attitudes toward giving smoking cessation advice among nursing staff at a long-term residential care facility. *Psychol Addict Behav*, **18**, 56–63.

24. Kerr, S., Whyte, R., Watson, H. *et al.* (2011) A mixed-methods evaluation of the effectiveness of tailored smoking cessation training for healthcare practitioners who work with older people. *Worldviews Evid Based Nurs*, **8**, 177–186.

Chapter 7

EPIDEMIOLOGY AND DEMOGRAPHY OF ALCOHOL AND THE OLDER PERSON

Stephan Arndt[1,2] and Susan K. Schultz[2]

[1] Iowa Consortium for Substance Abuse Research/University of Iowa, USA
[2] University of Iowa College of Medicine, USA

Introduction

The ageing of the 'baby boomers' is presenting new opportunities to understand how substance use presents in the elder years and how it may interact with other socioeconomic and health factors. This chapter reviews the epidemiology of substance use in older adults. While the concept of 'older' is often dependent on the context in which the term is used, for most of the studies described here the term refers to individuals over the age of 60 years, although when studies have used different thresholds, it is noted. When considering the research presented here, it is useful to recognize that across studies there may be a variety of descriptive terms used to define alcohol use that is occurring with sufficient magnitude to incur a risk for deleterious consequences. In many studies, the term 'misuse' is used, which refers either to alcohol use that is above a specified threshold for gender and age or use in situations that may lead to adverse outcomes, such as in the context of an existing medical condition. The terms 'immoderate', 'problematic', 'unhealthy' and 'hazardous' use are synonymous with this concept. In this chapter, the terms that were chosen by the researchers are used when discussing each individual study. Additionally, for each study described in this chapter, the threshold quantity of alcohol consumption that was used to designate the terms (e.g. 'misuse' or 'immoderate use') are also described. Because there are no universally accepted definitions for each of these thresholds, they are described here in a study-dependent manner.

It is also important to note that different epidemiologic results may be obtained depending on what consumption thresholds were used in each study. Most studies use a specific number of 'drinks' as a metric for determining the magnitude of use. A 'drink' is typically refers to one serving of 12 g of absolute alcohol, for example one 12-oz. (355 ml) beer, one 5-oz. (148 ml) glass of wine or one 1.5-oz. (44 ml) serving ('shot') of distilled spirits. Overall, the findings that are presented in this chapter tend to suggest in aggregate that overall alcohol use is reduced in older age groups. A comprehensive review is provided that demonstrates a range of estimates

Substance Use and Older People, First Edition.
Edited by Ilana B. Crome, Li-Tzy Wu, Rahul (Tony) Rao and Peter Crome.
© 2015 John Wiley & Sons, Ltd. Published 2015 by John Wiley & Sons, Ltd.

suggesting that between 4 and 14% of older adults may be in a hazardous drinking range. This chapter also reviews the demography of binge drinking (i.e. the consumption of substantial quantities of alcohol in one continuous episode typically lasting from a few hours to up to day in duration) and provides a review of current knowledge across a variety of data sources. In other sections of this chapter, there are terms employed such as a 'substance use disorder'. This is a diagnostic term that designates a category based on both magnitude of use as well as the presence of continued use of alcohol despite adverse consequences (e.g. social, occupational, medical etc.). This chapter reviews the findings observed by various studies that have applied diagnostic criteria to estimate substance use disorders in older adults. Finally, a review of demographic factors, such as socioeconomic status, gender, race and education, is discussed in relation to problematic use.

Main reviews

Epidemiological estimates of prevalence of alcohol use

When considering the current epidemiological data regarding alcohol use, it is helpful to be aware of the methods that are used in defining 'misuse', Studies of alcohol misuse in older adults use two typical strategies to identify problem use. The first strategy involves assessing the amount of alcohol consumed and the second strategy involves determining the presence of a clinical diagnosis of abuse or dependence. When using the strategy of quantifying the amount of alcohol consumption, the presence of hazardous drinking levels is assessed with questionnaires or interviews. When using the approach involving clinical diagnoses, typically structured interviews based on Diagnostic and Statistical Manual of Mental Disorders IV (DSM-IV) criteria are used to derive the diagnosis. While other methods are available, they are seldom used. For example, screening tools such as the Michigan Alcoholism Screening Test – Geriatric Version (MAST-G) [1], Alcohol Use Disorders Identification Test (AUDIT) [2] or CAGE questionnaire [3], quickly identify potential drinking problems and can be used with older populations. However, screening measures tend to be very sensitive and may 'overidentify' cases. Due to their excessive sensitivity, screening instruments may not be ideal for research that seeks to estimate the prevalence of problems in a population and, consequently, these screening tests are not used extensively in epidemiological studies. However, these instruments may be of great value in the clinical setting to provide a quick means of identifying a potential problem that may be further explored in the context of a clinical interview. In this way, these screening instruments can be used as intended and the clinical encounter can elicit the necessary information to add specificity to the diagnosis.

Estimates of alcohol problems based on amount of drinking

To understand the demography of alcohol use in the older adult, it is helpful to recognize that over 50% of the US adult population drinks alcohol at least monthly. The prevalence of people who drink any alcohol goes down with age. Figure 7.1

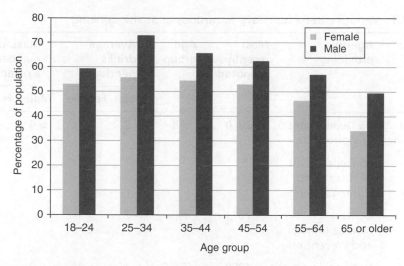

Figure 7.1 Any alcohol use in the past 30 days: US population all ages. (Estimates are based on the 2011 Behavioral Risk Factor Surveillance System, BRFSS [4]).

presents the percentage of men and women drinking in various age groups. These estimates are based on the 2011 Behavioral Risk Factor Surveillance System, BRFSS [4], a stratified random sample of the US population. The data set contains responses from 504 408 telephone interviews and includes questions about number of drinks, number of drinking days and other alcohol-related questions. There is a gradual but noticeable age-related decline in alcohol users, 40.7% of people 65 years of age or older drank some alcohol in the past month.

Different agencies have defined moderate versus hazardous use in a number of ways (Table 7.1). The terms 'heavy', 'high risk' and 'hazardous' reflect the terms used by the agencies which provide them. While it might be convenient to provide a gradation of severity, these terms are most commonly used interchangeably. The US Department of Agriculture and US Department of Health and Human Services define moderate use of alcohol as up to two drinks a day for men and up to one drink a day for women [5]. These agency's Dietary Guidelines for Americans 2010 define heavy or high risk drinking as more than three drinks on a given day or more than seven drinks a week for women and more than four drinks on a given day or 14 drinks a week for men. The Centers for Disease Control and Prevention (CDC) define 'heavy drinking' as more than two drinks a day for men and more than one drink per day for women, that is, anything more than moderate drinking [4]. Neither of these sources gives special consideration for older drinkers.

Older people may be substantially more sensitive to alcohol than younger people because of metabolic changes and increased use of medications and, in some medical conditions such as dementia in later life, any alcohol use at all may be problematic. Because of this, the National Institute on Alcohol Abuse and Alcoholism (NIAAA) and the Substance Abuse Mental Health Services Administration (SAMHSA) Center for Substance Abuse Treatment (CSAT) suggest revised criteria for moderate drinking

Table 7.1 Various criteria for heavy, hazardous or at-risk drinking

Label in text	Agency providing	Most recent year proposed	Age group	Average drinks per day[a]		Maximum number on a given day[a]	
				Male	Female	Male	Female
Dietary Guidelines	US Department of Agriculture	2010	All	> 2	> 1	> 4	> 3
	US Department of Health and Human Services						
CDC	Centers for Disease Control and Prevention	2011	All	> 2	> 1	–	–
NIAAA/ CSAT 1	National Institute on Alcohol Abuse and Alcoholism	1998	65+ / 60+	> 1	> 1	> 2	> 2
	Substance Abuse Mental Health Services Administration Center for Substance Abuse Treatment						
NIAAA/ CSAT 2	National Institute on Alcohol Abuse and Alcoholism	2012	65+	> 1	> 1	> 3	> 3
	Substance Abuse Mental Health Services Administration Center for Substance Abuse Treatment						

[a]Units are in terms of a 'drink', typically one serving of 12 g of absolute alcohol, e.g. one 12-oz. (355 ml) beer, one 5-oz. (148 ml) glass of wine, or one 1.5-oz. (44 ml) serving ('shot') of distilled spirits.

in older adults[6, 7]. The original NIAAA/CSAT 1 criterion for moderate drinking was: No more than one drink per day and no more than two drinks for any special occasion, for example weddings. CSAT also notes a somewhat lower but an unspecified limit for women. As a greater number of older adults are surviving into later life with substantial chronic medical conditions, there is a need for even more specialized methods to determine problematic use thresholds, yet there remain only very broad criteria. For example, the Center for Substance Abuse Treatment (CSAT), National Institute on Alcohol Abuse and Alcoholism (NIAAA) [8, 9], American

Public Health Association and National Highway Traffic Safety Administration [10] have more recently provided slightly more liberal criteria that includes older adults. Instead of a two drink maximum on a given day, the newer criteria allows for three drinks on a given day. Thus, the NIAAA/CSAT 2 criterion for hazardous drinking has become more than one drink per day on average or more than three drinks on a given day for those aged 65 or older. In contrast, the World Health Organization (WHO) does not explicitly give a number of units for harmful or hazardous use of alcohol. WHO defines harmful or hazardous use as any use that produces damage to one's health, either physical or mentally [11, 12]. While the WHO criteria may be more clinically sound and better reflect the diversity of medical health in late life, it is not easily measureable for epidemiological purposes.

While thresholds may not estimate individual vulnerabilities to problematic use, they do allow an assessment of magnitude of consumption by age. A decline in use with age is presented in Figure 7.2, which shows the 30-day prevalence for drinking more than one, two, three or four drinks per day in different age groups using the 2011 Behavioral Risk Factor Surveillance System data. These simple cut-off points do not consider the sex of the respondent nor the maximum number of drinks on a given day. The fairly steady decline in prevalence is apparent across all of the cut-off points, one or more through four or more. These findings of lower overall use are substantially less pronounced although still evident in the prevalence that is presented in Figure 7.2, which is based on the CDC average amount criterion that does consider sex. The difference between the two drink criteria and the CDC criteria reflects the added women who drink more than one drink per day. Interestingly, the proportion of men to women shifts over the age groups. The US Census Bureau's 2011 American Community Survey estimates the proportions of men and women

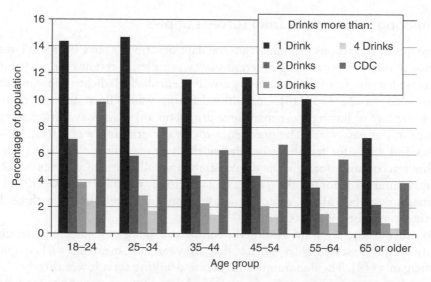

Figure 7.2 Average number of drinks per day for age groups compared to the CDC heavy drinking criterion. (Estimates are based on the 2011 Behavioral Risk Factor Surveillance System, BRFSS [4]. The CDC criterion considers sex (Male > 2 / Female > 1)).

in the youngest age group are 51.3 and 48.7%, respectively. In the 65 and older group, the proportions of men and women are 43.3 and 56.7%, respectively. Using the CDC sex adjusted criterion, more than two drinks for men and more than one drink for women, 3.9% (95% CI: 3.7%, 4.1%) of the population aged 65 or older are hazardous drinkers.

Importance of threshold selection for defining problem use

As evident thus far in these findings, the selection of the criterion threshold has substantial effects on the resulting estimates. For example, in analysing the Behavioral Risk Factor Surveillance System (2011 BRFSS data) using the 'more than one' criterion proposed by NIAAA and CSAT, the estimate goes up to 7.3% for 65 years or older adults that are hazardous or at-risk drinkers. In this analysis, only 3.5% (95% CI: 3.3%, 3.7%) of women fall into the hazardous drinking range, while 12.3% (95% CI: 11.8%, 12.8%) of men fall into it. Hence, this more conservative definition nearly doubles the number of older people considered hazardous drinkers.

The NIAAA/CSAT criteria also include a maximum number of drinks on an occasion. Including the maximum of two drinks in a given day substantially increases the number of 65 years or older adults falling into the hazardous drinking group, adding another 6.4% to the 7.3%, or 13.7%. Nearly one third (31.2%) of the additional hazardous drinkers 65 years or older reported having maximum of three drinks on a particular day. Thus, considering only the average drinks per day, 7.3% of 65 years or older adults are estimated hazardous drinkers but considering the no more than two on a given day, 13.7% are considered as such. Using the more than three drinks on a given day adds only 2.5% and results in 9.8% as the estimate for 65 years or older hazardous drinkers.

Estimating problem use from survey samples

Estimates of hazardous drinking from the data described above bear some resemblance to recent reports using different survey samples. A recent report used interviews with a sample of the community dwelling enrolled Medicare population aged 65 or older (n = 12 413) [13]. Unhealthy drinking was defined as more than one drink per day or having more than three drinks on any given day during a 'typical month in the past year'. The prevalence for heavy drinking was 9.0%, 16% for males and 4.0% for females. Considering the average number of drinks per day without accounting for episodic drinking, the overall estimate was 6.8%, 12.1% for males and 2.7% for females. These estimates closely resemble the BRFSS 2011 data estimates described above, especially considering this study's use of a three drink maximum number of drinks per day.

Another study, using the National Institute on Aging's Health and Retirement Study sample, assessed older (greater than 50 years old, mean age = 61) employed participants [14]. The definition of moderate drinking set a lower threshold, that is less than two drinks per day for men and less than one or more for women. Thus, an average of two drinks for men or one drink for women was considered (im)moderate, whereas these amounts would be considered moderate using the CDC criterion that require *greater than* two drinks for men or one drink for women. In this relatively young older group, 12.5% indicated (im)moderate drinking. A higher estimate of hazardous drinking is not surprising, given that the sample is younger and the definition more inclusive than the BRFSS or Medicare sample. To conclude this review of problem use, one report used the NIAAA National Epidemiologic Survey on Alcohol and Related Conditions (NESARC) 2001/2002 Wave 1 data [15]. This study focused on 8205 individuals 65 or older. Based on the sex-adjusted CRC criteria, the prevalence of heaving drinking among current drinkers (45.1%) was reported as 10.7% overall, 11.6% for men and 9.7% for women.

Summary of epidemiological estimates

In summary, between approximately 4 and 14% of older adults appear to be in a hazardous drinking range. Much of this difference occurs because of various definitions for hazardous use in this population. Adding a 'no more than' some number of drinks (e.g. two or three) on a given day can have a dramatic effect on the prevalence estimate. For example, an older person might drink rarely over the month but indulge in drinking three cans of beer or three glasses of wine on a special event. Using the average drinks per day, this person is well within the moderate use category. Adding a maximum of two drinks a day to the criterion makes the same person a hazardous drinker. Thus, the range, 4–14%, represents a continuum of hazard. Considering the actual number of affected people in the United States, there are between 1.6 million very hazardous to 5.6 million, at least, hazardous older drinkers.

Specific problematic drinking behaviours: binge drinking

Binge drinking poses additional concerns for older drinkers. Binge drinking, that is consuming large quantities of alcohol within a period, usually a day, is associated with numerous health and safety problems. This may be especially true for older adults. Furthermore, binge drinking is associated with increased risk for subsequent injury following spinal cord trauma [16]. A recent meta-analysis indicated a (nonlinear) dose response increase in alcohol consumption and injury (intentional and unintentional) injuries [17]. However, another study showed no correlation between binge drinking and falls in those aged 85 or more [18].

Binge drinking is usually defined by five or more drinks per setting, occasion or day for men and four or more drinks per day for women. This follows the 2004 NIAAA definition [19], which attempts to associate the number of drinks with a blood alcohol concentrations of 0.08 gram percent or above. The NIAAA newsletter also acknowledges that number of drinks for older people might be less but offers no quantification or estimate. SAMHSA, however, provides a cut-off of four drinks per occasion [20] regardless of sex. Elsewhere [21], SAMHSA defines binge drinking as five or more drinks on an occasion regardless of sex or age group. The CDC uses the NIAAA definition [4].

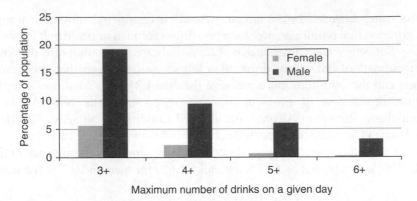

Figure 7.3 Percentage of men and women aged 65 or older who within the last 30 days drank more than the indicated number of drinks per day. (Estimates are based on the 2011 Behavioral Risk Factor Surveillance System, BRFSS [4]).

Regarding binge drinking in older adults, Figure 7.3 shows the estimated percentage of men and women aged 65 or older who within the last 30 days drank three or more drinks on a day, drank four or more drinks on a day and so on. These estimates use the BRFSS 2011. As with the average number of drinks per day, differing 30-day prevalence drops as the cut-off point increases; however, the sex difference is even more dramatic. Using the five or greater rule (regardless of sex or age) with the 2011 BRFSS data, 3.0% of people aged 65 or older binge drink. Only 6.1% of men and 0.7% of women drank five or more drinks within the last 30 days. Decreasing the criteria for women to four or more increases the estimate of binge drinking to 3.8% (6.1% for men and 2.2% for women). Using four or more drinks for both men and women results in an estimate of 5.3%, 9.5% for men and 2.2% for woman.

This pattern of observations in the above findings raises two key points regarding the demography of binge drinking. Firstly, binge drinking is clearly a male dominated problem. Secondly, the differing definitions only shift the overall prevalence estimates a few percentage points, from a low of 3.0% to a high of 5.3% considering both sexes. However small the shift in percentages, these translate into a significant number of people, between 1.2 million and 2.1 million elders in the Unite States, who binge drink based on these 2011 BRFSS data. There have been only a few reports in the literature specifically addressing binge drinking in older adults. One study used the Health and Retirement Study, waves 2004 and 2006 [14]. Respondents (n = 2902) were 50 years of age or older (mean = 60.4, SD = 7.14) and still employed. The prevalence of those who reported drinking five or more drinks on a single occasion was 2.65%. While the Health and Retirement study population was not necessarily representative of the general 65 or older population, the percentage of binge drinking is not far afield of the BRFSS estimates. However, the 2.65% estimate is a little lower than might be expected in a younger group, which may be due to selection factors, as only employed respondents were included.

Two studies addressing binge drinking used the National Survey on Drug Use and Health (NSDUH) data. One of these used data from the 2005 and 2006 NSDUH administrations and for those aged 65 or older (n = 4236), 14.5% of men and 3.3% of women reported drinking more than five drinks in a sitting [22]. More recently, using 2008–2009 NSDUH data, these same authors report an overall (both sexes) estimate of 9.2% as the binge drinking prevalence [23]. Using the 2011 data from the same NSDUH series, SAMHSA reports an 8.3% binge drinking (5 or more drinks in a sitting) for those aged 65 and older [21]. Using the highest number criterion of five or more drinks, estimates for binge drinking vary by data source. The BRFSS and Health and Retirement Study estimates are lower, generally around 5% or lower. The reports based on the NSDUH are higher, 8.3% or higher. It is difficult to suggest which is more accurate. Assuming the worst-case scenario, of 8 or 9%, then 3.2–3.6 million older adults binge drink.

Diagnoses of abuse or dependence

Diagnoses of alcohol abuse or dependence using DSM-IV criteria signal use reaching a level where the person has psychological, social or physical consequences and continues using at hazardous levels. There are issues with diagnoses in older people. For example, one criterion for dependence is increased tolerance, 'Did you need to use more alcohol than you used to in order to get the effect you wanted?' However, older people may have lower tolerance because of changes in their physiology or because of other medications. Other criteria for abuse or dependence involve degradation of the person's ability to perform in the person's social roles (e.g. work, family). These, too, change in older age and may be less prone to be 'degraded'. Finally, legal issues are a consequence leading to the identification of many people abusing alcohol. Older people, because of less exposure (e.g. driving fewer miles) may tend to have less contact with the criminal justice system and thus be underrepresented. Since diagnoses require more in-depth and costly interviews, they are less frequent in epidemiological studies. However, there are a few reports.

One report [24] uses the NESARC 2001/2002 Wave 1 data and combines DSM alcohol dependence and abuse into a single alcohol use disorder (AUD). With a relatively large sample size, 8205 respondents, the estimated prevalence was 1.5% for past 12-month AUD. Interestingly, the estimate of lifetime AUD was 16.1%, suggesting the difference, 14.6%, are in remission or recovery.

Although not nationally representative, the Massachusetts Medicare and Medicaid claims data were used to estimate AUD prevalence data [25]. In 2005 data with a sample size of 679 182 individuals, the 12-month prevalence for AUD was 1.2%. Mean age in this sample was 77.7 (SD = 8.7) and it was predominantly female (71.4%).

One other study is noteworthy. The National Comorbidity Survey–Replication study included 1461 respondents aged 65 or above. The mean age was 74 years and the interviews took place between 2001 and 2003. There were no cases (0%) of any substance use disorder in this group. Even though this is a relatively small sample, it is highly unlikely to find no cases even if the prevalence was as low as 0.5%. Although, it is possible that this is a reasonable sample and that the previous reports using larger samples were overestimating the prevalence of substance use disorder.

While it remains unclear why no cases were observed in the National Comorbidity Survey–Replication study, what can be said is that the diagnoses of abuse or dependence were extremely infrequent in its sample of respondents over age 65.

Thus, the above studies suggest a low prevalence of abuse or dependence among older adults, generally 1.5% or lower. This may be an underestimate because of issues with the diagnostic criteria in an older population, for example reduced tolerance, changing social roles, less exposure to legal consequences. Assuming the rate is 1–2%, between 400 000 and 800 000 of the US population aged 65 years or older may be affected with alcohol use disorder.

From a public health perspective and given the prevalence of hazardous or at risk drinking, binge drinking and AUD, it appears that the major problem lies with the amount consumed rather than formal diagnostic cases of AUD, at least in terms of the number of people affected. Too many older people drink too much alcohol consistently (hazardous/at risk drinking) and too much sporadically (binge). Older adults who binge do not drink consistently large amounts and vice versa. Using the BRFSS data, the correlation between constant and sporadic use is only about 0.4 (Pearson's r). Considering the prevalence of either hazardous/at-risk (constant) drinking or binge drinking, the number of affected people increases considerably.

Older substance abuse treatment populations

According to a more recently published study, slightly over 1% of the general population aged 50 or above sought help for drug or alcohol problems within the past year [26]. This study compared the NESARC (Wave 1, 2001–2002) data to an earlier but similar data set from 1992 (National Longitudinal Epidemiologic Survey, NLAES). A larger percentage (2.6%) were considering but not getting help. Both the percentage of people aged 50 or older who were getting help and the percentage of people considering getting help increased between the decade separating these two nationally representative samples.

A few studies have investigated the epidemiology of older problem drinkers in substance abuse treatment. These reports used SAMHSA's Treatment Episode Data Set (TEDS). SAMHSA publishes these de-identified data sets yearly. They include substance abuse admissions to treatment centres across the United States. Ideally, they include all treatment centres public and private, community based and hospital based. While they attempt to be inclusive, the coverage is probably near 100% in the publically funded community treatment centres and somewhat less so elsewhere. However, the overwhelming majority of admissions occur in these community centres. When building these data sets, SAMHSA's de-identification process categorizes client age. The oldest category is aged 55 or older, so studies are forced to define older adults using this group.

One early study used 1 101 983 admissions to treatment in 2001 [27]. Of these, 58 073 (5.3%) were aged 55 or older. Approximately 80% of the older admissions were male and represented more males than the younger admissions (69%). Additionally, the older admissions tended to be White (64%), widowed or divorced (45%), living independently (75%) and not in the labour force (62%) because of retirement or disability (44%). Over 21% of the older group were veterans. Alcohol was overwhelmingly the most frequent (76%) primary substance of abuse for the older treatment admissions. The older admissions were also far more likely to report only one substance of abuse than younger admissions (77% versus 46%).

A second study analysed SAMHSA's Treatment Episode Data Set (TEDS) admissions trends from 1992 to 2005 [28]. Notably, the percentage of 'alcohol only' older admissions declined over this period with concomitant increases in 'alcohol and drugs' and 'drugs only' admissions. There was as steady drop in alcohol as the primary substance of abuse from 84% in 1992 to 57% in 2005. Other notable changes in the demographics of older substance abuse admissions for alcohol included: a decrease in the percentage of males entering treatment, an increase in the percentage of Whites and an increase in the level of education.

More recently, another study analysed older first time admissions for treatment from 1998 to 2008 [29]. While older admissions for alcohol and drugs were increasing over this period, there was a dramatic decline in alcohol only admissions. Thus, the overall percentage of admissions where alcohol was mentioned declined. Even with the increase in drug admissions and the reduction of alcohol mentions, the majority of older people entering treatment mentioned alcohol as a problem, over 73% in 2008. As with the earlier study surveying 1992 to 2005, the more recent study noted increasing numbers of female admissions. There were also increasing percentages of older admissions and older first time clients entering treatment.

Special populations of older substance users

There is virtually no epidemiological literature on special populations within older persons, with the exception perhaps of older veterans. For example, there are no large-scale studies of elderly minority groups. There is also scant research on the older recovery community.

Reports on the epidemiology of alcohol use and problems among older veterans are inconsistent. One Australian study noted a much larger prevalence of high risk drinking in Vietnam veterans [30]. Approximately 90% of these veterans were aged 55 or older. Among the veterans, 58.6% were in the high risk category, more than four times that seen in the sex and aged matched general population. This study used the 2001 Australian National Health and Medical Research Council high risk criteria, seven or more drinks per day or 43 drinks per week [31]. Prevalence of alcohol use disorder (AUD) was associated with combat experience and post-traumatic stress disorder (PTSD). Another study from the United Kingdom found no relationship between military service and severe alcohol symptoms in an older population [32].

Using US national data and the BRFSS, Bohnert and colleagues found that veterans aged 41–60 years old were less likely to binge drink than nonveteran men [33]. Curiously, more veteran men aged 61–70 engaged in heavy drinking than similarly aged nonveteran men. Heavy drinking was defined as more than two drinks per day within the last 30 days. There is a fair amount of current literature on veterans' use of alcohol and the relation of PTSD and alcohol use, but little research on these effects on veterans in later life. The research that does exist in this area remains inconclusive with variable findings.

Demographic correlates of problem use

Aside from the prominent difference between men and women, correlates of problem alcohol use tend to have modest and inconsistent associations. Even the clear sex difference seems to have reasonably strong cohort effects, with later born men and, in particular, women exhibiting more drinking problems [34, 35]. In a recent review, Keyes and colleagues noted a reduction in the gender differences with increased problem drinking in women [36].

Higher education has been correlated with unhealthy alcohol use [13, 37, 38]. Income also has been frequently mentioned in the epidemiological literature, with higher income as a risk factor for alcohol problems [13, 37, 39]. However, not all studies have consistently found a significant association with education and income [24]. Where significant, these effect sizes have been small to modest.

Income is related to employment, and job status has been investigated as a correlate of alcohol problems in the older population. One study found that being employed was a risk factor for alcohol use disorders in women but not in men [39]. One study found no effect for employment [24] and another found the opposite effect: unemployment was associated with binge alcohol problems [40]. This is consistent with the literature on the effects of retirement on drinking. There does not seem to be a simple direct effect of retirement on drinking, either quantity or problems. Rather, whether or not the retirement was voluntary and the persons' social network after retirement appears to have an effect [41].

General health status is predictive of drinking, with healthier people having a higher likelihood of problem alcohol use [13, 37, 40]. However, another study found the opposite relationship [38]. Over a 20-year longitudinal study, acute health events predicted reduced drinking and abstinence [42]. Thus, the relationship between health and unhealthy drinking may not be entirely a simple one. A subset of older persons in good health tends to drink excessively. Once their health becomes problematic, they reduce their alcohol intake. However, there may also be a group who are unable to quit or reduce their intake. To further complicate the effects of general health on drinking problems, some studies suggest that having a painful condition affects drinking patterns and problems [42–44]. Those older people with painful conditions or those who used alcohol to manage their pain had more problems with alcohol. However, this same group sometimes tended to consume fewer drinks.

Other demographic factors include evidence for racial differences with alcohol problems. Among the general population, younger and older, alcohol issues are more frequently seen in Whites than in Blacks/African Americans [45–47]. This effect appears in older adults [13, 40]. However, the effect size varies considerably from study to study, has not been consistently significant [24, 48] or simple [39]. Marital status appears frequently as a predictor of alcohol problems. Being single (i.e. divorced, separated, single, never married) is a risk factor [13, 15, 22, 24, 37]. The effect size for marital status has been consistently small to moderate. Other factors, such as depression and psychological distress, have also shown positive although not entirely consistent correlation with alcohol problems [13, 38, 40, 42, 43]. Smoking, however, has been consistently strongly correlated with drinking and drinking problems [13, 43, 49, 50].

Discussion

The comprehensive review provided this far illustrates a number of differences in data collection methods that provide variation in the estimates of substance use and treatment in the older adult. Overall, the data suggest that approximately 4–14% of older adults appear to be in a hazardous drinking range. Regarding binge drinking, the data are quite variable and this is an understudied area. Rates range from as low as 2.2% for women to significantly higher, 9.5% in men, as binge drinking appears to be primarily a male problem. Assuming the worst-case scenario, of 8 or 9%, then 3.2 million to 3.6 million older adults binge drink. As we consider the rate of clinical diagnoses in older adults, there are issues with accurate clinical diagnoses in this population that occur due to a mismatch between the expected effects of alcohol and the actual vulnerability of older adults. For example alcohol tolerance may be influenced by multiple factors in the older adult due to changes in their physiology, comorbid illnesses or medications. Other criteria for abuse or dependence involving changes in social role or legal complications are also difficult to apply in the social context of retirement and other factors in late life. Consequently, studies suggest a low prevalence of abuse or dependence among older adults, generally 1.5% or lower. This may be an underestimate because of the issues mentioned with the diagnostic criteria in an older population. Assuming the rate is 1–2%, between 400 000 and 800 000 of the US population aged 65 years or older may be affected with alcohol use disorder. Regarding treatment, the landscape for older adults appears to be changing with time, with more women seeking treatment and more requests for treatment for both alcohol and other substance use, although older adults still predominantly seek alcohol only treatment admissions.

Conclusions and next steps

Without question, the importance of alcohol and other substance use among older adults will assume greater importance over time. While the findings discussed above suggest fairly low rates of problematic use and substance use diagnoses, the increased risk of medical co-morbidity and adverse outcomes for older adults may create a substantial public health burden as the proportion of older adults continues to grow. Furthermore, problems in detection that may relate to variation in thresholds for problematic use require continuing refinement over time to more accurately identify and track the scope of this problem. Many of the studies described above rely on community-based samples, yet many older adults may increasingly live in retirement facilities or other care environments such that they may not be adequately detected and evaluated in community-based study designs. Innovative sampling methods to best capture this problem will be needed in future studies, such as proactively seeking individuals who may be residing in settings that do not fall within the traditional 'community-based' designation.

References

1. Beresford, T.P. (1993) Alcoholism in the elderly. *International Review of Psychiatry*, 5(4), 477–483.
2. Babor, T.F., Higgins-Biddle, J.C., Saunders, J.B. and Monteiro, M.G. (2001) *The Alcohol Use Disorders Identification Test: Guidelines for Use in Primary Care*, 2nd edn. Department of Mental Health and Substance Dependence, World Health Organization, Geneva, Switzerland.
3. Ewing, J.A. (1994) Detecting alcoholism. The CAGE questionnaire. *JAMA*, 252(14), 1905–1907.
4. Centers for Disease Control and Prevention (CDC) (2011) *Behavioral Risk Factor Surveillance System Survey Data*. Centers for Disease Control and Prevention, US Department of Health and Human Services, Atlanta, GA.
5. US Department of Agriculture and US Department of Health and Human Services (2010) *Dietary Guidelines for Americans, 2010*, 7th edn. www.dietaryguidelines.gov (last accessed 1 April 2014).
6. Center for Substance Abuse Treatment (1998) *Substance Abuse Among Older Adults. Treatment Improvement Protocol (TIP) Series No. 26, Substance Abuse and Mental Health Services* Administration, Center for Substance Abuse Treatment, Rockville, MD.
7. National Institute on Alcohol Abuse and Alcoholism (1998) *Alcohol and Aging*. Alcohol Alert No 40, National Institute on Alcohol Abuse and Alcoholism, Rockville, MD.
8. National Institute on Alcohol Abuse and Alcoholism (2005) *Helping Patients Who Drink Too Much. A Clinical Guide*. National Institute on Alcohol Abuse and Alcoholism, Rockville, MD.
9. National Institute on Alcohol Abuse and Alcoholism (2012) *Alcohol & Health » Special Populations and Co-occurring Disorders » Older Adults*. National Institute on Alcohol Abuse and Alcoholism, Washington, DC. http://www.niaaa.nih.gov/alcohol-health/special-populations-co-occurring-disorders/older-adults (last accessed 1 April 2014).
10. American Public Health Association and Education Development Center (2008) *Alcohol Screening and Brief Intervention: A Guide for Public Health Practitioners*. National Highway Traffic Safety Administration, US Department of Transportation, Washington, DC.
11. WHO (World Health Organization) (2007) *Expert Committee on Problems Related to Alcohol Consumption. Second Report*. World Health Organization, Geneva, Switzerland.
12. WHO (World Health Organization) (2010) *Global Strategy to Reduce the Harmful Use of Alcohol*. World Health Organization, Geneva, Switzerland.
13. Merrick, E.L., Horgan, C.M., Hodgkin, D. *et al.* (2009) Unhealthy drinking patterns in older adults: prevalence and associated characteristics. *Journal of the American Geriatrics Society*, 56(2), 214–223.
14. Mezuk, B., Bohnert, A.S., Ratliff, S. and Zivin, K. (2011) Job strain, depressive symptoms, and drinking behavior among older adults: results from the health and retirement study. *The Journals of Gerontology Series B, Psychological Sciences and Social Sciences*, 66(4), 426–434.
15. Moore, A.A., Karno, M.P., Grella, C.E. *et al.* (2009) Alcohol, tobacco, and nonmedical drug use in older US adults: Data from the 2001/02 National Epidemiologic Survey

of Alcohol and Related Conditions. *Journal of the American Geriatrics Society*, **57**(12), 2275–2281.

16. Krause, J.S. (2010) Risk for Subsequent injuries after spinal cord injury: A 10-year longitudinal analysis. *Archives of Physical Medicine and Rehabilitation*, **91**(11), 1741–1746.

17. Taylor, B., Irving, H.M., Kanteres, F. *et al.* (2010) The more you drink, the harder you fall: A systematic review and meta-analysis of how acute alcohol consumption and injury or collision risk increase together. *Drug and Alcohol Dependence*, **110**(1–2), 108–116.

18. Grundstrom, A.C., Guse, C.E. and Layde, P.M. (2012) Risk factors for falls and fall-related injuries in adults 85 years of age and older. *Archives of Gerontology and Geriatrics*, **54**(3), 421–428.

19. National Institute on Alcohol Abuse and Alcoholism (2004) NIAAA council approves definition of binge drinking. *NIAAA Newsletter*, **2004**(3), 3.

20. Centers for Disease Control and Prevention (2012) *Fact Sheets: Alcohol and Public Health*. Centers for Disease Control and Prevention, Atlanta, GA. http://www.cdc.gov/alcohol/fact-sheets/alcohol-use.htm (last accessed 1 April 2014).

21. Substance Abuse and Mental Health Services Administration (2012) *Results from the 2011 National Survey on Drug Use and Health, Summary of National Findings*. NSDUH Series H-44, HHS Publication No. (SMA) 12-4713, Substance Abuse and Mental Health Services Administration, Rockville, MD.

22. Blazer, D.G. and Wu, L.-T. (2009) The epidemiology of substance use and disorders among middle aged and elderly community adults, national survey on drug use and health. *American Journal of Geriatric Psychiatry*, **17**(3), 237–245.

23. Blazer, D.G. and Wu, L.-T. (2012) Patterns of tobacco use and tobacco-related psychiatric morbidity and substance use among middle-aged and older adults in the United States. *Aging and Mental Health*, **16**(3), 296–304.

24. Lin, J.C., Karno, M.P., Grella, C.E *et al.* (2011) Alcohol, tobacco, and nonmedical drug use disorders in U.S. Adults aged 65 years and older: data from the 2001-2002 National Epidemiologic Survey of Alcohol and Related Conditions. *American Journal of Geriatric Psychiatry*, **19**(3), 292–299.

25. Lin, W.C., Zhang, J., Leung, G.Y. and Clark, R.E. (2011) Twelve-month diagnosed prevalence of behavioral health disorders among elderly medicare and medicaid members. *American Journal of Geriatric Psychiatry*, **19**(11), 970–979.

26. Sacco, P., Kuerbis, A., Goge, N. and Bucholz, K.K. (2012) Help seeking for drug and alcohol problems among adults age 50 and older: A comparison of the NLAES and NESARC surveys. *Drug and Alcohol Dependence*, **131**(1–2):157–161.

27. Arndt, S., Gunter, T.D. and Acion, L. (2005) Older admissions to substance abuse treatment in 2001. *American Journal of Geriatric Psychiatry*, **13**(5), 385–392.

28. Lofwall, M.R., Schuster, A. and Strain, E.C. (2008) Changing profile of abused substances by older persons entering treatment. *Journal of Nervous and Mental Disease*, **196**(12), 898–905.

29. Arndt, S., Clayton, R. and Schultz, S.K. (2011) Trends in substance abuse treatment 1998–2008: increasing older adult first-time admissions for illicit drugs. *American Journal of Geriatric Psychiatry*, **19**(8), 704–711.

30. O'Toole, B.I., Catts, S.V., Outram, S. *et al.* (2009) The physical and mental health of Australian Vietnam veterans 3 decades after the war and its relation to military service, combat, and post-traumatic stress disorder. *American Journal of Epidemiology*, **170**(3), 318–330.

31. National Health and Medical Research Council (2001) *Australian Alcohol Guidelines: Health Risks and Benefits*. National Health and Medical Research Council, Canberra, Australia.

32. Woodhead, C., Rona, R., Iversen, A. *et al.* (2011) Health of national service veterans: an analysis of a community-based sample using data from the 2007 Adult Psychiatric

Morbidity Survey of England. *Social Psychiatry and Psychiatric Epidemiology*, **46**(7), 559–566.

33. Bohnert, A.S., Ilgen, M.A., Bossarte, R.M. *et al.* (2012) Veteran status and alcohol use in men in the United States. *Military Medicine*, **177**(2), 198–203.

34. Grucza, R.A., Bucholz, K.K., Rice, J.P. and Bierut, L.J. (2008) Secular trends in the lifetime prevalence of alcohol dependence in the United States: a re-evaluation. *Alcoholism, Clinical and Experimental Research*, **32**(5), 763–770.

35. Kerr, W.C., Greenfield, T.K., Ye, Y. *et al.* (2013) Are the 1976–1985 birth cohorts heavier drinkers? Age-period-cohort analyses of the National Alcohol Surveys 1979–2010. *Addiction*, **108**(6), 1038–1048.

36. Keyes, K.M., Li, G. and Hasin, D.S. (2011) Birth cohort effects and gender differences in alcohol epidemiology: A review and synthesis. *Alcoholism: Clinical and Experimental Research*, **35**(12), 2101–2112.

37. Platt, A., Sloan, F.A. and Costanzo, P. (2010) Alcohol-consumption trajectories and associated characteristics among adults older than age 50. *Journal of Studies on Alcohol and Drugs*, **71**(2), 169.

38. St John, P.D., Montgomery, P.R. and Tyas, S.L. (2009) Alcohol misuse, gender and depressive symptoms in community-dwelling seniors. *International Journal of Geriatric Psychiatry*, **24**(4), 369–375.

39. Blazer, D.G. and Wu, L.-T. (2011) The epidemiology of alcohol use disorders and subthreshold dependence in a middle-aged and elderly community sample. *American Journal of Geriatric Psychiatry*, **19**(8), 685–694.

40. Bryant, A.N. and Kim, G. (2012) Racial/ethnic differences in prevalence and correlates of binge drinking among older adults. *Aging and Mental Health*, **16**(2), 208–217.

41. Kuerbis, A. and Sacco, P. (2012) The impact of retirement on the drinking patterns of older adults: a review. *Addictive Behaviors*, **37**(5), 587–595.

42. Moos, R.H., Brennan, P.L., Schutte, K.K. and Moos, B.S. (2010) Older adults' health and late-life drinking patterns: a 20-year perspective. *Aging and Mental Health*, **14**(1), 33–43.

43. Bobo, J.K., Greek, A.A., Klepinger, D.H. and Herting, J.R. (2013) Predicting 10-year alcohol use trajectories among men age 50 years and older. *American Journal of Geriatric Psychiatry*, **21**(2), 204–213.

44. Brennan, P.L., Schutte, K.K., SooHoo, S. and Moos, R.H. (2011) Painful medical conditions and alcohol use: a prospective study among older adults. *Pain Medicine*, **12**(7), 1049–1059.

45. Breslau, J., Kendler, K.S., Su, M. *et al.* (2005) Lifetime risk and persistence of psychiatric disorders across ethnic groups in the United States. *Psychological Medicine*, **35**(3), 317–327.

46. Grant, B.F. (1997) Prevalence and correlates of alcohol use and DSM-IV alcohol dependence in the United States: results of the National Longitudinal Alcohol Epidemiologic Survey. *Journal of Studies on Alcohol*, 1997, **58**(5), 464–473.

47. Schmidt, L.A., Ye, Y., Greenfield, T.K. and Bond, J. (2007) Ethnic disparities in clinical severity and services for alcohol problems: results from the National Alcohol Survey. *Alcoholism, Clinical and Experimental Research*, **31**(1), 48–56.

48. Han, B., Gfroerer, J.C., Colliver, J.D. and Penne, M.A. (2009) Substance use disorder among older adults in the United States in 2020. *Addiction*, **104**(1), 88–96.

49. Hser, Y.I., Hoffman, V., Grella, C.E. and Anglin, M.D. (2001) A 33-year follow-up of narcotics addicts. *Archives of General Psychiatry*, **58**(5), 503–508.

50. Schlaerth, K.R., Splawn, R.G., Ong, J. and Smith, S.D. (2004) Change in the pattern of illegal drug use in an inner city population over 50: an observational study. *Journal of Addictive Diseases*, **23**(2), 95–107.

Chapter 8

EPIDEMIOLOGY AND DEMOGRAPHY OF ILLICIT DRUG USE AND DRUG USE DISORDERS AMONG ADULTS AGED 50 AND OLDER

Shawna L. Carroll Chapman and Li-Tzy Wu

Department of Psychiatry and Behavioral Sciences, School of Medicine, Duke University Medical Center, USA

Introduction

The prevalence of illicit and nonmedical pharmaceutical drug use is on the rise among older populations (aged ≥50 years) and is projected to grow continuously as baby boomers, or persons born between 1946 and 1964, transition to their twilight years [1]. Estimates suggest the number of older substance abusers in the United States will reach five million in 2020, driven partly by illicit and nonmedical drug use [1]. Because 2020 is only the midpoint of when baby boomers will reach the age of 65, the estimated five million users are likely to underrepresent the true number of future older substance abusers [2]. This chapter focuses on use of illicit drugs (e.g. cannabis/marijuana, cocaine/crack, inhalants, hallucinogens, heroin, and stimulants/methamphetamine) and inhalants, discussing nonmedical prescription drug use only as it relates to illicit drug use. Nonmedical prescription drug use and abuse is addressed in Chapter 9. This introduction to the topic is concluded with a discussion of the reasons ageing baby boomers show an elevated likelihood of using illicit drugs. The extent and correlates of illicit drug use, abuse and dependence, as defined by the DSM-IV [3], in the older adult populations, including an overview of treatment need, are then reviewed. The chapter ends by outlining the next steps for future research.

Prevalences of illicit drug use will be likely to increase due to multiple factors. These include the large number of ageing baby boomers and popularity of substance use when baby boomers came of age [4, 5]. From 1980–2007, the proportion of Americans aged 45–64 increased from 20 to 25%, while the proportion of those aged under 18 fell from 28 to 25% [6]. This trend is projected to continue in the United States and similar trends exist in developed and developing nations [7, 8]. Because the proportion of older persons is already higher in developed nations due

Substance Use and Older People, First Edition.
Edited by Ilana B. Crome, Li-Tzy Wu, Rahul (Tony) Rao and Peter Crome.
© 2015 John Wiley & Sons, Ltd. Published 2015 by John Wiley & Sons, Ltd.

to past shifts in fertility and mortality, the trends may disproportionately affect developing nations [8]. Those who reach the age of greatest vulnerability for drug use initiation at a time when drugs were popular and available were at an elevated likelihood of use, which may continue throughout their lives [5]. Drugs were considered popular and available as baby boomers reached adolescence and early adulthood, and baby boomers have greater lifetime rates of drug use than previous generations [5].

The risk for illicit drug use also increases among those who engage in prescription-type nonmedical drug abuse and vice versa. The risk of nonmedical prescription drug use, abuse and dependence may increase with prolonged medical drug use [9]. Individuals misusing prescription drugs may also turn to illicit or street drugs when they are accessible [10]. Additionally, some illicit drug users who are aware of the psychoactive effects of prescription drugs may seek them out for nonmedical or recreational use [11]. It is suggested that a minimum of one out of four older adults has used a medication with the potential for abuse, a number that is likely to grow as baby boomers continue to age [12]. Prescription drugs are also more readily available now than in the past [13, 14]. Therefore, current and future elders may be at greater risk for nonmedical prescription drug use than elders in the past [15], which may potentially increase risk for illicit drug use [16].

Survey studies

This section includes studies conducted with data from the National Survey on Drug Use and Health (NSDUH) and the National Epidemiologic Survey on Alcohol and Related Conditions (NESARC) (Table 8.1). NSDUH is an annual national survey interviewing approximately 70 000 randomly selected noninstitutionalized, household individuals aged ≥12 years. It provides national and state-level data on substance use (i.e. tobacco, alcohol, illicit drug use and nonmedical pharmaceutical-type drug use) and is sponsored by the Substance Abuse and Mental Health Services Administration (SAMHSA), part of the US Department of Health and Human Services (DHHS). The NESARC includes data from a national sample of 43 093 adults aged ≥18 years surveyed in 2001/2002 (wave 1) and 2004/2005 (wave 2) regarding their tobacco, alcohol and illicit drug use and related mental disorders. The National Institute on Alcohol Abuse and Alcoholism (NIAAA) sponsored the NESARC to create a detailed and comprehensive data set related to substance use and co-morbid mental disorders. In addition, findings from the English National Survey of Psychiatric Morbidity (ENSPM), the Southeast London Community Health Survey (SLCHS) and the National Drug Treatment Monitoring System (NDTMS) in the United Kingdom are reviewed. This section begins with prevalences of illicit drug use among older adults aged ≥50 years [17, 18], continues with prevalences of drugs used most often [19, 20], changes in drug use patterns over time [5, 20] and variations in use based on age, gender, and race/ethnicity [17, 19, 21, 22]. This section finishes with information on correlates of drug use and a brief summary synthesizing the available information [17, 19, 21, 22].

Table 8.1 Studies of illicit drug use

Authors	Pub. Year	Data source	Sample/ Age (year)	Substances	Summary of findings
Fahmy et al. [25]	2012	2007 APMS and 2008–2010 SELCoH	N = 4296 ≥ 50 years	Drugs	• English Sample, Aged 50–64: lifetime cannabis 11.4%, past-year cannabis 1.8%, lifetime tranquilizers 2.3%, past-year tranquilizers 0.4%; • English Sample, Aged ≥ 65 years: lifetime cannabis 1.7%, past-year cannabis 0.4%, lifetime tranquilizers 1.5%, past-year tranquilizers 0.4%; • London Sample, Aged 50–64: lifetime cannabis 42.8%, past-year cannabis 9.0%, Lifetime LSD 14.9%, past-year tranquilizers 2.1%; • London Sample, Aged ≥ 65 years: Lifetime cannabis 9.4%, past-year cannabis 1.1%, lifetime tranquilizers 4.0%, past-year tranquilizers 0.7%. • There was a 10-fold increase in recent cannabis use by those aged 50–64 years from 1993 to 2007; • There was a twofold increase in recent cannabis use by those aged 65–74 from 2000 to 2007. • There was a 10-fold increase in lifetime use for cannabis, amphetamine, cocaine and LSD from 1993 to 2007.
Outlaw et al. [38]	2012	January 2005– October 2007 Treatment Knowledge Application Program	N = 199	Drugs	• Completers were more likely than noncompleters to decrease use of nonmedical prescription drugs, improve cognitive functioning, increase vitality, and decrease bodily pain. • Both groups had improved mental health but this was better for completers than noncompleters
White et al. [20]	2011	1985 and 2006 NSDUH	N = 1103 ≥ 50 years (1985) N = 5830 ≥ 50 years (2006)	Tobacco, alcohol, drug classes	• The proportion of older Americans who had used drugs in the past and currently used them was higher in 2006 than in 1985; • Current use was highest for marijuana (1.6 % vs. 0.3%; p < 0.001), cocaine (0.3% vs. 0.1%; p < 0.001), and inhalants (0.1% vs. 0%; p < 0.001).

(continued)

Table 8.1 (continued)

Authors	Pub. Year	Data source	Sample/ Age (year)	Substances	Summary of findings
Torres et al. [37]	2011	Southeast Houston, years not provided	N=227 Aged 45–80	Drugs	• Injecting drug users reported worse health status than national samples; • Participants also had high rates of sexually transmitted diseases, liver diseases, and stroke; • Almost one-third (31.3%) lacked health insurance; • 71.8% of participants endorsed tobacco use in the past 30 days; • Participants endorsed high rates of continuing drug use.
Lin et al. [22]	2011	2000–2001 NESARC	N=8205 ≥65 years	Alcohol Drugs	• Lifetime prevalence of any drug disorder 0.6%; past-year prevalence of any drug use disorder 0.2%; • Lifetime drug disorder: cannabis (0.21%), opioids (0.16%), tranquilizers (0.13%), amphetamines (0.11%), and sedatives (0.07%); • Correlates of lifetime drug disorder: ages 65–74 and divorced/separated
Moy et al. [35]	2011	1998–2005 (searched to 2007) PubMed, Cochrane Library, Medline, Project CORK, and EMBASE	N=16 studies that examined treatment trials	Nicotine, alcohol, drugs	• Only one study examined an illicit drug trial; • Most studies (13) were from the United States, with two from England and one from Canada; • Definition of older ages varied (range aged ≥50 years to ≥65 years), with most studies (9) focusing on patients aged ≥55 years.
Arndt et al. [30]	2011	1998–2008 TEDS	Treatment encounters N=258 542; ≥55 years	Alcohol Drugs	• Adults aged ≥55 years made up 2.9% of all first substance abuse admissions in 1998, which increased to 4.4% in 2008, notably among females, whites, and Blacks. • Alcohol admissions declined, but drug admissions increased (cocaine, marijuana, and heroin).
Beynon et al. [33]	2010	2003/2004– 2007/2008 England's NDTS and ONS	Cause of death N=504	Past drug use	• There was an increase in age at death from 36.46 in 2003/2004 to 41.38 in 2007/2008; • Those who died at age ≥40 years were more likely to die from a nondrug related death (OR 3.27, 95% CI 2.16–5.11).

Study	Year	Sample	Data source	Substance	Findings
Woo and Chen [32]	2010	N = 90 ≥65 years	2006–2007	Drugs	• Prevalence drug use among psychiatric emergency patients from urine toxicology screens: amphetamines (8.9%), benzodiazepines (6.7%), cocaine (6.7%), opiate (3.3%), and barbiturates (1.1%)
Han et al. [27]	2009	N > 25 000 aged ≥50 years	2002–2006 NSDUH	Drugs	• Substance use disorder among those aged ≥50 years would increase from 2.8 million (annual average) in 2002–2006 to 5.7 million in 2020; • Among Whites aged ≥50 years, the prevalence of substance use disorder would increase from 3.4% in 2002–2006 to 5.2% in 2020; • Among Blacks aged ≥50 years, the prevalence of substance use disorder would increase from 3.8% in 2002–2006 to 5.0% in 2020; • Among Hispanics aged ≥50 years, the prevalence of substance use disorder would increase from 3.2% in 2002–2006 to 4.4% in 2020.
Blazer and Wu [19]	2009	N = 10 953; ≥50 years	2005–2006 NSDUH	Alcohol Drug classes	• Past-year use of marijuana (2.6%), cocaine (0.4%), inhalants (0.1%), hallucinogens (0.1%), methamphetamine (0.1%), and heroin (0.05%). • Mean number of days using marijuana (81 days), cocaine (101 days), inhalants (41 days), hallucinogens (17 days), methamphetamine (96 days), and heroin (301 days). • Use of marijuana and cocaine were more prevalent in the 50–64 age group and in males. • Compared to those who used alcohol, marijuana and cocaine users were more likely to be separated, divorced, or widowed vs. married, and to have major depression in the past year. • Blacks were more likely to use alcohol and marijuana than Asian/Pacific Islanders/Native Hawaiians and to use cocaine than Whites.

(continued)

Table 8.1 (continued)

Authors	Pub. Year	Data source	Sample/ Age (year)	Substances	Summary of findings
Moore et al. [21]	2009	2000–2001 NESARC	N = 8205; ≥65 years	Alcohol Drugs	• Lifetime prevalences: 1.1% sedatives, 0.7% tranquilizers, 1.1% opioids, 0.4% amphetamines, 1.4% cannabis, 0.2% crack cocaine, 0.1% hallucinogens, 0.06% inhalants, and 0.01% heroin; • Past-year prevalences: 0.6% sedatives, 0.2% tranquilizers, 0.5% opioids, and 0.1% for cannabis.
Rajaratnam et al. [31]	2009	Year unavailable	N = 156 ≥24 years	Alcohol Drugs	• 29% (n = 46) of the sample were aged ≥55 years. • Past-month drug use among persons aged ≥55 (based on urinalysis): opioids (27.0%), benzodiazepines (35.1%), barbiturates (8.1%), cocaine (35.1%), amphetamines (2.7%), cannabis (2.7%).
Lofwall et al. [29]	2008	1992 and 2005 TEDS	Treatment encounter data; ≥50 years	Alcohol Drugs	• Between 1992 and 2005, the number of admissions for substance problems increased among persons aged 50–54 from 3.1% of the age group (47 361 admissions) to 6.0% (108 453 admissions) and increased among persons aged ≥55 years from 3.5% (55 344 admissions) to 4.2% (75 899 admissions). • Admissions for alcohol and drug problems and for drug problems increased, but admission for alcohol problems only decreased over time.
Johnson et al. [36]	2007	January 1994–June 1998	N = 1098	Alcohol Drugs	• Users were predominantly male (62%) and more likely than younger users to have never married; • 53% of older users endorsed alcohol abuse or dependence, 77% cocaine abuse or dependence, and 72% opiate abuse or dependence; • Older users had later onset of marijuana cocaine use, and crack; • Older users had earlier onset of heroin; • Older drug users were more likely than younger users to report a lack of recent sexual activity, but had a similar rate of sex trading compare to younger users, and more likely to have a history of a sexually transmitted disease than younger users.

Reference	Year	Survey	Type	N	Findings
Beynon et al. [26]	2007	1998–2004 NDTMS	Drugs	N = >10 000	• The median age of death rose from 30.8 years in 1998 to 34.9 in 2004–2005; • Of those aged 50–74 years, the majority of those receiving treatment were aged 50–54 years; • Between 1998 and 2004–2005 there was an increasing number of male and female drug users aged 55–59 years, and of males aged 60–64 years; • The proportion of adults aged 50–74 in contact with syringe exchange programs rose from 0.2% in 1992 to 3.8% in 2004; • The median age of problematic drug users in contact with syringe exchange programs rose from 27.0 in 1998 to 34.9 years in 2004–2005.
Colliver et al. [5]	2006	1999–2001 NSDUH	Drugs	Variable N (i.e. low-risk model any use N = 15 578, high risk model any use N = 2547)	From 1999–2001 to 2020: • The overall number of users is expected to increase from 719 000 to almost 3.3 million; • Use of any illicit drug will increase from 2.2 to 3.1%; • Past-year marijuana use in persons aged ≥50 years is projected to increase from 1.0 to 2.9%; • Non-medical use of prescription psychotherapeutics among those aged ≥50 years is projected to increase 190%; • The proportion of Black non-Hispanic users is expected to decrease from 8.5 to 5.9%; • The proportion of Hispanic older adult marijuana users is expected to increase from 1.0 to 4.9%.
Termorshuizen et al. [34]	2005	1985–2002 Amsterdam Cohort Study	Drugs	899	• Estimated prevalence of four months continuous abstinence 20 years after initiation was 27%; • Survival at 20 years post drug initiation was 73% or 84% when HIV/AIDS deaths were removed; • Older age of initiation, initiation before 1980, and Western European ethnic origin associated with greater abstinence.

NESARC: National Epidemiologic Survey on Alcohol and Related Conditions; NCS-R: National Comorbidity Survey-Replication; NDTMS: National Drug Treatment Monitoring System; NSDUH: National Survey on Drug Use and Health; QSHS: Quebec Survey on the Health of seniors; TEDS: Treatment Episode Data Sets.

Data from the 2011 NSDUH showed an age-related decline in prevalence of past-month illicit or nonmedical drug use (i.e. marijuana/hashish, cocaine/crack, heroin, hallucinogens, inhalants and nonmedical use of prescription-type psycho-therapeutics) (i.e., aged 50–54, 6.7% using illicit or nonmedical drugs; aged 55–59, 6.0%; aged 60–64, 2.7%; and aged ≥65 years, 1.0%) [18, 23]. However, any drug use was more prevalent in 2011 than it was in previous years for adults aged 50–59 (e.g. 2002 past-month use: aged 50–54, 3.4%; 55–59, 1.9%; 60–64, 2.5%; ≥65 years, 0.8%) [23, 24]. This pattern was also observed in the United Kingdom. Data for individuals aged ≥50 years from the ENSPM and SLCHS showed that lifetime use of cannabis, cocaine, amphetamine and lysergic acid diethylamide (LSD) increased for persons aged ≥50 years from 1993 to 2007 [25]. Beynon *et al.* (2007) [26] compared proportions of patients aged 11–49 to patients aged 50–74 in drug abuse treatment in two English counties from 1998 to 2004-2005. Beynon *et al.* (2007) [26] found increases in contact with treatment programmes for older adults aged 50–54, 55–59, 60–64 and ≥65 years. Taken together, these data suggest an increase in illicit drug use among adults aged ≥50 years.

Data from 2011 and 2007–2009 national surveys in the United States showed that marijuana was the illicit drug used most often (i.e. 2011 past-year use: a prevalence of 7.9% among adults aged 50–54, 7.0% aged 55–59, 4.4% aged 60-64 and 1.0% aged ≥65 years; and 2007–2009 past-year use by those aged ≥50 years, 3.2%; for those aged 50–59, 5.9% and aged ≥60, 1.1%) [17, 18]. In 2007–2009, past-year use of any illicit or nonmedical drug for adults aged ≥50 years was 5.2% [17]. In 2011, cocaine was the second most used drug by older adults (past-year use: 0.9% aged 50–54, 0.4% aged 55–59 and 0.4% aged 60–64) [18]. Earlier data showed similar patterns. Blazer and Wu [19] examined 2005–2006 NSDUH data for 10 953 individuals aged ≥50 years and found past-year prevalences of: marijuana 2.6%, cocaine 0.4%, inhalants 0.1%, hallucinogens 0.1%, methamphetamines 0.1% and heroin 0.05%. White *et al.* [20] compared 1985 and 2006 NSDUH data for adults aged ≥50 years (1985 n = 1103; 2006 n = 5830) and also found that illicit drugs used most were marijuana (past-year: 0.7 vs. 2.6%, respectively), cocaine (past-year: 0.1 vs. 0.5%, respectively) and inhalants (past-year: 0.0 vs. 0.2%, respectively). Although prevalences varied, marijuana and cocaine were the primary illicit drugs used by those aged ≥50 years. The low prevalence rate of marijuana use in 1985 (past-year: 0.7%) also suggested an increased use in recent years. In the United Kingdom, Fahmy *et al.* [25] found that lifetime drug use was less than 2% for persons aged ≥65 years, except for cannabis (9.4% in the London sample) and tranquilizers (4.0% in the London sample). Lifetime use was higher among adults aged 50–64 (not reported) and highest for cannabis (42.8% London sample) and LSD (14.9%). From 1993 to 2000, recent cannabis use increased for persons aged 50–64 and 65–74 years. From 1993 to 2007, lifetime use of cannabis, amphetamine, cocaine and LSD increased for persons aged ≥50 years.

While marijuana was consistently found to be used most, the overall pattern of drug use among older adults in the United States is changing. Analysing data from the 1999–2001 National Household Survey on Drug Abuse (NHSDA), Colliver *et al.* [5] estimated that, by 2020, the number of drug users aged ≥50 years would increase from 719 000 to nearly 3.3 million. Any illicit drug use would rise from 2.2 to 3.1% and marijuana use would increase from 1.0 to 2.9%. Han *et al.* [27] used 2002–2006 NSDUH data to estimate the prevalence of substance use disorder (alcohol or drugs) among those aged ≥50 years in 2020; the investigators estimated that the number of people aged ≥50 years with a substance use disorder would increase from 2.8 million (annual average) in 2002–2006 to 5.7 million in 2020. In an analysis of 1985 and 2006 NSDUH data, White *et al.* [20] found that the proportion of adults aged ≥50 years who had ever used illicit drugs (lifetime) increased for all categories examined (marijuana 5.5 to 26.1%, cocaine 1.7 to 8.3%, hallucinogens 0.5 to 8.5%, heroin 0.4 to 1.3%, inhalants 1.1 to 3.6% and PCP 0.3 to 2.3%, respectively). Current drug use among adults aged ≥50 years also increased for marijuana (0.3 to 1.6%, respectively) and cocaine (0.1 to 0.3%) as legal substance use (cigarettes and alcohol) either declined or remained stable [20].

When considering different ages, the shifting pattern of drug use is complex. 2007–2009 NSDUH data showed that most individuals aged ≥50 years used only one drug and that it was usually marijuana (45.2%). When not marijuana, it was a prescription-type drug used nonmedically (31.5%) [17]. Blazer and Wu [19] also found that marijuana and cocaine use occurred more among adults aged 50–64. However, data from the 2007–2009 NSDUH showed similar prevalences of marijuana and nonmedical prescription-type drug use among adults aged ≥60 years (1.2 and 1.1%, respectively) [17]. Collectively, these data suggest that drug use may shift from illicit to nonmedical pharmaceutical use as older adults age.

Comparing lifetime prevalences with past-year use prevalences also suggests occurrences of nonmedical use of prescription drugs among older adults aged ≥65 years. Moore *et al.* [21] analysed 2000–2001 NESARC data (n = 8205, aged ≥65 years) and found lifetime prevalences for illicit and nonmedical drug use were: 1.4% for cannabis, 1.1% for opioids, 1.1% for sedatives, 0.7% for tranquilizers, 0.4% for amphetamines, 0.2% for crack cocaine, 0.1% for hallucinogens, 0.06% for inhalants and 0.01% for heroin. However, past-year prevalences were 0.6% for sedatives, 0.5% for opioids, 0.2% for tranquilizers and 0.1% for cannabis. Lin *et al.* [22] also examined the NESARC data and found similar prevalences among older adults aged ≥65 years (i.e. lifetime use: cannabis 0.21%, followed by opioids 0.16%, tranquilizers 0.13%, amphetamine 0.11% and sedatives 0.07%). Overall, older adults aged ≥65 years appeared to use prescription-type drugs nonmedically.

The national survey data help to identify the representation of older marijuana users in a sample of noninstitutionalized adults. Lev-Ran *et al.* [28] examined the 2001–2002 NESARC data and found that respondents aged 45–64 made up 13.53% of all past-year cannabis users aged ≥18 years (13.88% male and 8.44% female). In addition, persons aged 45–64 made up 8.75% of all NESARC respondents aged ≥18 years with a cannabis use disorder (9.65% male and 6.28% female). Marijuana users aged ≥65 years were a small proportion of cannabis users aged ≥18 years (0.01%) and users with a cannabis use disorder (0.01%).

Like age, gender complicates the picture of drug use. Data from the 2007–2009 NSDUH showed that females aged ≥50 years had similar prevalences of marijuana and nonmedical prescription drug use (1.9 vs. 2.1%, respectively) [17]. Among women aged ≥60 years, marijuana use was lower than nonmedical prescription drug use (0.5 vs. 1.1%, respectively). The 2007–2009 NSDUH data showed that marijuana was used more by males aged ≥50 years than females aged ≥50 years [17]. Blazer and Wu [19] also found marijuana and cocaine use occurred more among males than females. Therefore, men and women may have different drug use patterns, with men using more illicit drugs than women.

A few studies examined the race/ethnicity of illicit drug users. Han *et al.* [27] used national data sources and estimated that, among Whites aged ≥50 years, the prevalence of substance use disorder would increase from 3.4% in 2002–2006 to 5.2% in 2020 among adults aged ≥50 years; the prevalence of Blacks aged ≥50 years with a substance use disorder would increase from 3.8% in 2002–2006 to 5.0% in 2020; and the prevalence of Hispanics with a substance use disorder would increase from 3.2% in 2002–2006 to 4.4% in 2020. Blazer and Wu [19] found that, among those aged ≥50 years, Blacks were more likely to use marijuana than Asian/Pacific Islanders/ Native Hawaiians and more likely to use cocaine than Whites. Moore *et al.* [21] found that, among adults aged ≥65 years, the odds of past-year illicit and nonmedical drug use were higher for Latinos (1.1%) when compared to Whites. Overall, studies suggest a greater prevalence of illicit drug use by non-Whites than Whites.

Multiple studies examined correlates of illicit drug use. In an analysis of older adults aged ≥50 years in the 2005–2006 NSDUH data, Blazer and Wu [19] found that marijuana and cocaine users were more likely than nonusers to be separated, divorced, or widowed versus married and to have had major depressive episodes in the past year. In an analysis of the 2000–2001 NESARC data, Moore *et al.* [21] found that the odds of past-year illicit and nonmedical drug use were higher for divorced/separated/widowed and never married persons when compared to those who were married or living with someone. Lin *et al.* [22] also found increased odds of drug use among those who were divorced or separated compared to those who were married as well as those of younger age (i.e. aged 65–74) compared to older adults (i.e. aged ≥75 years). Across studies, prevalence of drug use was lowest among currently married older adults.

In summary, reported prevalences for past-month any illicit or nonmedical drug use varied from 0.8% for those aged ≥65 years to 6.7% for those aged 50–54. Studies showed that marijuana was the drug used most by those aged ≥50 years (past-year prevalence range 0.7–7.9%) and followed by cocaine (past-year range 0.1–0.9%). Illicit drug use increased over time in the past decade. However, data also suggested that drug use patterns among older adults appeared to shift from illicit to nonmedical pharmaceutical-type drugs as they aged. Males were more likely than females to use illicit drugs, particularly marijuana, whereas females were more likely to use prescription-type pharmaceuticals nonmedically. Studies also suggested greater illicit drug use among non-Whites compared with Whites. Being divorced/separated/widowed or never married were associated with elevated odds of drug use.

Studies of treatment-seeking or clinical patients

Only a small fraction of Americans with a substance use disorder receive treatment. In 2011, 3.8 million, or 1.5% of the population aged 12 or older, received substance abuse treatment, while 21.6 million or 8.4% of the population were estimated to need treatment [23]. The analysis of treatment data can offer insight into shifting use patterns. Seven studies that focused on or had information specific to adults aged ≥50 years and provided information specific to treatment for illicit drug use were identified (Table 8.1). This section summarizes these studies. Two used the Treatment Episode Data Set (TEDS) data [29, 30]. TEDS is used to monitor substance abuse treatment admissions to facilities that have received public funds in the United States and is maintained by the Center for Behavioral Health Statistics and Quality, SAMHSA. TEDS includes information on admissions that receive state funds, including funds from federal block grants. Data may not differentiate multiple admissions for the same person. They also do not represent admissions to federal facilities (e.g. Veterans Administration), and differences in how States administer funds may affect data collection. This section also includes a study of patients aged ≥50 years receiving methadone treatment in New York [31], a study of patients aged ≥50 years receiving emergency psychiatric care at a large California hospital [32], a study of substance abuse treatment patients reported by the NDTMS in the United Kingdom [33], a study of drug users in the Amsterdam cohort study from The Netherlands [34] and a review of treatment trials [35].

TEDS data showed changes in admission patterns for individuals aged ≥50 years. Lofwall *et al.* [29] compared admission episode data from 1992 (n = 1.55 million) and 2005 (1.85 million) and found that the number of illicit drug abuse admissions significantly increased for those aged 50–54 and ≥55 years. In 1992, approximately 10% (provided by graph, exact number not given) of admissions for adults aged 50–54 involved an illicit drug, either alone or with alcohol. By 2005, the proportion had risen to 61%. In 1992, just under 10% (provided by graph, exact number not given) of admissions for adults aged ≥55 years involved an illicit drug. By 2005, the proportion had risen to 45%. Admissions for only alcohol use problems simultaneously declined. Daily substance use was highest among those aged ≥55 years. Illicit drugs used most often were heroin and cocaine, followed by nonmedical use of prescription opioids. From 1992–2005, cocaine use related admissions declined; in the 50–54-year-old age group, heroin related admissions reached the high point in 2002 (20.3%), but the rate was declining by 2005 (18.7%). Overall, increased admissions were seen for use or abuse of prescription opioids, marijuana and methamphetamines.

Also using the TEDS data, Arndt *et al.* [30] compared admission data in 1998 versus admission data in 2008 for the first-time (new) alcohol and drug abuse treatment admissions among adults aged 30–54 (n = 3 547 733) to those aged ≥55 years (n = 258 542) and found new admissions for those aged ≥55 years increased from 2.86% in 1998 to 4.42% in 2008. While alcohol was the primary substance for admissions among adults aged ≥55 years, admissions involving drugs were trending higher at a marked rate as alcohol problems only admissions declined (rates not reported, depicted in graph). Following alcohol, cocaine was the second common primary substance of abuse for admissions among adults aged ≥55 years. However, the proportion of cocaine-related admissions had declined for this age group by 2008. Marijuana, heroin and methamphetamine related admissions were on the rise, with heroin admissions showing the greatest increase in 2008.

Part of this increase in age may be because some drug users in contact with treatment providers are living longer and continuing to use drugs as they age. Beynon *et al.* [33] examined 2003/2004 to 2007/2008 cause of death data reported by the UK's Office of National Statistics for 504 persons known by the NDTMS. Investigators found an increase in age at death from median age 36.46 in 2003/2004 to median age 41.38 in 2007/2008. Persons aged ≥40 years at time of death were more likely to die from a nondrug-related cause. Termorshuizen *et al.* [34] found that, among 899 persons with a history of drug use in Amsterdam examined from 1985–2002, only 27% had maintained four months of continuous abstinence in 20 years since initiation. In addition, survival at 20 years after initiation was 73%. When those who died from HIV/AIDS were removed, 20-year survival rose to 84%. Abstinence correlated with older age at initiation, initiation before 1980 and a Western European ethnic origin.[34]

Two studies compared drug use by older adults (aged ≥55 years) and younger adults in drug use treatment. Rajaratnam *et al.* [31] evaluated 156 methadone treatment enrollees aged 24–68 years (29% aged ≥55 years) in New York and found the prevalences of past-month drug use for those aged ≥55 years was 35.1% for benzodiazepines, 35.1% for cocaine, 27.0% for opioids, 8.1% for barbiturates, 2.7% for amphetamines and 2.7% for cannabis. Methadone patients aged ≥55 years were less likely than patients aged 24–54 to report current heroin or overall drug use. Woo and Chen [32] analysed psychological screening assessments of 5914 emergency psychiatric patients aged 18–64 and 104 emergency psychiatric patients aged ≥65 years in 2006–2007 at a California hospital. They found that the positive urine toxicology rate was 31.5% for patients aged 18–64 and 26.7% for patients aged ≥65 years. Among the 26.7% patients aged ≥65 years who screened positive: 8.9% were positive for amphetamines, 6.7% for benzodiazepine, 6.7% for cocaine, 3.3% for opiates and 1.1% for barbiturates. These findings reveal a lower prevalence of drug use among older patients than younger patients, a pattern consistent with the survey data.

Studies that analysed the TEDS data also examined the racial characteristics of alcohol/drug related admissions among adults aged ≥50 years. Lofwall *et al.* [29] found that, for all admissions among adults aged ≥55 years, White admissions for combined drugs and alcohol treatment dropped from 53.7% in 1992 to 46.7% in 2005. For Whites aged 50–54, drug-only admissions rose from 37.8% in 1992 to 46.8% in 2005; for Whites aged ≥55 years drug-only admissions rose from 40.7% to 45.8%. In 2005, 61% of drug only admissions were White for all age groups, and 24% were Black. Black admissions for drugs only did not increase for Blacks aged 50–54 but rose from 33.3% in 1992 to 39.7% in 2005 for Blacks aged ≥55 years. In addition, for Blacks aged ≥55 years, combined drugs and alcohol related treatment increased from 34.2% in 1992 to 40.7% in 2005. In 2005, admissions related to alcohol use only remained the primarily problem among Whites. Between 1998 and 2008, Arndt *et al.* [30] found that the proportions of alcohol or drug abuse treatment admissions for individuals aged ≥55 years increased more among Blacks than Whites but less among Latinos than non-Latinos. Taken together, the findings suggest that drug abuse admissions were disproportionately high among Blacks compared to Whites.

Studies also explored characteristics of adults aged ≥50 years seeking or in illicit drug abuse treatment. Of methadone patients aged ≥55 years, Rajaratnam *et al.* [31] found that when compared to patients aged 24–54, patients aged ≥55 years were more likely to have a history of co-morbid alcohol use, less impulsiveness, hostility, paranoia and interpersonal sensitivity, more chronic medical problems, greater use of medication for medical problems and a more liberal take home medication schedules. However, only 7.1% of patients aged ≥55 years had regular contact with a physician, which did not differ significantly from patients aged 24–54 and was slightly less than what was found for the overall population. These findings demonstrate poor medical health among older drug users.

One study identified changes in age of drug use initiation. Using the TEDS data, Arndt *et al.* [30] found that from 1998 to 2008 the median age for first cocaine use among older users decreased from 40–44 years to 30–34 years for patients aged ≥55 years. In addition, the median age for first heroin use decreased from 21–24 years to 18–20 years among those aged ≥55 years. While the data are limited, they suggest an earlier age of first drug use among older drug users seeking substance abuse treatment.

One study examined studies of older adult substance treatment. In a systematic review of studies that examined substance (e.g. drugs, alcohol and nicotine) treatment trials for or including patients aged ≥50 years and published from 1984 to 2005, Moy *et al.* [35] found 11 studies related to alcohol dependence, three to nicotine dependence, one to opiate dependence and one to prescription medications. Only three came from outside the United States, two came from the United Kingdom and one from Canada. Ages considered varied, with two examining those aged ≥50 years, nine aged ≥55 years, two aged ≥60 years and three aged ≥65 years. In 15 of the 16 studies, the majority of subjects were White. Overall, older people responded to treatment and sometimes have better outcomes than younger patients. This review suggests that more studies are needed on illicit drug abuse treatment.

In summary, TEDS data showed that treatment admissions for illicit drug use were on the rise, with a more than fourfold increase in the proportion of admissions involving drug use or abuse from 1992–2005 for those aged 50–54 (~10–61%) and aged ≥55 years (just under 10–45%). Increased age of drug admissions may relate to drug users in treatment living longer. However, alcohol admissions were simultaneously on the decline. Cocaine was the primary illicit drug used by older adults seeking substance abuse treatment. However, cocaine admissions appeared to have declined recently as marijuana and methamphetamine related admissions have increased. Drugs used most in smaller studies varied but cocaine remained one of the three (cocaine, benzodiazepines and amphetamines) drugs used most.

For individuals aged ≥55 years, illicit drug related admissions increased for Whites and Blacks but proportionally more among Blacks than Whites.

Health implications

Three studies examined health implications of drug use by older (aged ≥50 years) drug users. Johnson *et al.* [36] analysed data for 1098 (8% aged ≥50 years, 16% aged 45–49 years) Black participants collected from the St. Louis *EachOneTeachOne* project between January 1994 and June 1998. Johnson *et al.* combined the aged 45–49 and ≥50 years categories for analysis and found that those aged ≥45 years were three times more likely than younger respondents to be male. Older users were twice as likely to report a lack of recent sexual activity compared to younger users. However, sexual risk behaviours by older users were substantial, with no difference in age groups among those who reported trading sex for drugs (13% of 1220 respondents). Frequency of sex partners and having a partner that was an injecting drug user did not vary between age groups. Older users were also more likely to report a history of infection with a sexually transmitted disease and to intermingle substances with sexual activity. Being male, having a sexual dysfunction, a history of sexually transmitted disease, alcohol abuse, cocaine abuse, opiate dependence and having two or more recent sex partners enhanced perception of risk for HIV/AIDS among older drug users. Older drug users may have substantial HIV/AIDS risk.

Torres *et al.* [37] examined health consequences of long-term injecting drug use on 227 Mexican American injecting heroin users (IDU) aged 45–80. Injecting drug users reported worse health status than national samples (e.g. *fair health*: IDU 49.3%, NESARC 18.3%, NSDUH 16.8%; *poor health*: IDU 17.2%, NESARC 8.5%, NSDUH 6.5%). These injecting drug users also had high rates of sexually transmitted diseases (Gonorrhoea 20.7%, Syphilis 11.5%), liver diseases (Hepatitis-C 55.1%, Cirrhosis 9.7%, Hepatitis-B 7.9%) and stroke (4.0%). Almost one-third (31.3%) lacked health insurance. In addition, 71.8% of participants reported tobacco use in the past 30 days, higher than national samples (21.9% NESARC, 18.5% NSDUH), and participants endorsed high rates of continuing drug use. Overall, findings indicate that older injecting drug users have multiple health risks.

One study also showed better overall treatment outcomes for older substance abusers (aged ≥50 years) in treatment. Outlaw *et al.* [38] examined 199 adults aged 50–89 with a substance use disorder who participated in a cognitive-behavioural/self-management treatment programme from January 2005 to October 2007. Of all participants, 58% failed to complete at least 75% of the programme. From intake to six-month follow-up, completers reported greater reduction in the number of nonmedical prescription drug use days and number of days experiencing trouble understanding, concentrating and remembering not due to alcohol or drug use. Over time there was also reduced bodily pain for completers but increased pain for noncompleters. Both groups had improved mental health but this was better for completers than noncompleters.

Discussion

Illicit drug use prevalence was higher among younger adults (aged 50–54) than older adults aged ≥55 years. Past-month illicit or nonmedical drug use prevalences ranged from 0.8% for those aged ≥65 years to 6.7% for adults aged 50–54. Survey data showed drug use was on the rise, which corresponded to treatment data. In TEDS, approximately 10% of substance abuse treatment admissions for adults aged 50–54 involved drug use in 1992; 61% of substance abuse treatment admissions involved drugs in 2005. In 1992, just under 10% of substance abuse treatment admissions for adults aged ≥55 years involved drugs; and, in 2005, 45% of substance abuse treatment admissions for those aged ≥55 years involved drugs. It appeared that the increased prevalence of illicit drug use in the older population is influenced by long-term, chronic drug users as well as later-onset older drug users.

Marijuana was the drug used most often by adults aged ≥50 years (past-year prevalence range 0.7% among adults aged ≥50 years to 7.9% among adults aged 50–54), followed by cocaine (past-year range 0.1% aged ≥50 years to 0.9% among adults aged 50–54). Marijuana was used more by males than females and younger elders (aged 50–54) than older adults (aged ≥55 years). Females and elders (aged ≥65 years) tended to use nonmedical pharmaceutical-type drugs. The primary illicit drug identified from treatment admission data in TEDS was cocaine. However, cocaine admissions declined recently as marijuana and methamphetamine related admissions increased, suggesting a changing pattern of illicit drug use or abuse.

Illicit drug use was proportionally higher among non-Whites when compared to Whites aged ≥65 years, which was echoed in treatment data where illicit drug use related admissions for adults aged ≥55 years had increased proportionally more among Blacks than Whites. While Moore et al. [21] found past-year illicit and nonmedical drug use were higher for Latinos than Whites, Arndt et al. [30] found that admissions for individuals aged ≥55 years increased less among Latinos than non-Latinos. This discrepancy could suggest that Latinos might not have accessed substance abuse treatment.

Historically, most substance abuse prevention has focused on adolescents and young adults, with little attention on how to best prevent drug abuse among the elderly [5]. Elder adults face unique consequences to drug use. For example, the chronic health conditions and related medication use observed among participants in treatment studies could exacerbate drug effects or cause negative reactions [31, 32]. Reasons for elder substance abuse also likely differ from those for adolescent and young adult use [5]. Adolescents may begin or engage in substance use for peer approval [39]. However, older adults may engage in substance use for reasons of anxiety, loneliness or depression [40]. The reliable demographic correlate of drug use found in reported research is being unmarried, and it is possible that correlates are changing as the cohort of elder substance abusers transitions to the baby boomer generation.

Next steps

Additional research is needed to better characterize correlates of drug use, abuse and dependence among older adults and to differentiate patterns of use based on age, race/ethnicity and gender. There is a continuous need to monitor shifting patterns of drug use and to examine how shifting patterns affect elders by age, race/ethnicity and gender, as well as by characteristics found more often among the elderly, such as living in a care facility. Future studies need to include Latinos, one of the fastest growing segments of the population. More focused research is also needed on ageing illicit drug abusers who have used prolonged treatment to ensure their treatment needs continue to be met as they age.

References

1. Gfroerer, J., Penne, M., Pemberton, M. and Folsom, R. (2003) Substance abuse treatment need among older adults in 2020: the impact of the aging baby-boom cohort. *Drug Alcohol Depend*, **69**, 127–135.
2. Johnson, P.B. and Sung, H.E. (2009) Substance abuse among aging baby boomers: Health and treatment implications. *J Addict Nurs*, **20**, 124–126.
3. American Psychiatric Association (2000) *Diagnostic and Statistical Manual of Mental Disorders*, 4th edn. American Psychiatric Association, Washington, DC.
4. Vincent, G.K. and Velkoff, V.A. (2010) The Next Four Decades, the Older Population in the United States: 2010 to 2050. Current Population Reports, P25-1138, US Census Bureau, Washington, DC.
5. Colliver, J.D., Compton, W.M., Gfroerer, J.C. and Condon, T. (2006) Projecting drug use among aging baby boomers in 2020. *Ann Epidemiol*, **16**, 257–265.
6. Centers for Disease Control and Prevention (2010) Health, United States, 2009: With Special Feature on Medical Technology. National Center for Health Statistics, US Department of Health and Human Services, Atlanta, GA.
7. Kinsella, K. and He, W. (2009) *An Aging World: 2008*. US Census Bureau, International Population Reports P95/09-1, US Government Printing Office, Washington, DC.
8. Mirkin, B. and Weinberger, M.B. (2001) *The Demography of Population Aging. Technical Meeting on Population Aging and Living Arrangements of Older Persons: Critical Issues and Policy Responses*. United Nations Population Bulletin, Special Issue Nos. 42/43.
9. Voyer, P., Preville, M., Cohen, D. *et al.* (2010) The prevalence of benzodiazepine dependence among community-dwelling older adult users in Quebec according to typical and atypical criteria. *Can J Aging*, **29**(2), 205–213.
10. Pollini, R.A., Banta-Green, C.J., Cuevas-Mota, J. *et al.* (2011) Problematic use of prescription-type opioids prior to heroin use among young heroin injectors. *Subst Abuse and Rehabil*, **2**, 173–180.
11. Davis, W.R. and Johnson, B.D. (2008) Prescription opioid use, misuse, and diversion among street drug users in New York City. *Drug Alcohol Depend*, **92**, 267–276.
12. Simoni-Wastila, L. and Yang, H.K. (2006) Psychoactive drug abuse in older adults. *Am J Geriatr Pharmacother*, **4**, 380–394.
13. Manchikanti, L. (2006) Prescription drug abuse: What is being done to address this new drug epidemic? Testimony before the Subcommittee on Criminal Justice, Drug Policy and Human Resources. *Pain Physician*, **9**, 287–321.
14. Manchikanti, L. (2007) National drug control policy and prescription drug abuse: Facts and fallacies. *Pain Physician*, **10**, 399–424.

15. Wu, L.-T. and Blazer, D.G. (2011) Illicit and nonmedical drug use among older adults: A review. *J Aging Health*, **223**, 481–504.
16. Blazer, D.G. and Wu, L.-T. (2009) Nonprescription use of pain relievers by middle-aged and elderly community-living adults: National Survey on Drug Use and Health. *J Am Geriatr Soc*, **57**, 1252–1257.
17. Center for Behavioral Health Statistics and Quality (2011) *The NSDUH Report: Illicit Drug Use among Older Adults*. Substance Abuse and Mental Health Services Administration, Rockville, MD.
18. Center for Behavioral Health Statistics and Quality (2012) *Results from the 2011 National Survey on Drug Use and Health: Mental Health Detailed Tables*. Substance Abuse and Mental Health Services Administration, Rockville MD.
19. Blazer, D.G. and Wu, L.-T. (2009) The epidemiology of substance use and disorders among middle aged and elderly community adults: National Survey on Drug Use and Health (NSDUH). *Am J Geriatr Psychiatry*, **17**, 237–245.
20. White, J.B., Duncan, D.F., Bradley, D. *et al.* (2011) Generational shift and drug abuse in older Americans. *J Soc Behav Health Sci*, **5**, 58–66.
21. Moore, A.A., Karno, M.P., Grella, C.E. *et al.* (2009) Alcohol, tobacco, and nonmedical drug use in older U.S. adults: Data from the 2001/02 National Epidemiologic Survey of Alcohol and Related Conditions. *J Am Geriatr Soc*, **57**, 2275–2281.
22. Lin, J.C., Karno, M.P., Grella, C.E. *et al.* (2011) Alcohol, tobacco, and non-medical drug use disorders in U.S. adults aged 65 and older: Data from the 2001-2002 National Epidemiologic Survey of Alcohol and Related Conditions. *Am J Geriatr Psychiatry*, **19**, 292–299.
23. Center for Behavioral Health Statistics and Quality (2012) *Results from the 2011 National Survey on Drug Use and Health: Summary of National Findings*. NSDUH Series H-44, HHS Publication No. (SMA) 12-4713. Substance Abuse and Mental Health Services Administration, Rockville, MD.
24. Center for Behavioral Health Statistics and Quality (2003) *Results from the 2002 National Survey on Drug Use and Health: Mental Health Detailed Tables*. Substance Abuse and Mental Health Services Administration, Rockville MD.
25. Fahmy, V., Hatch, .SL., Hotopf, M. and Stewart, R. (2012) Prevalences of illicit drug use in people aged 50 years and over from two surveys. *Age Ageing*, **41**(4), 553–556.
26. Beynon, C.M., McVeigh, J. and Roe, B. (2007) Problematic drug use, ageing and older people: Trends in the age of drug users in northwest England. *Ageing Soc*, **27**, 799–810.
27. Han, B., Gfroerer, J.C., Colliver, J.D. and Penne, M.A. (2009) Substance use disorder among older adults in the United States in 2020. *Addiction*, **104**, 88–96.
28. Lev-Ran, S., Imtiaz, S., Taylor, B.J. *et al.* (2012) Gender differences in health-related quality of life among cannabis users: Results from the national epidemiologic survey on alcohol and related conditions. *Drug Alcohol Depend*, **123**, 190–200.
29. Lofwall, M.R., Schuster, A. and Strain, E.C. (2008) Changing profile of abused substances by older persons entering treatment. *J Nerv Ment Dis*, **196**, 898–905.
30. Arndt, S., Clayton, R. and Schultz, S.K. (2011) Trends in substance abuse treatment 1998-2008: Increasing older adult first-time admissions for illicit drugs. *Am J Geriatr Psychiatry*, **19**, 704–711.
31. Rajaratnam, R., Sivesind, D., Todman, M. *et al.* (2009) The aging methadone maintenance patient: Treatment adjustment, long-term success, and quality of life. *J Opioid Manag*, **5**, 27–37.
32. Woo, B.K.P. and Chen, W. (2010) Substance misuse among older patients in psychiatric emergency service. *Gen Hosp Psychiatry*, **32**, 99–101.
33. Beynon, C., McVeigh, J., Hurst, A. and Marr, A. (2010) Changing mortality of drug users in treatment in North West England. *Int J Drug Policy*, **21**, 429–431.

34. Termorshuizen, F., Krol, A., Prins, M. and van Ameijden, E.J.C. (2005) Long-term outcome of chronic drug use: The Amsterdam cohort study among drug users. *Am J Epidemiol*, **161**, 271–279.
35. Moy, I., Crome, P., Crome, I. and Fisher, M. (2011) Systematic and narrative review of treatment for older people with substance problems. *Eur Geriatr Med*, **2**, 212–236.
36. Johnson, S.D., Striley, C. and Cottler, L.B. (2007) Comorbid substance use and HIV risk in older African American drug users. *J Aging Health*, **19**, 646–658.
37. Torres, L.R., Kaplan, C. and Valdez, A. (2011) Health consequences of long-term injection heroin use among aging Mexican American men. *J Aging Health*, **23**, 912–932.
38. Outlaw, F.H., Marquart, J.M., Roy, A. *et al.* (2012) Treatment outcomes for older adults who abuse substances. *J Appl Gerontol*, **31**, 78–100.
39. Trucco, E.M., Colder, C.R. and Wieczorek, W.F. (2011) Vulnerability to peer influence: A moderated mediation study of early adolescent alcohol use initiation. *Addict Behav*, **36**, 729–736.
40. Christie, M.M., Bamber, D., Powell, C. *et al.* (2012) Older adult problem drinkers: Who presents for alcohol treatment. *Aging Ment Health*, **17**(1), 24–32.

Chapter 9

EPIDEMIOLOGY AND DEMOGRAPHY OF NONMEDICAL PRESCRIPTION DRUG USE

Jane Carlisle Maxwell

Addiction Research Institute, Center for Social Work Research, The University of Texas at Austin, USA

Introduction

This chapter provides data on the nonmedical use of prescription drugs by an older adult population. The focus of this chapter is on recent information drawn from four US large-scale data sets which are available for analysis. Comparisons are made of the characteristics of the ageing populations as seen in these four major data sets.

1. The National Household Survey on Drug Use and Health (NSDUH) of the federal Substance Abuse and Mental Health Services Administration (SAMHSA) provides national data on the use of tobacco, alcohol, illicit drugs (including nonmedical use of prescription drugs) and mental health in the United States [1].
2. The Drug Abuse Warning Network (DAWN) of SAMHSA provides demographic and visit-level information on emergency department (ED) visits. DAWN uses an annual probability sample of hospitals to produce estimates of drug-related emergency department visits for the United States [2].
3. The Treatment Episode Data set (TEDS) of SAMHSA collects information on the demographic and substance abuse problems of admissions to treatment for individuals aged 12 and older. The facilities report to individual State administrative data systems [3].
4. The Mortality Multiple Cause public use data file of the National Center for Health Statistics (NCHS), Centers for Disease Control and Prevention, enables users to access and analyse data from all birth and death certificates in the United States. There are 2.4 million death certificate records reported annually, and this chapter uses data on deaths due to accidental poisoning and exposure to noxious substances [4].

Substance Use and Older People, First Edition.
Edited by Ilana B. Crome, Li-Tzy Wu, Rahul (Tony) Rao and Peter Crome.
© 2015 John Wiley & Sons, Ltd. Published 2015 by John Wiley & Sons, Ltd.

The data sets report age groups differently, with 65 years and over being the oldest age category in NSDUH and DAWN, 55 and over the oldest age category for TEDS and ten-year groups through age 85 and older for NCHS. When data permit, the age, gender and race/ethnic groups are compared to highlight the differences and serve as the basis of projections of special needs into the future.

Findings

The size of the ageing population in the United States is continuing to grow. Between 2000 and 2010, the number of persons 50 years and older increased from 76.9 million to 99 million, and the number of persons 65 years and older increased from 35 million to 40 million. In 1900, the population of those 65 and older comprised 4.1% of the total population; in 2010 it was 13% [5].

National surveys

The National Survey on Drug Use and Health (NSDUH), an annual survey of over 70 000 respondents in the civilian population of the United States aged 12 years old or older, reports the prevalence of use of various drugs, including the nonmedical use of any prescription-type pain reliever, tranquilizer or sedative. Nonmedical use is defined as use of a medication without a prescription belonging to the respondent or use that occurred simply for the experience or feeling the drug caused. Over-the-counter substances are not included in these estimates. Persons living in nursing homes, mental institutions, prisons, the homeless not living in a shelter and those in other institutional group quarters are not surveyed.

Due to the increasing population of older adults and high substance use rate of the baby boomer generation born between 1946 and 1964, the number of adults ages 50 or older with a substance use disorder (SUD) is projected to double from 2.8 million in 2002–2006 to 5.7 million in 2020 [6]. Almost 90% of these ageing past-year users began their drug use before age 30 and about 1 in 7 of those with a past history of ever using drugs (lifetime users) reported still using drugs in the past year at ages 50–59 [7].

Those who initiated alcohol use by age 16 were twice as likely to have a SUD and those who initiated illicit drug use by that age were more than four times as likely to have a past-year SUD. Males in their fifties who had ever used drugs and also reported using them in the past year were 2.32 times more likely to have past-year SUD than their female counterparts, and past-year SUD was also associated with being unmarried, low education and income, unemployed due to disability and, in the past year, using alcohol and tobacco, having a major depressive episode and not attending religious services [7].

In 2011, 13.3% of all NSDUH respondents ages 12 and older had used a prescription pain reliever such as codeine, oxycodone or hydrocodone nonmedically. Additionally, 8.4% reported having used tranquilizers such as benzodiazepines and 2.9% reported having used sedatives such as sleep medications nonmedically [8].

However, the prevalence rates of nonmedical use of prescription drugs decrease with age. The influence of the baby boomers on drug use prevalence is shown by the finding that lifetime use of pain relievers by those 50–54 was more than five times higher than those 65 and older (Figure 9.1).

Table 9.1 shows race/ethnic and gender distribution of past-year users of prescription pain relievers (opioids), tranquilizers and sedatives, as well as of those who used any illicit drug (hallucinogens, heroin, marijuana, cocaine, inhalants) or any prescription drugs (pain relievers/opioids, tranquilizers, stimulants or sedatives). Females were more likely to report use of tranquilizers and sedatives; more Whites reported use of tranquilizers and Hispanics reported higher use of sedatives (Table 9.1).

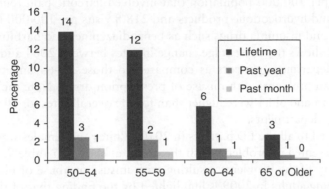

Figure 9.1 Lifetime, past-year and past-month nonmedical use of pain relievers: NSDUH 2011 [1].
Notes: Nonmedical use is defined as use of a medication without a prescription belonging to the respondent or use that occurred simply for the experience or feeling the drug caused. Pain relievers include hydrocodone, methadone, morphine, oxycodone, tramadol and similar drugs.

Table 9.1 Characteristics of past-year users aged 50 and older: NSDUH 2011 [9]

	White (%)	Black (%)	Hispanic (%)	Male (%)	Female (%)
Used pain relievers	77.9	10.1	9.4	50.6	49.4
Used tranquilizers	86.1	3.9	9.8	39.0	61.0
Used sedatives	71.2	*	28.8	25.5	74.5
Used any illicit drugs	79.0	9.7	7.5	46.6	53.4

*Unreliable
Notes: Pain relievers include codeine, oxycodone, or hydrocodone used nonmedically.
Tranquilizers include benzodiazepines, meprobamate products and muscle relaxers used nonmedically.
Sedatives include temazepam, flurazepam, triazolam and any barbiturate used nonmedically.
Illicit drugs include marijuana/hashish, cocaine (including crack), heroin, hallucinogens, inhalants or prescription-type psychotherapeutics used nonmedically.

Emergency department cases

The Drug Abuse Warning Network (DAWN) provides demographic information on emergency department visits between 2004 and 2011 resulting from substance misuse or abuse, adverse reactions to drugs taken as prescribed, accidental ingestion of drugs, drug-related suicide attempts and other drug-related medical emergencies. Included are all types of drugs: illegal drugs, prescription and over-the-counter pharmaceuticals (e.g. dietary supplements, cough medicine), and substances inhaled for their psychoactive effects.

In 2011 there were 5.1 million drug-related ED visits, with 1.6 million involving pharmaceuticals, 1.3 million involving illicit drugs, 0.6 million involving alcohol in combination with drugs and 0.1 million involving underage drinking. There were 221.7 visits per 100 000 population that involved narcotic pain relievers such as oxycodone and hydrocodone products and 218.8 visits per 100 000 that involved anti-anxiety and insomnia drugs such as benzodiazepines and barbiturates [10].

Figure 9.2 shows the percentage change in rates between 2004 and 2011 for all emergency department patients as compared to those 55–64 and those 65 and older who had problems with misuse of prescription drugs. Note the rates for the populations 55 and older were higher than for the overall rates for all patients seen in emergency departments.

As compared to all the ED patients in 2010, Whites and females were disproportionally represented in problems with the drugs, as shown in Table 9.2.

The severity of the problems resulting with misuse or abuse of pharmaceutical drugs by ageing adults in 2009 is highlighted by the finding that of those aged 50 and older treated in the ED, 54% were treated and released and 36% were admitted to the hospital. Of those admitted to the hospital, 66% were admitted to an inpatient unit, 24% were admitted to an intensive care unit and 10% were admitted to a chemical dependence, detoxification or psychiatric unit [12].

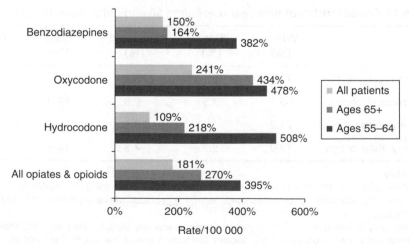

Figure 9.2 Change in rates for emergency department patients: DAWN 2004–2011 [9].

Table 9.2 Characteristics of emergency department patients aged 55 and over: DAWN 2010 [11]

	White (%)	Black (%)	Hispanic (%)	Male (%)	Female (%)
Opiates/opioids	84.7	9.6	4.0	43.4	56.6
Hydrocodone/combinations	83.2	8.2	5.8	40.4	59.6
Oxycodone/combinations	86.1	9.5	2.6	39.8	60.2
Benzodiazepines	85.7	7.5	5.6	39.0	61.0
All misuse and abuse episodes	60.1	32.3	6.4	58.8	41.2

Notes: Other opiates and synthetics include buprenorphine, codeine, hydrocodone, hydromorphone, meperidine, morphine, opium, oxycodone, pentazocine, propoxyphene, tramadol and any other drug with morphine-like effects. Benzodiazepines include alprazolam, chlordiazepoxide, clonazepam, clorazepate, diazepam, flunitrazepam, flurazepam, halazepam, lorazepam, oxazepam, prazepam, temazepam, triazolam and other unspecified benzodiazepines.

Treatment admissions

The Treatment Episode Data Set (TEDS) collects admission and discharge data from the States on patients treated in publicly-funded substance abuse programmes that can provide detoxification, residential and outpatient settings as well as medication-assisted therapies such as methadone and buprenorphine. In some States, private programmes that do not receive governmental funding may also be included in the TEDS data set. In 2010, there were 1.8 million treatment admissions reported to TEDS.

TEDS substance problem categories include 'Other Opiates and Synthetics', such as buprenorphine, codeine, hydrocodone, hydromorphone, meperidine, morphine, opium, oxycodone, pentazocine, propoxyphene, tramadol and any other drug with morphine-like effects.

Of all patients entering treatment for substance abuse, the proportion of those aged 45 and older with a primary problem with other opiates increased from 1.3 to 15.5% between 1992 and 2010 (Figure 9.3). Less than 1% of the patients over the age of 45 had a primary problem with benzodiazepines. In comparison, the most common substance abused was alcohol (57% of all patients over the age of 45).

Table 9.3 shows that in the 2010 admissions for these two drug groups, Whites, and females were overrepresented, as compared to admissions for all drugs.

The combination of benzodiazepines and narcotic pain relievers is a growing problem, with treatment admissions for use of these two drugs in combination increasing nearly six times between 2000 and 2010. Those using these drugs together were more likely to be White, female and better educated than patients who used other drugs. They used these two drugs in combination on a daily basis and 46% reported a co-occurring psychiatric disorder. They were more likely to be self-referred to treatment and to need detoxification and short-term residential treatment. Although 67% of the admissions were among younger patients aged 18–35, 3% were aged 45–54 and 2.6% were aged 55–64 [15].

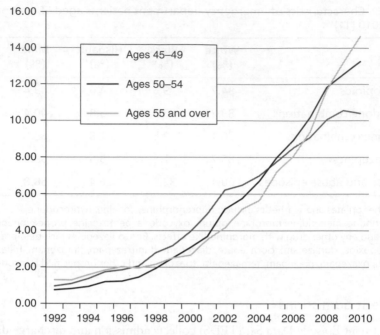

Figure 9.3 Proportion of treatment admissions aged 45 and over with primary problems with other opiates and synthetics: TEDS 1992–2010 [13].
Note: Other opiates and synthetics include buprenorphine, codeine, hydrocodone, hydromorphone, meperidine, morphine, opium, oxycodone, pentazocine, propoxyphene, tramadol and any other drug with morphine-like effects.

Table 9.3 Characteristics of treatment admissions aged 55 and older: TEDS 2010 [14]

	White (%)	Black (%)	Hispanic (%)	Male (%)	Female (%)
Other opiates	80.9	10.1	5.1	54.7	45.3
Benzodiazepines	81.4	6.9	9.7	53.9	46.1
All substances	56.2	28.4	11.1	77.1	22.9

Drug poisoning deaths

Each year the National Center for Health Statistics (NCHS) provides data on the number of deaths due to accidental poisoning and exposure to noxious substances including methadone, natural and semi-synthetic opioids (e.g. morphine, oxycodone, hydrocodone), synthetic opioid analgesics (fentanyl), methadone, cocaine, benzodiazepines and heroin. Because of the way the drugs are categorized in the International Classification of Diseases, Tenth Revision (ICD-10) [16], more detailed information on the specific drugs in these categories cannot be reported.

Between 1999 and 2010, the drug poisoning death rate for all drugs increased among all age groups (Figure 9.4). Since 2005, the drug poisoning death rate has been highest among those aged 45–54 and lowest among those 65 and older. Between 1999 and 2010, the death rate for those aged 55–64 increased from 4.2 per 100 000 to 15.0 per 100 000. For those 65 and older, the death rate increased from 2.7 per 100 000 to 4.3 per 100 000 during the same time period.

The drug poisoning death rates vary by specific drug category and by age group (Figure 9.5). The rate involving natural and semi-synthetic opioids, such as

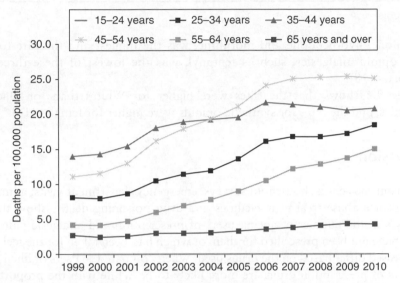

Figure 9.4 Drug poisoning death rates by age: United States, 1999–2010 [17].

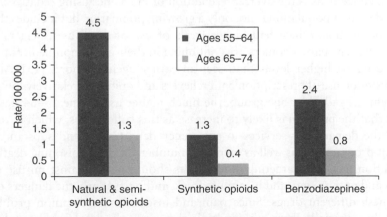

Figure 9.5 Drug poisoning death rates by age group: NCHS 2010 [13].
Note: The International Classification of Diseases-10 definition of natural and semi-synthetic opioid analgesics includes morphine, oxycodone, and hydrocodone. Synthetic opioid analgesics include fentanyl.

Table 9.4 Drug poisoning deaths per 100 000 aged 55–64: CDC 2010 [13]

	White	Black	Hispanic	Male	Female
Natural and semi-synthetic opioids	5.2	2.5	2.3	5.1	3.9
Synthetic opioids	1.5	0.8	*	1.2	2.2
Benzodiazepines	2.9	0.8	1	2.7	2.2
All drug poisoning	18	20.2	9.8	20	14.1

*Unreliable

oxycodone, hydrocodone and morphine, was the highest and the rate for synthetic opioid analgesics, such as fentanyl, was the lowest of these three drug categories [18].

Table 9.4 shows that the rates were higher for Whites than for Blacks or Hispanics, and the rates for synthetic opioids were higher for females [18].

Discussion

Data from the census, household surveys, emergency department visits, admissions to substance abuse treatment facilities and drug poisoning deaths show that the increases in the number of ageing users of prescription and analgesic pain drugs which have not been prescribed for them or which had been taken for the feeling the drug caused differ based on the drugs used. When compared to users of illicit drugs, misusers of prescription drugs are more likely to be White with the proportion of male and female varying by data set and drug, although the finding that higher proportions of females are reporting use of these drugs compared to use of most other drugs is a concern, as is the overrepresentation of Hispanics using sedatives.

The older adult population is not only a growing population but includes the baby boomer population, which had higher levels of use of drugs as teenagers and as young adults. The baby boomers are continuing in their use of nonmedical pharmaceutical drugs at higher levels than seen in earlier ageing cohorts [19]. Although nonprescription use of prescription pain relievers and opioids is relatively low among the current 65 and older age group, the much higher use by the 55–64 age group suggests that the problem is likely to increase as this cohort ages, which in turn will increase the demand for services in emergency departments and substance abuse treatment programmes, as well as increased numbers of drug poisoning deaths [20].

Prevention messages targeting older adults should warn against misuse of pain relievers and anti-anxiety and insomnia drugs, and particularly the dangers of combining these different drugs. Since pain and insomnia are common problems in older adults, especially those with multiple chronic medical conditions, and require multiple medications, efforts should be focused on educating these older adults on better pain and insomnia management options rather than depending on prescription and over-the-counter (OTC) pain relievers [21].

Medical personnel as well as behavioural health specialists should monitor for warning signs of prescription drug misuse and the abuse of multiple drugs and alcohol by older adults [22], especially since older adults have been found to have inadequate knowledge of prescription drug safety and interactions with alcohol [23]. Given older adults may be taking medications prescribed by different physicians for different conditions, each physician should obtain and maintain updated lists of all medications. Since recall may be an issue for some patients, physicians should have all medication containers brought in at each visit and pharmacists should be proactive in warning each patient of the potential interactions as well as warning the prescribing physician of other medications used by the patient.

Furthermore, inappropriate prescribing, for example concomitant use of ≥3 psychotropic/opioid drugs and drug combinations, including nonsteroid anti-inflammatory drugs (NSAIDs), is a serious problem in medically ill older adults [24], which underscores the importance of evaluation and monitoring of medications by physicians. These evaluations should consider not only the pharmacological properties of the drugs but also clinical, epidemiological, social, cultural and economic factors of the older patients [25], as well as the patterns of use by gender.

Benzodiazepines can potentiate the effects of narcotic pain relievers even when taken as prescribed. They can cause confusion, night wandering, amnesia, ataxia and hangover effects because ageing bodies metabolize drugs less efficiently and the effects of the drugs can last longer. Factors associated with dependence on benzodiazepines are being female, dosing level, having cognitive impairment, panic disorders, suicidal ideations and a degree of embarrassment in seeking help for emotional problems [26]. Likewise, ageing users are more likely to be affected by opioids because of changes in body composition, including reduction in total body water, reduced hepatic and renal functions and respiratory depression, among other side effects [27]. In addition, benzodiazepines and opioids can increase the risk of falls and hip fractures, with resulting hospitalization and disability [28]. The common pattern of using prescription and nonprescription medications together means that nearly 1 in 25 ageing individuals is potentially at risk of a major drug–drug interaction such as increased risk of bleeding, rhabdomyolysis or decreased effectiveness of the drugs [29].

Caregivers for older adults, including their adult children [30], and especially those caring for older adults with dementia or other forms of cognitive impairment, should be aware that these drugs can further impair cognitive functioning. Thorpe *et al.* found that older adults with dementia on average took more medications, such as muscle relaxants/antispasmodics, fluoxetine, short–acting nifedipine and doxazosin, than did those without dementia [31].

Use of benzodiazepines and pain relievers alone or in combination can also lead to a treatment-resistant population because of the severe withdrawal symptoms and the pattern of daily use, which may be difficult to change. Providing medical and supportive services to mitigate the severe withdrawal effects may be critical to avoid treatment attrition and relapse [32], but most substance abuse treatment programme protocols were designed for adolescents and young adults, and new approaches are needed for older adults. Only 6% of substance abuse treatment facilities in 2011 reported having a programme or group designed specifically for seniors [33], although older adults with SUD have been shown to respond well to age-specific, supportive and nonconfrontational group treatment. These individuals can recover and maintain an improved quality of life [34].

Conclusions

The US population aged 50 and older is growing in numbers and in nonmedical use of prescription drugs. Compared to users of illicit drugs, the misusers of prescription drugs tend to be White and female, with differences based on the specific prescription drugs. Implementation of prevention and treatment efforts targeted to the older adult population can help decrease adverse events that lead to functional disability, more hospitalizations and premature death.

Acknowledgement

The author wishes to thank Dr Namkee Choi for her careful and constructive comments on this paper.

References

1. SAMHSA (2012) Results from the 2011 National Survey on Drug Use and Health: Summary of National Findings. NSDUH Series H-44, HHS Publication No. (SMA) 12-4713, Substance Abuse and Mental Health Services Administration (SAMHSA), Rockville, MD.
2. Drug Abuse Warning Network (2012) 2011: Selected Tables of National Estimates of Drug-Related Emergency Department Visits. Center for Behavioral Health Statistics and Quality, Substance Abuse and Mental Health Services Administration (SAMHSA), Rockville, MD.
3. SAMHSA (2012) Treatment Episode Data Set (TEDS): 2000–2010. National Admissions to Substance Abuse Treatment Services. DASIS Series S-61, HHS Publication No. (SMA) 12-4701, Center for Behavioral Health Statistics and Quality, Substance Abuse and Mental Health Services Administration (SAMHSA), Rockville, MD.
4. Murphy, S.L., Xu, J. and Kochanek, K.D. (2013) Deaths: Final Data for 2010. National Vital Statistics Reports, Vol. 61, No. 4, US Department of Health and Human Services. http://www.cdc.gov/nchs/data/nvsr/nvsr61/nvsr61_04.pdf (last accessed 3 April 2014).
5. Werner, C.A. (2011) The Older Population: 2010, 2010 Census Briefs. US Census Bureau. http://www.census.gov/prod/cen2010/briefs/c2010br-09.pdf (last accessed 3 April 2014).
6. Han, B., Gfroerer, J.C., Colliver, J.D. and Penne, M.A. (2008) Substance use disorder among older adults in the United States in 2020. Addiction, 104, 88–96.
7. Han, B., Gfroerer, J.C. and Colliver, J.D. (2009) An examination of trends in illicit drug use among adults aged 50 to 59 in the United States: OAS Data Review, Office of Applied Studies, Substance Abuse and Mental Health Services Administration (SAMHSA), Rockville, MD. http://www.samhsa.gov/data/2k11/DataReview/OAS_data_review_OlderAdults.pdf (last accessed 3 April 2014).

8. SAMHSA, National Survey on Drug Use and Health, 2010 and 2011, Table 1.1B. Substance Abuse and Mental Health Services Administration (SAMHSA), Rockville, MD.
9. SAMHSA (2012) National Survey on Drug Use and Health 2011. Center for Substance Abuse Treatment, Substance Abuse and Mental Health Services Administration (SAMHSA), Rockville, MD. [Computer file]. ICPSR34481-v1. Research Triangle Institute, Research Triangle Park, NC [producer]. Inter-university Consortium for Political and Social Research, Ann Arbor, MI [distributor].
10. Drug Abuse Warning Network (2011) National Estimates of Drug-related Emergency Department Visits, 2004–2011. Center for Behavioral Health Statistics and Quality, Substance Abuse and Mental Health Services Administration (SAMHSA), Rockville, MD.
11. SAMHSA (2012) Drug Abuse Warning Network (DAWN), 2010. Center for Substance Abuse Treatment, Substance Abuse and Mental Health Services Administration (SAMHSA), Rockville, MD. ICPSR34083-v1. Inter-university Consortium for Political and Social Research, Ann Arbor, MI [distributor]. doi:10.3886/ICPSR34083.v1.
12. SAMHSA (2012) The DAWN Report: Drug-Related Emergency Department Visits Involving Pharmaceutical Misuse or Abuse by Older Adults: 2009. Center for Behavioral Health Statistics and Quality, Substance Abuse and Mental Health Services Administration (SAMHSA), Rockville, MD.
13. SAMHSA (2012) Treatment Episode Data Set – Admissions (TEDS-A) – Concatenated, 1992–2010. Office of Applied Studies, Substance Abuse and Mental Health Services Administration (SAMHSA). ICPSR25221-v5. Inter-university Consortium for Political and Social Research, Ann Arbor, MI [distributor]. doi:10.3886/ICPSR25221.v5.
14. SAMHSA (2012) Treatment Episode Data Set – Admissions (TEDS-A), 2010. Center for Behavioral Health Statistics and Quality, Substance Abuse and Mental Health Services Administration (SAMHSA). ICPSR33261-v1. Inter-university Consortium for Political and Social Research, Ann Arbor, MI [distributor]. doi:10.3886/ICPSR33261.v1.
15. SAMHSA (2012) The TEDS Report: Admissions Reporting Benzodiazepine and Narcotic Pain Reliever Abuse at Treatment Entry. Center for Behavioral Health Statistics and Quality, Substance Abuse and Mental Health Services Administration (SAMHSA), Rockville, MD.
16. WHO (2008) International Statistical Classification of Diseases and Related Health Problems, 10th Revision. World Health Organization (WHO), Geneva, Switzerland.
17. Warner, M., Chen, L.H., Makuc, D.M. et al. (2011) Drug poisoning deaths in the United States, 1980–2008. NCHS Data Brief, No. 81, National Center for Health Statistics, Hyattsville, MD. http://www.cdc.gov/nchs/data/databriefs/db81.htm (last accessed 3 April 2014).
18. Centers for Disease Control (2010) National Vital Statistics Report (NVSR). Deaths: Final Data for 2010, 61(4). http://www.cdc.gov/nchs/data_access/Vitalstatsonline.htm (last accessed 3 April 2014).
19. Colliver, J.D., Compton, W.M., Gfroerer, J.C. and Condon, T. (2006) Projecting drug use among aging baby boomers in 2020. Annals of Epidemiology, 16, 257–265.
20. Blazer, D.G. and Wu, L.-T. (2009) Nonprescription use of pain relievers by middle-aged and elderly community-living adults: National Survey on Drug Use and Health. Journal of the American Geriatric Society, 57, 1252–1257.
21. Qato, D.M., Alexander, G.C., Conti, R.M. et al. (2008) Use of prescription and over-the-counter medications and dietary supplements among older adults in the United States. JAMA, 300(24): 2867–2878.
22. SAMHSA (2012) The DAWN Report: Drug-Related Emergency Department Visits Involving Pharmaceutical Misuse or Abuse by Older Adults: 2009. Center for Behavioral Health Statistics and Quality, Substance Abuse and Mental Health Services Administration (SAMHSA), Rockville, MD.

23. Zanjani, F., Hoogland, A. and Downer, B. (2013) Alcohol and prescription drug safety in older adults. *Drug, Healthcare and Patient Safety*, **5**, 13–27.
24. Peron, E.P., Marcum, Z.A., Boyce, R. *et al.* (2011) Year in review: medication mishaps in the elderly. *American Journal of Geriatric Pharmacotherapy*, **9**, 1–10.
25. Boparai, M.K. and Korc-Grodzicki, B. (2011) Prescribing for older adults. *Mount Sinai Journal of Medicine*, **78**, 613–626.
26. Voyer, P., Preville, M., Roussel, M.-E. *et al.* (2009) Factors associated with benzodiazepine dependence among community-dwelling seniors. *Journal of Community Health Nursing*, **26**, 101–113.
27. Wang, P.S., Bohn, R.L., Glynn, R.J. *et al.* (2001) Hazardous benzodiazepine regimens in the elderly: Effects of half-life, dosage, and duration on risk of hip fracture. *American Journal of Psychiatry*, **158**, 892–898; Miller, M., Stuermer, T., Azrael, D. *et al.* (2011) opioid analgesics and the risk of fractures in older adults with arthritis. *Journal of the American Geriatrics Society*, **59**, 430–443; Huang, A.R. and Mallet, L. (2012) Prescribing opioids in older people. *Maturitas*, **74**, 123–129; Solomon, D.H., Rassen, J.A., Glynn, R.J. *et al.* (2010) The comparative safety of opioids for nonmalignant pain in older adults. *Archives of Internal Medicine*, **170**, 1979–1986; Benyamin, R., Trescot, A.M., Datta, S. *et al.* (2008) Opioid complications and side effects, *Pain Physician*, **11** (2 Suppl), S105–S120.
28. Albert, S.M., Colombi, A. and Hanlon, J. (2010) Potentially inappropriate medications and risk of hospitalization in retirees. *Drugs and Aging*, **27**, 407–415.
29. Qato, D.M., Alexander, G.C., Conti, R.M. *et al.* (2008) Use of prescription and over-the-counter medications and dietary supplements among older adults in the United States. *JAMA*, **300** (24), 2867–2878.
30. Thorpe, J.M., Thorpe, C.T., Kennelty, K.A. *et al.* (2012) The impact of family caregivers on potentially inappropriate medication use in noninstitutionalised older adults with dementia. *The American Journal of Geriatric Pharmacotherapy*, **10**(4), 230–241.
31. Lau, D.T., Mercaldo, N.D., Harfis, A.T. *et al.* (2010) Polypharmacy and potentially inappropriate medication use among community-dwelling elders with dementia. *Alzheimer Disease and Associated Disorders*, **24**, 56–63.
32. De Wet, C., Reed, L., Glasper, A. *et al.* (2004) Benzodiazepine co-dependence exacerbates the opiate withdrawal syndrome. *Drug and Alcohol Dependence*, **76**, 31–35.
33. SAMHSA (2012) National Survey of Substance Abuse Treatment Services (N-SSATS): 2011. Data on Substance Abuse Treatment Facilities. BHSIS Series S-64, HHS Publication No. (SMA) 12-4730, Center for Behavioral Health Statistics and Quality. Substance Abuse and Mental Health Services Administration (SAMHSA), Rockville, MD.
34. Lynskey, M.T., Day, C. and Hall, W. (2003) Alcohol and other drug use disorders among older-aged people. *Drug and Alcohol Review*, **22**, 125–133. Peterson, M. and Zimberg, S. (1996) Treating alcoholism: an age-specific intervention that works for older patients, *Geriatrics*, **51**, 45–49. Blow, F.C., Walton, M.A., Chermack, S.T. *et al.* (2000) Older adult treatment outcome following elder-specific inpatient alcoholism treatment. *Journal of Substance Abuse Treatment*, **19**, 67–75.SAMHSA (1998) *Substance Abuse Among Older Adults*. Treatment Improvement Protocol (TIP) Series, No. 26, Center for Substance Abuse Treatment, Substance Abuse and Mental Health Services Administration (SAMHSA), Rockville, MD. http://www.ncbi.nlm.nih.gov/books/NBK64411/ (last accessed 3 April 2014).

LONGITUDINAL STUDIES OF AGEING AND SUBSTANCE ABUSE

Chapter 10
AGEING AND THE DEVELOPMENT OF ALCOHOL USE AND MISUSE

Marja Aartsen

Faculty of Social Sciences, VU University Amsterdam, The Netherlands

Background

Substance use and misuse is typically associated with younger age groups. The increasing number of older people needing treatment for substance use problems, however, requires a readjustment of that image. The prevalence rates of alcohol problems in older adults, aged 65 and over, in Europe is expected to more than double between 2001 and 2020 [1], and for the United States an increase from 1.7 million people in 2000 to 4.4 million in 2020 who are in need of treatment for addiction is anticipated [2]. However, knowledge about substance use and misuse in older adults is still fairly limited compared to younger age groups. Existing evidence mainly stems from cross-sectional studies in western societies, which limits generalizability and conclusions about developments in substance use with ageing [3]. As far as studies have been conducted, they mainly focus on alcohol use and misuse, as alcohol is the principal substance of abuse in older adults [4]. Very few studies have been done on other substances such as cannabis, heroin and cocaine. The European Monitoring Centre for Drugs and Drug Addiction characterized substance use among older adults as a 'neglected problem' [1]. This chapter summarizes current knowledge about the natural course of substance use and misuse in noninstitutionalized older adults aged 55 and over. In addressing the aim of this chapter, two databases (PubMed and PsychINFO) and Google Scholar have been used to search for longitudinal studies on developments in substance use and misuse in older adults.

Before turning to the literature, some comments on limitations of review studies on substance use are warranted. The first is that social norms and customs about substance use may differ across countries which may cause differences in definitions of misuse. For example, any alcoholic consumption in Islamic countries is seen as misuse whereas drinking wine at dinner even for younger people is common practice in France. The use of cannabis is tolerated in The Netherlands, whereas other countries often consider it a violation of the

Substance Use and Older People, First Edition.
Edited by Ilana B. Crome, Li-Tzy Wu, Rahul (Tony) Rao and Peter Crome.
© 2015 John Wiley & Sons, Ltd. Published 2015 by John Wiley & Sons, Ltd.

law. Social classification schemes such as heavy and risk-full use or misuse may, therefore, not be very helpful to distinguish hazardous use from use that is not harmful. In addition, people generally underreport alcohol consumption [5]; alcohol problems often remain undetected by general practitioners or other healthcare professionals [6, 7]. Screening instruments to assess harmful/ heavy alcohol use and alcohol use disorders may lack sufficient sensitiveness for older adults, since they are often developed for use with younger people. Older people differ from younger people in various ways, such as the symptoms, which are less specific in older adults, lower levels of use at which intoxication may occur and the concomitant use of medicines that do not tolerate alcohol [8, 9]. Finally, research results and community programmes may lead to enhanced awareness among healthcare professionals of substance use problems in older adults, which probably leads to higher detection rates. Prevalence rates of alcohol use and misuse, therefore, should be viewed with caution, since the actual levels of alcohol use and the number of older people with an alcohol use disorder in the general population may differ from observed levels, but is likely to be much higher.

Results

Based on existing studies, epidemiological and demographic aspects of changes in alcohol use and misuse with ageing can be examined. According to the World Health Organization, the prevalence of lifetime abstention is the lowest in the European Region (13% men, 25% women) and the Americas – including the United States, Canada, Central and South America – (15% men, 27% women) and highest in South East Asia Region (68% men and 93% women) [10]. Among drinkers, the highest prevalence of heavy episodic drinking, defined as drinking at least 60 grammes or more of pure alcohol on at least one occasion in the past seven days, is found in the African and Eastern Mediterranean regions (Table 10.1). Heavy episodic drinking is harmful as it leads to serious health problems and is particularly associated with injury [10].

A U-shaped relation between alcohol use and various health outcomes is consistently found [11]. In general, moderate alcohol users are healthier than high-risk users and abstainers [12–15], although in women the mortality from breast cancer was 30% higher among women reporting at least one drink daily than among nondrinkers [16]. The better health in moderate users not necessarily implies that moderate drinking is beneficial for health. That abstainers are worse than moderate users is possibly explained on the basis of the great heterogeneity in the nonusing group. Not drinking may be associated with certain medications, which indicates the presence of diseases, a previous alcohol dependence and also a healthy lifestyle [3]. Higher education is associated with more but also risk-full alcohol use [17–21]. Alcohol users smoke more than nonusers [22, 23], and alcoholics often live alone [24, 25].

Table 10.1 Drinking patterns by sex and World Health Organization region (all ages)

	Men (%)	Women (%)
Lifetime abstainers		
African Region	49.1	65.2
Region of the Americas	15.2	27.4
Eastern Mediterranean Region	82.4	93.4
European Region	12.6	24.6
South-East Asian Region	68.4	92.8
Western Pacific Region	14.3	44.5
Heavy episodic drinkers among drinkers		
African Region	30.5	16.2
Region of the Americas	17.9	4.5
Eastern Mediterranean Region	24.9	17.9
European Region	16.8	4.6
South-East Asian Region	23.0	12.9
Western Pacific Region	11.6	1.3

Source: WHO 2011 [10]

Differences in alcohol use across cohorts

A general picture that emerges from the literature is that the level of substance use in current older people differs from that of earlier born cohorts of the same age. In a Finnish study based on 5870 men and 5883 women aged between 65 and 79, it was found that younger birth cohorts have higher levels of alcohol use than earlier born cohorts of the same age. This was found in both men and women [26]. In The Netherlands, the proportion of heavy drinkers (i.e. >3 glasses/day for men and >2 glasses /day for women) aged between 55 and 65 years in 1992 increased from 12 to 20% in 2002 [27]. Research in the United States among 600 people, with according to DSM-IV criteria for a lifetime alcohol dependence [28], shows that in the cohort born between 1940 and 1951, 33% of the men and 6% of the women met a lifetime diagnosis of alcohol dependence. In the later-born cohort (born between 1952 and 1960) this prevalence rose to 40% for men and 13% for women. The recent increase in the number of older adults who need treatment for alcohol problems is mainly caused by the baby boom generation (defined as people born between 1946 and 1964) who have less healthy life styles and higher levels of alcohol use than older generations, of which the first now reach the age of 65 [30, 31].

Developments in alcohol use within people

To describe developments of alcohol use with ageing, longitudinal studies are needed since cross-sectional studies do not differentiate between age and cohort effects. However, longitudinal studies on alcohol use in older adults in the general population are fairly limited. Most studies found that people generally reduce the number of drinks consumed as they age [26, 32–37]. In a study in the United States, a mean decline from 0.60 glasses on average per day at baseline to 0.36 glasses per day 15 years later was found [33]. In a Dutch study, a mean decline of 1.23 glasses per day for men to 1.13 ten years later was found, but not for women who on average drank 0.5 glasses per day [38].

Gender differences

Several studies indicate a gender effect, although findings are inconclusive. Brennan and colleagues [37] found that on average alcohol consumption declined in older men (aged between 55 and 65 at baseline) somewhat later than it did in older women. However, the reversed gender difference is seen among heavily drinking older people. Men who drink heavily reduce drinking over time while women who drink heavily remained stable in alcohol consumption [17]. In line with this is a study by Aartsen and Comijs [38], who found that heavily drinking older men (aged 65–85 at baseline) that reported having health problems at baseline significantly reduced the number of glasses consumed per week from 26 to 14 in the ten years of follow-up. Heavily drinking women (aged 65–85 at baseline) and healthy men do not reduce the level of alcohol intake during follow-up. In Finland, men born in 1926–1946 do not seem to decrease drinking while ageing either [39].

Different trajectories

A relatively new development in addiction research is the focus on homogenous subgroups of people with similar trajectories of substance use to better understand how addiction behaviour develops over time and how factors affect the shape of the trajectory. Latent class growth models [40] enabled researchers to identify heterogeneity in developments or trajectories in alcohol use over time, and to identify factors that enhances the likelihood for certain trajectories. In a sample of 6787 American people, aged between 51 and 61 years, Platt and colleagues [33] distinguished sporadic drinkers (30.0%), steady drinkers (20.7%), decreasing drinkers (18.4%) and increasing drinkers (2.2%) from abstinent people (28.8%). People who had a history of problem drinking before baseline were more likely to increase drinking at follow-up. Increasing drinkers were also more often highly educated and likely to be male, white, unmarried and less religious, and in excellent to good health [33]. In a Japanese study among 2566 adults aged 60 to 96 and followed from 1987 to 1999 three drinking trajectories were found: stable trajectory (37.8%), curvilinear trajectory (13.7%) and decline (10.6%). Thirty-eight percent of the Japanese older people were abstinent. Compared to abstainers, people with a decline trajectory in drinking were more often men, and more likely to be employed and healthy at baseline. It was suggested that the decline in drinking may be caused by leaving the workforce. Drinking at work is often stimulated in Japan. Compared to abstainers, the stable group was less likely to have functional limitations while the group with a curvilinear trajectory more often encountered the death of a loved one [35].

Age and onset of problem drinking

The categorization in age of onset of alcohol-related problems is gaining prominence among clinicians [41]. Older adults with drinking problems constitute a heterogeneous group with people who have the first alcoholic episode before the age of 25 (early onset), and those with the first episode after the age of 25 (late onset). Almost one-third of the older alcoholics have a late onset of problem drinking [42]. These groups are likely to represent different disorders with respect to aetiology, course, prevention strategies and treatment needs. Factors associated with the early age of onset are antisocial personality disorder, being homeless, a family history of alcohol problems and low socioeconomic status [43]. Late onset is associated with female gender, higher socioeconomic status [44] and stressful life events [45].

Discussion

Explanations for age differences in alcohol use

Different explanations for the lower drinking levels in older than in younger people have been put forward [46]. The first is the cohort hypothesis, suggesting that exposures to factors influencing the level of substance use differ across birth cohorts or other subgroups of people. As discussed in the previous paragraphs, cohort effects have been observed and studies that distinguish cohort from age effects indicate that current older adults are heavier consumers of alcohol than older cohorts of older people. According to Neve and colleagues, cohort differences may be caused by 'endogenous' and 'exogenous' mechanisms [47]. Endogenous mechanisms are, for example, social norms and values, such as the belief of baby boomers that alcohol intake improves health [30]. Exogenous mechanisms are, for example, policies about the age at which buying alcohol is allowed, penalties for driving after drinking and openings hours of stores for alcohol. A study among 30 countries in Europe, Asia, North America and Australia revealed a clear inverse relationship between policy strength and alcohol consumption [48]. Since effects of alcohol policy on levels of consumption are found to differ across age groups [49–51], age differences in alcohol use are likely. The stabilization of heavy drinking in women [17, 38] may be partly explained by the increased exposure to risk factors such as losing a partner and living alone.

The mortality hypothesis states that the prevalence of heavy drinking and alcoholism appears to be lower among older age strata, since older people who have been drinking excessive levels of alcohol during their life die at an earlier age. Much evidence is available for a relationship between lowered mortality in moderately drinking men and women and increased mortality in men and women at six or more drinks per day [52, 53], suggesting that reported age differences in average drinking levels in cross-sectional studies indeed reflect mortality differences rather than decreasing drinking levels with age.

The morbidity hypothesis assumes that due to the increased prevalence of chronic diseases older adults increasingly reduce alcohol consumption due to adverse interactions between medication and alcohol, which may aggravate their medical conditions. Evidence for this hypothesis is found in the study by Aartsen and Comijs [38], who found that only older men who are excessive users and who had other health problems, such as more depressive symptoms, higher levels of anxiety and more chronic diseases at baseline, significantly reduced the number of glasses consumed per week. However, in the health and retirement study among 11 191 US residents aged 50 years and over, no relation with psychiatric co-morbidity was found. Only people who drank excessively while having diabetes or lung disease significantly reduced drinking over time [54].

The biological hypothesis proposes that due to less efficient liver metabolism and decreases in lean body mass and total body water with ageing smaller amounts of substance use may lead to intoxication and organ damage [42]. Therefore, older adults are likely to reduce the amount of alcohol that they can comfortably consume. Women are more susceptible to the negative effects of increased alcohol consumption than men due to the less lean muscle mass [55, 56], which may lead to gender differences in rates of decline of substance use with age. Evidence for the biological hypothesis is mixed, however, especially when it comes to problem drinkers. Men with health problems who drink heavily on average limit drinking, whereas women who drink heavily do not reduce the level of alcohol intake with ageing [38]. Moderate drinkers, that is less than three glasses per day for men and less than one glass per day for women, reduce the number of drinks when they age; women do so sooner in life than men.

Conclusions

Older men and women who drink moderate amounts of alcohol generally reduce alcohol use when they become older to adjust for the bodily changes that limit the ability to metabolize alcohol. However, as ageing is almost by definition a heterogeneous process causing increasing differences between older people, so are changes in alcohol use with ageing. Various explanations have been put forward and all partly contribute to the understanding of age-related changes in alcohol consumption. Physical changes in ability to metabolize alcohol, changing policies toward alcohol use, the higher exposure to risk factors that may induce problem drinking and increased morbidity all may contribute to the heterogeneity of trajectories in alcohol use among older adults.

A worrisome development is the evident increase in alcohol use in younger generations of older adults, specifically the baby boomers. They consume more alcohol and encounter more alcohol-related problems than previous generations of older adults, which warrant increased attention for older problem drinkers. However, due to the scarcity of longitudinal studies in the general population, still many questions are unanswered, such as 'How can we prevent older people becoming heavy or dependent users?'. Other issues yet to be solved are: the gender difference in speed at which alcohol use declines with age; why older men who suffer from health limitations are more inclined to lower drinking levels than healthy but heavy drinking men; whether drinking moderate amounts of alcohol indeed leads to better health outcomes or whether it is only a spurious association; whether the aetiology for alcohol dependence is the same as for heavy or risky use. Finally, more insight is needed in the effect of strict policies on alcohol use to reduce risk-full drinking in older. To solve these issues, additional in-depth research is needed in the general population, as well as in patient populations. It is up to policy makers, healthcare professionals and researchers to stimulate research and further develop screening instruments and prevention programmes that are tuned to the specific situation of older adults.

References

1. Gossop, M. (2008) *Substance Use among Older Adults: A Neglected Problem*. European Monitoring Centre for Drugs and Drug Addiction, Lisbon. http://www.emcdda.europa. eu/attachements.cfm/att_50566_EN_TDAD08001ENC_web.pdf (last accessed 4 April 2014).
2. Gfroerer, J., Penne, M., Pemberton, M. *et al.* (2003) Substance abuse treatment need among older adults in 2020. The impact of the aging baby-boom cohort. *Drug and Alcohol Dependence*, **69**, 127–135.
3. Aartsen, M.J. (2011) Substance use and abuse among older adults: a state of the art. In: *Psychiatric Disorders: Trends and Developments* (ed. T. Uehara). InTech, Rijeka, Croatia, pp. 389–403.
4. Blazer, D.G. and Wu, L.-T. (2009) The epidemiology of substance use and disorders among middle aged and elderly community adults: national survey on drug use and health. *American Journal of Geriatric Psychiatry*, **17**, 237–245.
5. Boniface, S. and Shelton, N. (2013) How is alcohol consumption affected if we account for under-reporting? A hypothetical scenario. *European Journal of Public Health*. First published online: 26 February 2013. doi:10.1093/eurpub/ckt016.
6. Brower, K.J., Mudd, S., Blow, F.C. *et al.* (1994) Severity and treatment of alcohol withdrawal in elderly versus younger patients. *Alcoholism: Clinical and Experimental Research*, **18**, 196–201.
7. Stewart, D. and Oslin, D.W. (2001) Recognition and treatment of late-life addictions in medical settings. *Journal of Clinical Geropsychology*, **7**, 145–158.
8. Beullens, J. and Aertgeerts, B. (2004) Screening for alcohol abuse and dependence in older people using DSM criteria: a review. *Aging & Mental Health*, **8**, 76–82.
9. Dehart, S.S. and Hoffmann, N.G. (1995) Screening and diagnosis of "alcohol abuse and dependence" in older adults. *Substance Use & Misuse*, **30**, 1717–1747.
10. WHO (World Health Organization) (2011) *Global Status Report on Alcohol and Health*. World Health Organization, Geneva, Switzerland.
11. Chen, L.Y. and Hardy, C.L. (2009) Alcohol consumption and health status in older adults a longitudinal analysis. *Journal of Aging and Health*, **21**, 824–847.

12. Rodgers, B., Windsor, T.D., Anstey, K.J. *et al.* (2005) Non-linear relationships between cognitive function and alcohol consumption in young, middle-aged and older adults: the PATH Through Life Project. *Addiction*, **100**, 1280–1290.

13. Blow, F.C., Walton, M.A., Barry, K.L. *et al.* (2000) The relationship between alcohol problems and health functioning of older adults in primary care settings. *Journal of the American Geriatric Society*, **48**, 769–774.

14. Bridevaux, I.P., Bradley, K.A., Bryson, C.L. *et al.* (2004) Alcohol screening results in elderly male veterans: association with health status and mortality. *Journal of the American Geriatric Society*, **52**, 1510–1517.

15. Mukamal, K.J., Longstreth, W.T., Mittleman, M.A. *et al.* (2001) Alcohol consumption and subclinical findings on magnetic resonance imaging of the brain in older adults: the cardiovascular health study. *Stroke*, **32**, 1939–1946.

16. Thun, M.J., Peto, R., Lopez, A.D. *et al.* (1997) Alcohol consumption and mortality among middle-aged and elderly US adults. *New England Journal of Medicine*, **337**, 1705–1714.

17. Breslow, R.A., Faden, V.B. and Smothers, B. (2003) Alcohol consumption by elderly Americans. *Journal of Studies on Alcohol*, **64**, 884–892.

18. Merrick, E., Horgan, C.M., Hodgkin, D. *et al.* (2008) Unhealthy drinking patterns in older adults: prevalence and associated characteristics. *Journal of American Geriatrics Society*, **56**, 214–223.

19. Forster, L.E., Pollow, R. and Stoller, E.P. (1993) Alcohol use and potential risk for alcohol related adverse drug reactions among community-based elderly. *Journal of Community Health*, **18**, 225–239.

20. Goodwin, J.S., Sanchez, C.J., Thomas, P. *et al.* (1987) Alcohol intake in a healthy elderly population. *American Journal of Public Health*, **77**, 173–177.

21. Ruchlin, H.S. (1997) Prevalence and correlates of alcohol use among older adults. *Preventive Medicine*, **26**, 651–657.

22. Ganry, O., Baudoin, C., Fardellone, P. *et al.* (2001) Alcohol consumption by non-institutionalized elderly women: the EPIDOS Study. *Public Health*, **115**, 186–191.

23. Mirand, A.L. and Welte, J.W. (1996) Alcohol consumption among the elderly in a general population, Erie County, New York. *American Journal of Public Health*, **86**, 978–984.

24. Brennan, P.L. (2005) Functioning and health service use among elderly nursing home residents with alcohol use disorders: findings from the National Nursing Home Survey. *American Journal of Geriatric Psychiatry*, **13**, 475–483.

25. Onen, S.H., Onen, F., Mangeon, J.P. *et al.* (2005) Alcohol abuse and dependence in elderly emergency department patients. *Archives of Gerontology and Geriatrics*, **41**, 191–200.

26. Sulander, T., Helakorpi, S., Rahkonen, O. *et al.* (2004) Smoking and alcohol consumption among the elderly: trends and associations, 1985–2001. *Preventive Medicine*, **39**, 413–418.

27. Comijs, H.C., Aartsen, M.J., Visser, M. *et al.* (2012) Alcoholgebruik onder 55-plussers in Nederland [Alcohol use among 55-plus in The Netherlands]. *Tijdschrift voor Gerontologie en Geriatrie*, **43**, 115–126.

28. Holdcraft, L.C. and Iacono, W.G. (2002) Cohort effects on gender differences in alcohol dependence. *Addiction*, **97**, 1025–1036.

29. Grant, B.F. (1996) Prevalence and correlates of drug use and DSM-IV drug dependence in the United States: results of the National Longitudinal Alcohol Epidemiologic Survey. *Journal of Substance Abuse*, **8**, 195–210.

30. Heuberger, R.A. (2009) Alcohol and the older adult: A comprehensive review. *Journal of Nutrition for the Elderly*, **28**, 203–235.

31. Volfson, E. and Oslin, D.W. (2011) Addiction. In: *Textbook of Geriatric Neuropsychiatry* (eds C.E. Coffey and J.L. Cummings), 3rd edn. American Psychiatric Publishing, Arlington, VA, pp. 427–441.

32. Moos, R.H., Schutte, K.K., Brennan, P.L. *et al.* (2009) Older adults' alcohol consumption and late-life drinking problems: a 20-year perspective. *Addiction,* 104, 1293–1302.

33. Platt, A., Sloan, F.A., Costanzo, P. (2010) Alcohol-consumption trajectories and associated characteristics among adults older than age 50. *Journal of Studies on Alcohol and Drugs,* 71, 169–79.

34. Adams, W.L., Garry, P.J., Rhyne, R. *et al.* (1990) Alcohol intake in the healthy elderly. Changes with age in a cross-sectional and longitudinal study. *Journal of American Geriatric Society,* 38, 211–116.

35. Gee, G.C., Liang, J., Bennett, J. *et al.* (2007) Trajectories of alcohol consumption among older Japanese followed from 1987–1999. *Research on Aging,* 29, 323–347.

36. Bobo, J.K. and Greek, A.A. (2011) Increasing and decreasing alcohol use trajectories among older women in the US across a 10-year interval. *International Journal of Environmental Research and Public Health,* 8, 3263–3276.

37. Brennan, P.L., Schutte, K.K., Moos, B.S. *et al.* (2011) Twenty-year alcohol-consumption and drinking-problem trajectories of older men and women. *Journal of Studies on Alcohol and Drugs,* 72, 308–321.

38. Aartsen, M.J. and Comijs, H.C. (2012) Alcoholgebruik en depressieve symptomen bij ouderen: Resultaten van de Longitudinal Aging Study Amsterdam [Alcohol use and depressive symptoms in older adults: Results of the Longitudinal Aging Study Amsterdam]. *Tijdschrift voor Gerontologie en Geriatrie,* 43, 127–137.

39. Ilomäki, J., Korhonen, M.J., Lavikainen, P. *et al.* (2010) Changes in alcohol consumption and drinking patterns during 11 years of follow-up among ageing men: the FinDrink study. *The European Journal of Public Health,* 20, 133–138.

40. Jung, T. and Wickrama, K.A.S. (2008) An introduction to latent class growth analysis and growth mixture modeling. *Social and Personality Psychology Compass,* 2, 302–317.

41. Liberto, J.G. and Oslin, D.W. (1995) Early versus late onset alcohol disorder in the elderly. *International Journal of Addiction,* 130, 1799–1818.

42. Dufour, M. and Fuller, R.K. (1995) Alcohol in the elderly. *Annual Review of Medicine,* 46, 123–132.

43. Watson, C.G., Hancock, M.B.A., Gearhart, L.P.M. *et al.* (1997) A comparison of the symptoms associated with early and late onset alcohol dependence. *Journal of Nervous and Mental Disease,* 185, 507–509.

44. Atkinson, R.M., Tolson, R. and Turner, J.A. (1990) Late versus early onset problem drinking in older men. *Alcoholism: Clinical and Experimental Research,* 14, 574–579.

45. Hurt, R.D., Finlayson, R.E., Morse, R.M. *et al.* (1988) Alcoholism in elderly persons: Medical aspects and prognosis of 216 inpatients. *Mayo Clinic Procedures,* 63, 753–760.

46. Stall, R. (1987) Research issues concerning alcohol consumption among aging populations. *Drug and Alcohol Dependence,* 19, 195–213.

47. Neve, R.J., Diederiks, J.P., Knibbe, R.A. *et al.* (1993) Developments in drinking behavior in The Netherlands from 1958 to 1989, a cohort analysis. *Addiction,* 88, 611–621.

48. Brand, D.A., Saisana, M., Rynn, L.A. *et al.* (2007) Comparative analysis of alcohol control policies in 30 countries. *PLoS Medicine,* 4, e151. doi:10.1371/journal.pmed.0040151.

49. Bloomfield, K., Wicki, M., Gustafsson, N.K. *et al.* (2010) Changes in alcohol-related problems after alcohol policy changes in Denmark, Finland, and Sweden. *Journal of Studies on Alcohol and Drugs,* 71, 32–40.

50. Chaloupka, F.J., Grossman, M. and Saffer, H. (2002) Effects of price on alcohol consumption and alcohol-related problems. *Alcohol Research & Health,* 26, 22–34.

51. Kuo, M., Heeb, J.L., Gmel, G. *et al.* (2003) Does price matter? The effect of decreased price on spirits consumption in Switzerland. *Alcoholism: Clinical and Experimental Research*, **27**, 720–725.
52. Vogel, R.A. (2002) Alcohol, heart disease, and mortality: a review. *Reviews in Cardiovascular Medicine*, **3**, 7–13.
53. Holman, C.D., English, D.R., Milne, E. et al. (1996) Meta-analysis of alcohol and all-cause mortality: a validation of NHMRC recommendations. *The Medical Journal of Australia*, **164**, 141–145.
54. Newsom, J.T., Huguet, N., McCarthy, M.J. *et al.* (2012) Health behavior change following chronic illness in middle and later life. *The Journals of Gerontology Series B: Psychological Sciences and Social Sciences*, **67**, 279–288.
55. Morgan, M.Y. and Sherlock, S. (1997) Sex-related differences among 100 patients with alcoholic liver disease. *British Medical Journal*, **1**, 939–941.
56. Mann, K., Batra, A., Günthner, A. *et al.* (1992) Do women develop alcoholic brain damage more readily than men? *Alcoholism: Clinical and Experimental Research*, **16**, 1052–1056.

Chapter 11

PROGRESSION FROM SUBSTANCE USE TO THE DEVELOPMENT OF SUBSTANCE USE DISORDERS

Carla L. Storr[1] and Kerry M. Green[2]

[1] Department of Family & Community Health, University of Maryland School of Nursing, USA
[2] Department of Behavioral and Community Health, University of Maryland School of Public Health, USA

Introduction

Substance use is common among older adults [1–3] and yet little is known about what constitutes risky substance use behaviours in older adults or even the trajectory of substance use disorders (SUD) in this population. Changes in substance using behaviours, as reflected in Figure 11.1, denote the substance use progression process – specifically, how substance use can progress from beneficial use, such as the taking of prescribed medication or moderate drinking of alcohol in social situations, to misuse. Substance misuse can progress to undesirable physical, social and psychological consequences. Healthcare providers look for emerging problematic signs and symptoms in making a determination that an individual has developed a SUD and is in need of treatment.

Substances most commonly misused by older individuals that increase their risk of developing a SUD include alcohol, tobacco products and various classes of prescription drugs (e.g. opioids, stimulants and benzodiazepines) [4–7]. This misuse of substances may be continued from earlier life stages or even be initiated among individuals advancing into their later years. Alcohol use can be especially problematic for elderly persons. Alcohol, medical problems and prescription medications are likely to come together in the elderly, putting seniors at risk of problems resulting from combined effects. As is addressed later in this chapter, the specific substance and an individual's personal history are some of the many factors that influence substance use progression.

Understanding the substance use progression process among older adults is critical, as forecasts project increased service needs for substance use problems among the elderly in many countries around the globe. It has been estimated that between 2000 and 2020, the number of older adults aged 50 years or older in the United States and aged 65 and older in Europe with substance use problems or in need of treatment for

Substance Use and Older People, First Edition.
Edited by Ilana B. Crome, Li-Tzy Wu, Rahul (Tony) Rao and Peter Crome.
© 2015 John Wiley & Sons, Ltd. Published 2015 by John Wiley & Sons, Ltd.

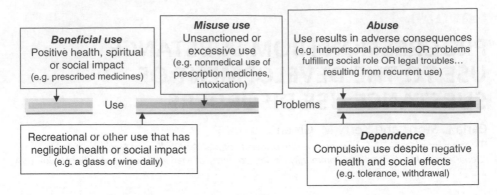

Figure 11.1   Psychoactive substance use spectrum.

a SUD is expected to more than double [8–10]. The increase is no doubt attributed in part to the increase in the sheer numbers of older adults in the population, as well as the conditions that come with ageing (e.g. emotional, social and medical problems) that can increase the risk for substance misuse. However, social and environmental changes over time may have also intensified the situation of increasing need. Previous substance use experiences and current attitudes among current ageing adults differ from previous generations of ageing adults and affect the substance use progression process. Further, major advances in medicine have included more reliance on pharmacological agents, including increased use of multiple psychotropic medications [11–13], increasing the availability to use for nonmedical purposes [14].

This chapter begins by introducing a framework for understanding the progression from substance use to SUDs. After briefly characterizing various stages of substance use involvement, several factors that may increase the risk of progression to SUDs are reviewed and potential adverse effects of substance misuse or signs of substance use problems are summarized. Furthermore, the challenges to studying substance use progression among older populations and the approaches several recent studies have taken are discussed. Given the likely impact of substance use problems in older people on social and healthcare services, as well as on their own quality of life, there is a need for a better understanding of the substance use progression process in older adults. Thus, the chapter concludes with recommendations for future research.

Substance use progression process

Substance use at any age can lead to serious problems and/or addiction. The pathway towards a SUD involves changes in substance use behaviours and factors that influence the progression into further involvement with alcohol and drugs [15, 16]. A model depicting a framework of the development of addiction via four stereotypic stages of substance use and how progression may be affected by the typical public health host–agent–environment triad – labeled as individual-level

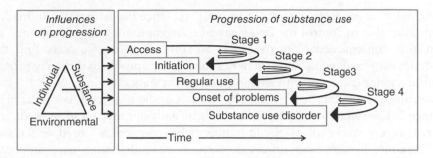

Figure 11.2 Framework of progression from substance use to substance use disorders.

susceptibility (e.g. genetic vulnerability), substance properties (e.g. biologically and pharmacologically reinforcing properties) and environmental factors (e.g. prescribing practices) – is illustrated in Figure 11.2. This is a general framework that can apply to the study of substance abuse among individuals at any age and is used here to guide the materials presented in this chapter to better understand substance use progression among older people. Advanced age itself is an individual factor that interacts with environmental and substance properties to influence progression. Time and duration of use, two factors that are highly correlated with age, are relevant for the stages portion of the framework.

As shown in Figure 11.2, the development of drug and alcohol use addiction is conceptualized as a series of advancement through several stages. Each stage is an integral part of a complex continuous progression of further drug involvement and behaviour change but can also be a discrete endpoint in and of itself, as not everyone progresses to problematic stages. In general, transitions to the next phases (e.g. from regular use to onset of problems) are for the most part conditional upon the previous stage(s). Thus, initiation should be considered as a risk factor for further use and continued use as a risk factor for developing problems. Reciprocal relationships or feedback loops with earlier stages also occur. For example, users may seek out new avenues of access and features of SUD, such as tolerance and dependence, promote further use. Most individuals who initiate substance use do not progress to developing a SUD [17, 18]; however, individuals do not need to use large quantities or be heavy users to develop problems related to substance use. The criteria for SUDs have more to do with the adverse consequences of the use rather than the amount of substance consumed or even the frequency of use.

While the patterns of progression from use to addiction are not always consistent or predictable, most often the pattern involves the continuum of use shown in Figure 11.2 involving one type of substance. It starts with an occasion or opportunity to use. While cost and expectations can influence subjective and social availability that engages initiation, in order to use a substance an individual requires physical accessibility [19]. Access to prescription drugs with abuse and dependency potential is not rare among older adults, as approximately a quarter of older adults are prescribed them; for others access can occur via sharing among their social network [3, 20]. Thus, in the first stage of progression, access is a condition for an individual to move from abstinence to use [21]. Once use is initiated individuals are usually able to control the frequency of consumption or can discontinue use. Damaging consequences (e.g. overdose) are rare. However, if users find their substance use is making them feel better or solving their problems they may progress to more regular use, thereby moving on to the next stage.

Continued use, often on a regular basis, or episodic heavy use is characteristic of Stage 2. Consumption may not necessarily be daily but may occur in predictable patterns (every weekend) or circumstances (whenever lonely, bored or stressed). For example, psychoactive drug use, such as benzodiazepine use, supposedly recommended for a limited time period may turn into persistent use over extended time among elderly individuals [22]. Frequent or chronic long-term use often leads to tolerance (e.g. quantity or dose increases). Stage 3 is where misuse of prescription drugs may occur as individuals start using more often or in quantities not prescribed. Users may not realize their consumption has escalated, or they may even try to hide their substance use at this point, but others in their social network may suspect problems through mood and behaviour changes of the user. In Stage 3, legal, emotional, physical or social problems resulting from regular use (often daily and heavy use) appear. Effects are unpredictable, but sometimes severe, and the individual often no longer can hide problems. In Stage 4, severe consequences are very likely because substance use becomes compulsive and out of control. Multiple problems occur at the same time reflecting progression and development of a SUD. Someone who has a SUD will continue regular use despite the harm. Progression to this stage makes the cycle of use even more difficult to interrupt, and treatment/medical intervention is warranted so that recovery can occur.

Another type of progression worth noting involves the use of multiple substances and whether an individual starts with one and substitutes or moves on to another type. A consistent sequence of which substances are used, beginning with tobacco and alcohol, progressing to cannabis and then other illicit drugs is common among adolescents and young adults [23, 24]. Studies among adults find the ordering is not always consistent and drug availability and social environmental factors may influence the patterns of drug use [25, 26]. Unusual sequencing has not been found to increase the risk of developing dependence [27, 28]. However, regular use of one substance may make it easier to use another substance as the abstinence barrier has already been crossed. For example, nonmedical use of psychoactive drugs has been found to be associated with current alcohol, tobacco and cannabis use [2], and tobacco use is strongly associated with binge drinking and illicit or nonmedical drug use in older American adults residing in the community [29]. Multiple substances can be used complementarily or the drug of choice may change over time [30]. Often, individuals may mix or move to other substances that have similar pharmacological effects (e.g. using benzodiazepines to avoid alcohol withdrawal or Oxycontin users turning to heroin). Sometimes the substitution of another substance yields less adverse effects and withdrawal [31].

There is a possibility that the use of multiple substances will influence consumption patterns and the development of dependence. For example, elderly individuals (≥75 years) with a regular pattern of use of multiple drugs (e.g. antidepressants, antipsychotics, benzodiazepines) have been found to be more susceptible to persistent chronic drug use compared to those using only one drug as needed [22]. Studies have also shown a highly co-morbid relationship between alcohol use and drug use disorders though, to date, this overlap has been found to be more common among younger age groups yet still significant in older populations [32, 33]. Therefore, in considering progression to a substance use disorder, it is important to take into consideration an individual's substance use history, past and present, and any combination of substances.

Risk factors influencing substance use progression

The second part of the framework focuses on influences (or risk factors) for progression that may arise from properties of the substance, environment and individual susceptibility (the left portion of Figure 11.1), which interact with one another to affect risk of progression. Little research has focused on identifying risk factors or situations that may be unique for older individuals. This section highlights some of the most relevant factors.

Individual factors

It is important to note that not all individuals are equally vulnerable to the development of substance use disorders. Many of the potential personal risk factors for substance use and progression to SUDs among older adults include influences often found among the general population, as well as factors unique to older populations. A list of common risk factors is provided in Table 11.1. For example, there is substantial evidence that family history and genetics are important in the development of SUDs throughout the lifespan [34, 35]. Genes involved in vulnerability to SUDs include those that alter drug metabolism or the function of a drug receptor

Table 11.1 Influences on substance use and the progression of substance use to disorders

- Cognitive impairment and change
- Poor health (chronic pain, disabilities, sensory deficits)
- Insomnia
- Previous and/or concurrent psychiatric co-morbidities (i.e. depression)
- Change in social status/activity (retirement, reduced mobility/ability to function, boredom)
- Bereavement
- Stress and/or reduced coping skills (family conflict, financial resources)
- Previous substance use disorder and/or concurrent substance use
- Family history of substance use disorders
- Properties of the substance (use of multiple substances)
- Social isolation (living alone, loss of family and friends, living in a rural area)
- Nonmedical use and dangerous prescribing practices

as well as those involved in general mechanisms of modulating stress response, emotion and behavioural control [36]. Twin studies indicate that there is both a substantial heritability of substance-specific addictions (highest for opiates and cocaine) and a genetic overlap across addiction to different substances [37]. Furthermore, findings suggest heritability can vary over the lifespan and that there is a genetic basis to each stage of substance involvement [37–39]. Heritable factors appear to be more important among adults than among youth, possibly because of an accumulation of genetic influences overtime, as well greater flexibility as one ages to create and choose environments that may interact with or promote one's genetic predisposition [35]. Early stages of progression seem to be influenced more by family environmental factors and to be less heritable, whereas heritable factors seem to strongly influence progression to later stages, such as problem use and dependence with evidence for the heritability of nicotine dependence, alcohol disorders and drug disorders, as well as other substances [37, 40, 41].

Differences are also seen depending on the personal history of involvement with substances. Studies suggest that those who begin substance use in early adolescence (often termed early onset users) may be most vulnerable to negative consequences throughout the course of their life [42, 43]. In terms of alcohol problems, studies have identified two types of problem users – long-term abusers with early onset abuse and late-onset abusers (onset after age 50) [44, 45]. Early-onset abusers tend to have a greater family history of alcoholism [46, 47], while late-onset abusers are suspected of developing drinking problems as a reaction to the life changes as a result of ageing, such as the loss of social support [48, 49]. While early-onset abusers are the more common pattern of alcohol abuse among the elderly, studies have found that approximately one-third or more of the elderly with drinking problems developed these problems in old age or have a recurrence of problems after a lengthy interval of remission [50, 51]. Thus, personal history with substance use is an important individual factor that drives substance use progression in the elderly.

Implications of brain changes and age-related pharmacokinetic/dynamic changes among older adults may impact the course of substance use problems. The ageing process, in particular, affects neurotransmitter systems (predominantly dopaminergic, serotonergic and glutamatergic systems) and neural circuits involved in both the reward and pain processing systems [52]. Ageing affects the process by which the substance is absorbed, distributed, metabolized and eliminated by the body. The same amount of alcohol that previously had little effect can now cause intoxication and intensify problems associated with insomnia, incontinence and gastrointestinal problems among older adults.

As health problems and disabilities increase with age, chronic illnesses can make older adults more vulnerable to substance use [53]. Prescribed medications can interact with psychoactive substances and chronic medical or psychological conditions can be triggered or worsened by substance use. In general, the use and misuse of alcohol and illegal drugs declines with advancing age [54, 55]. However, older adults are frequent users of prescribed and over-the-counter medications, which have significant abuse potential, especially if use increases overtime [3, 52, 56]. These substances can be abused by being used in greater quantity or in a manner not prescribed. Self-medication may occur in response to stressful conditions, as well as to physical or mental health conditions, such as anxiety, low mood and psychotic symptoms. The self-medication hypothesis postulates that individuals may use substances that have short-term analgesic-like effects (e.g. alcohol or cannabis) or other psychoactive substances to cope with these mental health, physical health or stressful conditions [57]. This self-medication (e.g. the use of alcohol to cope with depression and/or anxiety) can lead to SUDs [58]. Men and women often react to stressful and health conditions differently, including the type of substance used as they age, and, therefore, gender plays an important role in the particulars of self-medication. In general, studies indicate that older men are much more likely than older women to have alcohol-related problems [52] but older women have been found to be at greater risk for prescription drug abuse [3].

Most older adults are able to cope with life stresses and are aided in this by social supports from family and friends. However, elderly who have more chronic, continuing sources of stress, coupled with a lack of social network supports and resources, may be more likely to be excessive drinkers [54]. Thus, changes in social networks and social roles (e.g. retirement) may influence the substance use progression in older populations. For example, substance misuse may be a coping mechanism to deal with the death of a spouse or other difficulties, such as family conflict or financial strain.

Factors that reduce the risk of the progression of substance use have not been studied in depth among older populations. However, many of the protective factors found in younger populations [59, 60] may also be relevant to this age group and require further study. Potential factors that protect against substance use and progression to other stages of substance involvement among the elderly that have been identified include being married, never using alcohol or tobacco and attending religious services regularly [61, 62].

Substance properties

Psychoactive substances are essential to the substance use progression process as they alter neurochemical activity. After crossing the blood–brain barrier, these substances act primarily upon the central nervous system, affecting brain function, altering perceptions, mood, consciousness, cognition and behaviour. Evidence from animal models indicates that expression of the effects may become more prominent in older individuals [63, 64]. The response to a substance depends upon specific drug effects, as well as nonspecific effects based more on a person's experience, mood and expectations. Nonspecific effects may explain why, sometimes, the user may experience pleasant feelings yet other times more depressed, melancholy feelings with the use of the same amount of the same substance. Reinforcing effects (e.g. euphoria, alertness) may encourage sustained use, which escalates in frequency and quantity as tolerance develops. For example, regular drinkers generally are able to tolerate larger amounts of alcohol on repeated use and may need to consume more to produce the same effect. Additionally, sleeping pills and tranquillizers may be particularly suited to misuse, as their properties often cause them to be used over a significant period of time, despite being recommended by physicians for short-term use only during times of stress.

With the advent of both technological and pharmacological innovations, similar substances can be administered in various ways [65]. How the substance is used and individual differences both determine how quickly a drug effect occurs, the concentration that reaches its site of action and the duration of drug action, all of which may influence the substance use progression process. Inhalation, which includes smoking, allows quick absorption by the lungs. Other methods that cross mucus membranes, such as topical applications, provide localized action but may also lead to widespread effects through absorption into the general circulation. Other drugs that cross membrane barriers, including patches or rectal suppository/enema, can provide controlled prolonged effects. Oral ingestion in beverage or tablet/capsule form is probably the most appealing route of administration to older adults because of the ease of administration. However, this route is less efficient (variable absorption) as the substance must first pass digestive processes and metabolism influences, which produce less predictable plasma levels. Differences in age, gender, nutrition, kidney and liver function, and genetics in addition to substance specific clearance characteristics (half-life) influence degradation and elimination rates.

Substances more commonly used by older adults are among those with a high tendency to induce dependence and are associated with physical harm to the user (propensity to damage organs, change physiological functions, result in illness or death) and serious consequences for families, communities and society (intoxication ramifications, impairment to social life, healthcare costs) [66]. The potentiating effect of one substance on another can be considerable (e.g. use of alcohol and nicotine paired with psychoactive substances). Ageing-related changes can elevate the risk for severe neurotoxicity and substance-related adverse consequences [52]. However, the effectiveness of one substance may be diminished by the repeated use of another. This cross-tolerance or cross-dependence usually occurs among substances of the same type but may also occur with drugs that have similar pharmacological effects that are in different categories. Therefore, when considering the progression along the substance use continuum, the specific substance (or substances) is an important consideration.

Environmental influences

In addition to individual factors and substance properties, physical and social environmental factors affect the risk for progression in the substance use process. Many older adults live alone or in rural communities with less access to others. This social isolation may make an individual vulnerable to developing a SUD as there are fewer restraints on use [67]. Isolated environments may also cause problem behaviours to go undetected and untreated.

The environment, including policies and norms, often influences our attitudes and behaviours. Upon retirement, for example, the constraint against substance use enforced via workplace policies and the cultural premise to not engage in these kinds of behaviours to uphold workplace safety and productivity are lost [68].

Factors related to where one lives may also promote substance use or serve a protective function if others monitor behaviours. Neighbourhoods with more adverse conditions have been found to be associated with more binge drinking [69]. Social events with alcohol, 'sharing' of prescribed medications and other practices in group living environments may all increase the risk of substance use progression. In these settings, women and the most socially outgoing are likely to have high rates of consumption. The responsiveness to social conditions suggests that problem substance use among the elderly may well increase with the ageing of younger and more tolerant cohorts.

The misuse of psychoactive substances can also be influenced by societal messages and the healthcare system. The lack of media attention given to substance abuse among older individuals compared to that targeting adolescents and young adults creates social stigma and lack of awareness about substance use disorders in older populations. Media campaigns for prescribed medications aimed at older populations could be encouraging adoption without considering long-term consequences or addiction potential [70–72]. Increased awareness of prescribing practices for older people and avoidance of certain medical practices may dampen the use and abuse of psychoactive substances that are contraindicated among the elderly [73, 74]. These practices include: (i) prescribing medications without adequate diagnoses; (ii) prescribing a drug at a higher dose and/or for a longer duration than recommended without adequate patient monitoring; (iii) failing to determine alcohol consumption behaviours, the use of other substances with abuse potential and the use of other medications that may interact with any newly prescribe medications; and (iv) failing to provide adequate and comprehensible instructions for patients regarding proper use and side effects to expect and report. Especially troublesome is that one half of all drugs taken by the elderly can interact with alcohol, and such interactions are especially associated with the drugs the elderly take most frequently [75]. Contributing to many adverse interactions are over-the-counter preparations, of which many contain alcohol and are not viewed as 'drugs' [76].

Miscommunication among providers and patients contributes to prospects of misuse, as does lack of coordination and follow-up of care. The older adult often has sensory and cognitive deficits that make understanding medication instructions difficult, and they may fail to fully report symptoms and side effects. Family and care providers should closely monitor for signs of underlying causes or symptoms that encourage the misuse of psychoactive substances, such as disruptions of daily activities due to pain [77], sleep disturbances [78] and self-medicating with over-the-counter nonprescription substances [56].

Future direction

Hampering the study of progression of substance use to SUD among elderly are detection and provider recognition issues. Traditional medical evaluations often do not identify older adults at risk of substance use problems because standard recommendations of safe levels of use are lacking and diagnostic criteria often include

Table 11.2 Typical symptoms of drug use progression among the elderly

- Loss of coordination (recurrent falls and unexplained bruises)
- Irritability if questioned about alcohol or drug use
- A loss of interest in activities once enjoyed
- Withdrawal from social activities
- Neglect of personal grooming and hygiene
- Irrational or secretive behaviour
- Cognitive dysfunction (trouble concentrating, memory problems and blackouts)
- Changes in eating and sleeping habits (malnutrition, sleep disturbances)
- Increasing financial or legal problems
- Depression, negativity and labile moods
- Hangovers
- Evidence of withdrawal symptoms, such as the early morning shakes

indicators more relevant for younger people [7, 79, 80]. In addition, it can be difficult to diagnose potential adverse effects of substance use or the development of substance use problems among the elderly, especially among those living alone. Signs of abuse and problems resulting from substance use among the elderly may be dismissed or mistaken for symptoms of ageing problems, such as depression, dementia and self-neglect (Table 11.2). Friends and family may be reluctant to consider that there may be a problem because addiction is stereotyped as being a problem affecting younger people and side effects while taking prescription type drugs are thought to be monitored by the healthcare system. Older people can be particularly unwilling to admit to misusing drugs because they may be ashamed or may not even recognize the problem. There may also be attitudinal issues in which substance abuse is not viewed as a priority because of more pressing health problems.

There are numerous gaps in our understanding of the progression of substance use among older populations as this topic is difficult to study. Evidence quantifying the number of elderly in different stages of substance involvement has, for the most part, been reliant on estimates from surveys of small samples of older adults, especially older than 65 years of age. While it is possible to begin to formulate a characterization of progression of substance use among elderly from cross-sectional surveys of different people at different ages, this characterization has several limitations. Findings may lack generalizability; for example, segments of older adults (e.g. those living in nursing homes and residential care facilities) are often excluded from national surveys, whose sampling frames focus on noninstitutionalized civilian populations and community dwelling residents. Cross-sectional designs cannot capture cohort effects, which is critical in studying substance use, as studies have found variation in substance use patterns for different birth cohorts [28, 81]. The male–female gap of being involved with different substances is closing in more recent cohorts [81]. Surveys are also limited in scope as they tend not to collect detailed information on the source, quantity, frequency, route of administration and continuity in relation to use of each drug (e.g. sporadically over the years since first use versus those who consumed continuously on a daily basis year in and year out). Recall bias is a great threat for information needed to understand progression of use. Thus, survey estimates represent no more than snapshots and are only the initial steps in the study of the time course from first access to SUDs. Therefore, future research using longitudinal studies with multiple assessments over the life course is critical for elucidating the substance use progression process. Advanced statistical techniques have been used to begin to model substance use trajectories among late-middle aged individuals followed up over time [82–85]; however, what is lacking and an area of future research is studies that examine factors that influence these trajectories and change the course of progression. Unfortunately, these studies are costly, time consuming and entail difficulties retaining samples over time due to high rates of morbidity and mortality in older populations. Despite difficulties, longitudinal studies would greatly contribute to the understanding of the substance use progression process.

Conclusions

Older adults are at risk of developing SUDs. Substance use, including the progression to heavier and more harmful use, is a precondition and contributor to developing a SUD. Different levels of use or stages of progression can occur within one substance, as well as across the use of different substances. The progression from substance use to a SUD has more to do with the consequences of use than the amount or frequency consumed, as heavy or regular use alone does not define diagnostic criteria for a substance use disorder. Tobacco, alcohol and prescribed psychoactive substances are the most frequently misused substances among older individuals.

Individual factors, substance use properties and environmental influences all contribute to the progression of use to SUDs. These aspects interact with one another to make it more (or less) likely that an individual will progress through the continuum. Key individual risk factors involve prior history of substance use involvement, physiological changes, multiple health problems and possible genetic predispositions. Key properties of the substance (or substances) include the biologically and pharmacologically reinforcing properties (leading to tolerance and dependence), as well as the consumption pattern, such as frequency and quantity. Key environmental influences are stigma, advertising targeted to ageing populations, prescribing practices leading to misuse and social isolation. Different factors may be influential at different stages along the use spectrum.

While progress has been made in understanding SUDs among older populations in recent years, there is still much to be learned about progression. Hampering the study of progression of substance use to SUD among the elderly are study design and recognition issues. Specifically, data are limited by a reliance on cross-sectional designs, underrepresentation of high-risk populations (e.g. physically ill, disabled, long-term care residents) and the lack of necessary details on substance usage and problems. In terms of recognition issues, physicians and other caregivers may be more attuned to the physical health problems of older populations, ignoring the signs and symptoms of a SUD. Patients and their families, in particular, need to be educated about the dangers of using medications that were not prescribed or using them in ways other than prescribed. It is also critical to provide education to caregivers of older populations to identify early symptoms. Potential signs of substance use progressing into problems include falls, fractures, decreased mobility and cognitive decline, all common among older adults already and thus difficult to determine if they are a consequence of a SUD or part of physical decline. The realities of demographic change and the increasing service needs of ageing substance misusers stress the need for a better understanding of substance use behaviours and trajectories, and influences or risk factors for progression among older adults.

Acknowledgement

Funds from a grant from the National Institute of Drug abuse (DA026863) provided support for the contributions of Dr Green.

References

1. Moore, A.A., Karno, M.P., Grella, C.E. *et al.* (2009) Alcohol, tobacco, and nonmedical drug use in older U.S. Adults: Data from the 2001/02 National Epidemiologic Survey of Alcohol and Related Conditions. *J Am Geriatr Soc*, 57(12) 2275–2281.
2. Zarba, A., Storr, C.L. and Wagner, F.A. (2005) Carrying habits into old age: prescription drug use without medical advice by older American adults. *J Am Geriatr Soc,* 53(1), 170–171.
3. Simoni-Wastila, L. and Yang, H.K. (2006) Psychoactive drug abuse in older adults. *Am J Geriatr Pharmacother*, 4(4), 380–394.
4. Moore, A.A., Hays, R.D., Greendale, G.A. *et al.* (1999) Drinking habits among older persons: Findings from the NHANES I Epidemiologic Followup Study (1982–84). National Health and Nutrition Examination Survey. *J Am Geriatr Soc*, 47(4), 412–416.
5. Lin, J.C., Karno, M.P., Grella, C.E. *et al.* (2011) Alcohol, tobacco, and nonmedical drug use disorders in U.S. Adults aged 65 years and older: Data from the 2001–2002 National Epidemiologic Survey of Alcohol and Related Conditions. *Am J Geriatr Psychiatry*, 19(3), 292–299.
6. Kalapatapu, R.K. and Sullivan, M.A. (2010) Prescription use disorders in older adults. *Am J Addict*, 19(6), 515–522.
7. Holmwood, C. (2011) Alcohol and drug problems in older people. *BMJ*, 343, d6761.
8. EMCDDA (European Monitoring Centre for Drugs and Drug Addiction) (2008) *Substance Use Among Older Adults: A Neglected Problem.* Drugs in Focus issue 18, Office for Official Publications of the European Communities, Lisbon.
9. Gfroerer, J., Penne, M., Pemberton, M. and Folsom, R. (2003) Substance abuse treatment need among older adults in 2020: The impact of the aging baby-boom cohort. *Drug Alcohol Depend*, 69(2), 127–135.
10. Han, B., Gfroerer, J.C., Colliver, J.D. and Penne, M.A. (2009) Substance use disorder among older adults in the United States in 2020. *Addiction*, 104(1), 88–96.
11. Mojtabai, R. and Olfson, M. (2010) National trends in psychotropic medication polypharmacy in office-based psychiatry. *Arch Gen Psychiatry*, 67(1), 26–36.
12. Ruths, S., Sørensen, P.H., Kirkevold, Ø. *et al.* (2012) Trends in psychotropic drug prescribing in Norwegian nursing homes from 1997 to 2009: A comparison of six cohorts. *Int J Geriatr Psychiatry*, 28(8), 868–876. doi: 10.1002/gps.3902.

13. Jyrkkä, J., Enlund, H., Korhonen, M.J. *et al.* (2009) Patterns of drug use and factors associated with polypharmacy and excessive polypharmacy in elderly persons: results of the Kuopio 75+ study: a cross-sectional analysis. *Drugs Aging*, **26**(6), 493–503.

14. Moore, A.A., Giuli, L., Gould, R. *et al.* (2006) Alcohol use, comorbidity, and mortality. *J Am Geriatr Soc*, **54**(5), 757–762.

15. Wagner, F.A. and Anthony, J.C. (2002) From first drug use to drug dependence: developmental periods of risk for dependence upon marijuana, cocaine and alcohol. *Neuropsychopharmacology*, **26**, 479–488.

16. Anthony, J.C. and Helzer, J.E. (1995) Epidemiology of drug dependence. In: *Textbook in Psychiatric Epidemiology* (eds M.T. Tsuang, M. Tohen, G.E. Zahner). Wiley–Liss, New York, pp. 361 406.

17. Anthony, J.C., Warner, L.A. and Kessler, R.C. (1994) Comparative epidemiology of dependence on tobacco, alcohol, controlled substances, and inhalants: Basic findings from the National Comorbidity Survey. *Exp Clin Psychopharmacol*, **2**, 244–268.

18. Kalaydjian, A., Swendsen, J., Chiu, W.T. *et al.* (2009) Sociodemographic predictors of transitions across stages of alcohol use, disorders, and remission in the National Comorbidity Survey Replication. *Compr Psychiatry*, **50**(4), 299–306.

19. US Congress, Office of Technology Assessment (1994) *Technologies for Understanding and Preventing Substance Abuse and Addiction*. OTA-HER-597, US Government Printing Office, Washington, DC.

20. De Wilde, S., Carey, I.M., Harris, T. *et al.* (2007) Trends in potentially inappropriate prescribing amongst older UK primary care patients. *Pharmacoepidemiol Drug Saf*, **16**(6), 658–667.

21. Van Etten, M.L. and Anthony, J.C. (1999) Comparative epidemiology of initial drug opportunities and transitions to first use: marijuana, cocaine, hallucinogen and heroin. *Drug Alcohol Depend*, **54**, 117–125.

22. Rikala, M., Korhonen, M.J., Sulkava, R. and Hartikainen, S. (2011) Psychotropic drug use in community-dwelling elderly people-characteristics of persistent and incident users. *Eur J Clin Pharmacol*, **67**(7), 731–739.

23. Kandel, D.B., Yamaguchi, K. and Klein, L.C. (2006) Testing the gateway hypothesis. *Addiction*, **101**(4), 470–472.

24. Stenbacka, M., Allebeck, P. and Romelsjo, A. (1993) Initiation into drug abuse: the pathway from being offered drug to trying cannabis and progression to intravenous drug abuse. *Scand J Soc Med*, **21**, 31–39.

25. Degenhardt, L., Dierker, L., Chiu, W.T. *et al.* (2010) Evaluating the drug use "gateway" theory using cross-national data: consistency and associations of the order of initiation of drug use among participants in the WHO World Mental Health Surveys. *Drug Alcohol Depend*, **108**(1–2), 84–97.

26. Myers, B., van Heerden, M.S., Grimsrud, A. *et al.* (2011) Prevalence and correlates of atypical patterns of drug use progression: findings from the South African Stress and Health Study. *Afr J Psychiatry* (Johannesbg), **14**(1), 38–44.

27. Wells, J.E. and McGee, M.A. (2008) Violations of the usual sequence of drug initiation: prevalence and associations with the development of dependence in the New Zealand Mental Health Survey. *J Stud Alcohol Drugs*, **69**(6), 789–795.

28. Degenhardt, L., Chiu, W.T., Conway, K. *et al.* (2009) Does the 'gateway' matter? Associations between the order of drug use initiation and the development of drug dependence in the National Comorbidity Study Replication. *Psychol Med*, **39**(1), 157–167.

29. Blazer, D.G., Wu, L.-T. (2012) Patterns of tobacco use and tobacco-related psychiatric morbidity and substance use among middle-aged and older adults in the United States. *Aging Ment Health*, **16**(3), 296–304.

30. Petry, N. (2001) A behavioural economic analysis of polydrug abuse in alcoholics: asymmetrical substitution of alcohol and cocaine. *Drug Alcohol Depend*, **62**, 31–39.
31. Reiman, A. (2009) Cannabis as a substitute for alcohol and other drugs. *Harm Reduct J*, **6**, 35.
32. Stinson, F.S., Grant, B.F., Dawson, D.A. *et al.* (2006) Comorbidity between DSM-IV alcohol and specific drug use disorders in the United States, Results from the National Epidemiologic Survey on Alcohol and Related Conditions. *Alcohol Research & Health*, **29**(2), 94–106.
33. Finlayson, R.E. and Davis, L.J. (1994) Prescription drug dependence in the elderly population: demographic and clinical features of 100 inpatients. *Mayo Clinic Proceedings*, **69**, 1137–1145.
34. Merikangas, K.R., Stolar, M., Stevens, D.E. *et al.* (1998) Familial transmission of substance use disorders. *Arch Gen Psychiatry*, **55**(11), 973–979.
35. Urbanoski, K.A. and Kelly, J.F. (2012) Understanding genetic risk for substance use and addiction: A guide for non-geneticists. *Clin Psychol Rev*, **32**(1), 60–70.
36. Ducci, F. and Goldman, D. (2012) The genetic basis of addictive disorders. *Psychiatr Clin North Am*, **35**(2), 495–519.
37. Agrawal, A., Verweij, K.J., Gillespie, N.A. *et al.* (2012) The genetics of addiction-a translational perspective. *Transl Psychiatry*, **2**, e140.
38. Agrawal, A. and Lynskey, M.T. (2006) The genetic epidemiology of cannabis use, abuse and dependence. *Addiction*, **101**(6), 801–812.
39. Kendler, K.S., Schmitt, E., Aggen, S.H. and Prescott, C.A. (2008) Genetic and environmental influences on alcohol, caffeine, cannabis, and nicotine use from early adolescence to middle adulthood. *Arch Gen Psychiatry*, **65**(6), 674–682.
40. Schuckit, M.A. (2009) An overview of genetic influences in alcoholism. *J Subst Abuse Treat*, **36**, S5–S14.
41. Agrawal, A. and Lynskey, M.T. (2008) Are there genetic influences on addiction: Evidence from family, adoption, and twin studies. *Addiction*, **103**, 1069–1081.
42. Fergusson, D.M. and Horwood, L.J. (1997) Early onset cannabis use and psychosocial adjustment in young adults. *Addiction*, **92**(3), 279–296.
43. Lynskey, M.T., Heath, A.C., Bucholz, K.K. *et al.* (2003) Escalation of drug use in early-onset cannabis users vs co-twin controls. *JAMA*, **289**(4), 427–433.
44. Schuckit, M.A. (1997) Geriatric alcoholism and drug abuse. *Gerontologist*, **17**, 168–174.
45. Atkinson, R.M. (1994) Late onset problem drinking in older adults. *Int J Geriat Psychiatry*, **9**, 321–326.
46. Kofoed, L.L., Tolsom, R.L., Atkinson, R.M. *et al.* (1984) Elderly groups in an alcoholism clinic. In: *Alcohol and Drug Abuse in Old Age* (ed. R.M. Atkinson). American Psychiatric Press, Inc., Washington, DC, pp. 35–48.
47. Atkinson, R.M., Turner, J.A., Kofoed L.L. and Tolson, R.L. (1984) Early versus late onset alcoholism in older persons: preliminary findings. *Alcohol Clin Exp Res*, **9**, 513–515.
48. Dupree, L.W., Broskowski, H. and Schonfeld, L. (1984) The Gerontology Alcohol Project: A behavioural treatment program for elderly alcohol abusers. *Gerontologist*, **24**, 510–516.
49. Zimberg, S. (1974) The elderly alcoholic. *Gerontologist*, **14**, 221–224.
50. Gomberg, E.S.L. (1990) Drugs, alcohol, and aging. In: *Research Advances in Alcohol and Drug Problems*, Vol. 10 (eds L.T. Kozlowski, H.M. Annis, H.D. Cappell *et al.*). Plenum Press, New York, pp. 171–213.
51. Rigler, S.K. (2000) Alcoholism in the elderly. *Am Fam Physician*, **61**, 1710–1716.
52. Dowling, G.J., Weiss, S.R.B. and Condon, T.P. (2008) Drugs of abuse and the aging brain. *Neuropsychopharm*, **33**(2), 209–218.

53. Kaiser, R.M. (2009) Physiological and clinical considerations of geriatric care. In: *The American Psychiatric Publishing Textbook of Geriatric Psychiatry* (eds D.G. Blazer and D.C. Steffens). American Psychiatric Publishing, Washington, DC, pp. 45–62.

54. Moos, R.H., Schutte, K.K., Brennan, P.L. and Moos, B.S. (2010) Late-life and life history predictors of older adults' high risk alcohol consumption and drinking problems. *Drug Alcohol Depend*, **108**(1–2), 13–20.

55. Grant, B.F. (1997) Prevalence and correlates of alcohol use and DSM-IV alcohol dependence in the United States: Results of the National Longitudinal Alcohol Epidemiologic Survey. *J Stud Alcohol*, **58**(5), 464–473.

56. Conca, A.J. and Worthen, D.R. (2012) Nonprescription drug abuse. *J Pharm Pract*, **25**(1), 13–21.

57. Aira, M., Hartikaninen, S. and Sulkava, R. (2008) Drinking alcohol for medicinal purposes by people aged over 75: a community-based interview study. *Fam Pract*, **25**(6), 445–449.

58. Crum, R.M., Mojtabai, R., Lazareck, S. *et al.* (2013) A prospective assessment of reports of drinking to self-medicate mood symptoms with the incidence and persistence of alcohol dependence. *JAMA Psychiatry*, **1**, 1–9.

59. Hawkins, J.D., Catalano, R.F. and Miller, J.Y. (1992) Risk and protective factors for alcohol and other drug problems in adolescence and early adulthood: implications for substance abuse prevention. *Psychol Bull*, **112**(1), 64–105.

60. Newcomb, M.D. and Felix-Ortiz, M. (1992) Multiple protective and risk factors for drug use and abuse: cross-sectional and prospective findings. *J Pers Soc Psychol*, **63**(2), 280–296.

61. Blazer, D.G. and Wu, L.-T. (2009) The epidemiology of substance use and disorders among middle-aged and elderly community adults: National survey on drug use and health. *Am J Geriatric Psych*, **17**, 237–245.

62. Han, B., Gfroerer, J.C. and Colliver, J.D. (2009) *An Examination of Trends in Illicit Drug Use Among Adults Aged 50 to 59 in the United States*. Substance Abuse and Mental Health Administration, Office of Applied Studies, Rockville, MD.

63. Van Skike, C.E., Botta, P., Chin, V.S. *et al.* (2010) Behavioural effects of ethanol in cerebellum are age dependent: potential system and molecular mechanisms. *Alcohol Clin Exp Res*, **34**(12), 2070–2080.

64. Spear, L.P. (2001) Acute, rapid, and chronic tolerance during ontogeny: observations when equating ethanol perturbation across age. *Alcohol Clin Exp Res*, **25**(9), 1301–1308.

65. Rigler, S.K., Shireman, T.I. and Kallenbach, L. (2007) Predictors of long-acting opioid use and oral versus transdermal route among older Medicaid beneficiaries. *Am J Geriatr Pharmacother*, **5**(2), 91–99.

66. Nutt, D., King, L.A., Saulsbury, W. and Blakemore, C. (2007) Development of a rational scale to assess the harm of drugs of potential misuse. *Lancet*, **369**(9566), 1047–1053.

67. Fink, A., Hays, R.D., Moore, A.A. and Beck, J.C. (1996) Alcohol-related problems in older persons: Determinants, consequences, and screening. *Arch Intern Med*, **156**(11), 1150–1156.

68. Kuerbis, A. and Sacco, P. (2012) The impact of retirement on the drinking patterns of older adults: a review. *Addict Behav*, **37**(5), 587–595.

69. Rudolph, K.E., Glass, T.A., Crum, R.M. and Schwartz, B.S. (2013) Neighborhood psychosocial hazards and binge drinking among late middle-aged adults. *J Urban Health*, **90**(5), 970–982.

70. Mintzes, B., Barer, M.L., Kravitz, R.L. *et al.* (2003) How does direct-to-consumer advertising (DTCA) affect prescribing? A survey in primary care environments with and without legal DTCA. *CMAJ*, **169**(5), 405–412.

71. Hall, D.V. and Jones, S.C. (2008) Australian consumer responses to DTCA and other pharmaceutical company sponsored advertisements. *Aust NZ J Public Health*, **32**(5), 471–478.

72. Frosch, D.L., May, S.G., Tietbohl, C. and Pagán, J.A. (2011) Living in the "land of no"? Consumer perceptions of healthy lifestyle portrayals in direct-to-consumer advertisements of prescription drugs. *Soc Sci Med*, **73**(7), 995–1002.

73. Keith, S.W., Maio, V., Dudash, K. *et al.* (2013) A physician-focused intervention to reduce potentially inappropriate medication prescribing in older people. *Drugs & Aging*, **30**(2), 119–127.

74. Royal College of Psychiatrists (2011) *Our Invisible Addicts: First Report of the Older Persons' Substance Misuse Working Group of the Royal College of Psychiatrists*. College Report CR165, Royal College of Psychiatrists, London. http://rcpsych.ac.uk/files/pdfversion/CR165.pdf (last accessed 7 April 2014).

75. Lamy, P. (1998) Actions of alcohol and drugs in older people. *Generations*, **12**(4), 9–13.

76. Coons, S.J., Hendricks, J. and Sheahan, S. (1998) Self-medication with nonprescription drugs. *Generations*, **12**(4), 22–26.

77. Brennan, P.L., Schutte, K.K. and Moos, R.H. (2005) Pain and use of alcohol to manage pain: prevalence and 3-year outcomes among older problem and non-problem drinkers. *Addiction*, **100**(6), 777–786.

78. Hairston, I.S. (2012) Sleep and hazardous drinking in the elderly: a clarion call for increased clinical and translational research. *J Addict Res Ther*, **3**, 3.

79. Center for Substance Abuse Treatment (1998) *Substance Abuse Among Older Adults*. Treatment Improvement Protocol (TIP) Series, No. 26, Substance Abuse and Mental Health Services Administration, Rockville, MD. http://www.ncbi.nlm.nih.gov/books/NBK6441 (last accessed 7 April 2014).

80. Moore, A.A., Morton, S.C., Beck, J.C. *et al.* (1999) A new paradigm for alcohol use in older persons. *Med Care*, **37**(2), 165–179.

81. Degenhardt, L., Chiu, W.T., Sampson, N. *et al.* (2008) Toward a global view of alcohol, tobacco, cannabis, and cocaine use: findings from the WHO World Mental Health Surveys. *PLoS Med*, **5**(7), e141.

82. Brennan, P.L., Schutte, K.K., SooHoo, S. and Moos, R.H. (2011) Painful medical conditions and alcohol use: a prospective study among older adults. *Pain Med*, **12**(7), 1049–1059.

83. Brennan, P.L., Schutte, K.K., Moos, B.S. and Moos, R.H. (2011) Twenty-year alcohol-consumption and drinking-problem trajectories of older men and women. *J Stud Alcohol Drugs*, **72**(2), 308–321.

84. Bobo, J.K., Greek, A.A., Klepinger, D.H. and Herting, J.R. (2010) Alcohol use trajectories in two cohorts of U.S. women aged 50 to 65 at baseline. *J Am Geriatr Soc*, **58**(12), 2375–2380.

85. Bobo, J.K., Greek, A.A., Klepinger, D.H. and Herting, J.R. (2013) Predicting 10-year alcohol use trajectories among men age 50 years and older. *Am J Geriatr Psychiatry*, **21**(2), 204–213.

Chapter 12

PSYCHOPHARMACOLOGY AND THE CONSEQUENCES OF ALCOHOL AND DRUG INTERACTIONS

Vijay A. Ramchandani[1], Patricia W. Slattum[2], Ashwin A. Patkar[3,4], Li-Tzy Wu[4], Jonathan C. Lee[5,6], Maitreyee Mohanty[2], Marion Coe[1] and Ting-Kai Li[4]

[1] *Laboratory of Clinical and Translational Studies, National Institute on Alcohol Abuse and Alcoholism, National Institutes of Health, USA*
[2] *Virginia Commonwealth University, USA*
[3] *Duke Addictions Program & Center for Addictive Behavior and Change, School of Medicine, Duke University Medical Center, USA*
[4] *Department of Psychiatry and Behavioral Sciences, School of Medicine, Duke University Medical Center, USA*
[5] *The Farley Center at Williamsburg Place, USA*
[6] *Brody School of Medicine, East Carolina University, USA*

The extent of alcohol and drug misuse among older adults

Substance misuse in the general population

The use and abuse of alcohol and other drugs is a growing concern in the older population, with roughly 40% of the total US population now at age 45 or older [1]. Because of the large proportion of the middle aged and older population and prevalent rate of substance use in the middle aged group, the number of Americans aged 50 years and older with alcohol or drug related disorders has been projected to double from 2.8 million in 2002–2006 to 5.7 million in 2020 [2]. Alcohol is the primary substance of use and abuse in later life. The US National Surveys of Drug Use and Health (NSDUH) estimates that 60% of adults aged 50 and older used alcohol in the past year (65.6% in adults aged 50–64; 51.9% in adults aged 65 and older), with 8.3% reporting binge drinking and 1.7% reporting heavy drinking patterns. An estimated 5% of these alcohol users (or 3% of adults aged 50 and older) suffered an alcohol use disorder in the past year [3]. In a national sample of 10 953 adults aged 50 and older, Blazer and Wu [4] found prevalent rates of current at-risk (≥2 drinks per day in the past month) and binge (≥5 drinks on the same occasion in the past month) alcohol use, respectively, among adults aged 50 and older in both men (16.7% and 19.6%, respectively) and women (10.9% and 6.3%, respectively). Binge drinking among men was significantly associated

Substance Use and Older People, First Edition.
Edited by Ilana B. Crome, Li-Tzy Wu, Rahul (Tony) Rao and Peter Crome.
© 2015 John Wiley & Sons, Ltd. Published 2015 by John Wiley & Sons, Ltd.

with use of tobacco and illicit drugs in past-year reports. Binge drinking among women not only was significantly associated with use of tobacco and illicit drugs, but also with nonmedical prescription drugs (opioids, sedatives, tranquilizers, stimulants) in past-year reports [4]. Survey of Medicare beneficiaries aged 65 years or older reported that 75.2% of the drinkers consumed 30 or fewer drinks per month (e.g. whiskey or gin, mixed drinks, wine, beer and any other type of alcoholic beverage) and that 10% of the drinkers consumed more than 30 drinks per month. The survey also recorded that 14.8% of the subjects indulged in heavy episodic drinking (four or more drinks in a single day) [5]. While prevalence estimates of alcohol use vary depending on the setting of the study and the measure of alcohol consumption available data suggest that use of one substance increases the likelihood of using another substance, that use of multiple substances is an emerging concern among middle-aged and older substance misusers [4, 6].

Although illicit and nonmedical drug use is less common among older adults, it has increasingly become a public health concern as the size of older populations continues to rise [6]. In the general population, an estimated 5.2% of American adults aged 50 and older used illicit drugs or nonmedical prescription drugs in the past year [7]. Marijuana use (3.2%) was more common than nonmedical use of prescription psychoactive drugs (2.3%), including opioids, sedatives, tranquilizers and stimulants. Similar to binge drinking, illicit and nonmedical drug use was more prevalent among adults aged 50–59 (9.0% versus 2.3% in adults aged 60 and older) and men aged 60 and older (6.9% versus 3.8% in women aged 50 and older) [7]. Among illicit drug users aged 50 and older, more than one in nine (11.7%) reported a drug use disorder in the past year [3]. Among nonmedical users of opioid pain killers aged 50 and older, close to one in ten (9.4%) experienced dependence symptoms consistent with opioid use disorder in the past year [8]. In summary, a sizable proportion of older adults are recent or active users of psychoactive substances, and a subset of substance misusers appears to have used or misused multiple substances.

Substance misuse or addiction in clinical settings

The Treatment Episode Data Set (TEDS) systematically collects annual substance abuse treatment admissions to treatment facilities that receive State alcohol and/or drug agency funds for the provision of substance abuse treatment. Data from the 2005 TEDS showed that, among adults aged 50 and older, alcohol was the most frequently reported primary substance of abuse at the time of admission and that the proportions of alcohol-related admissions increase with age [9]. Among adults aged 50–69, 55–62% of all substance abuse treatment admissions reported alcohol as the primary substance of abuse; the proportions rose to more than 70% (71–76%) among adults aged 60 and older. Opioids and cocaine ranked second and third as the most commonly reported primary substances of abuse; less than 10% of admissions reported other drugs (e.g. marijuana, stimulants, other drugs) as primary substances of abuse at the time of admission [9]. More recent data from the TEDS revealed a significant increase in benzodiazepine-related admissions [10]. Moreover, the vast majority of benzodiazepine-related admissions (about 90% of adults aged 55 and older) involved abuse of multiple substances, mainly opiates and alcohol.

The Drug Abuse Warning Network (DAWN) gathers annual visit-level information on emergency department (ED) visits resulting from substance misuse or abuse, adverse reactions to drugs taken as prescribed, accidental ingestion of drugs, drug-related suicide attempts and other drug-related medical emergencies [11]. In 2008, an estimated 118 495 ED visits involved illicit drug use by older adults aged 50 and older [11]. Cocaine (63% of all admissions) was the most commonly reported illicit drug in these ED visits, followed by heroin (26.5%), marijuana (18.5%) and amphetamines (5.3%). The findings further indicated that cocaine was more frequently involved among ED visits by blacks and Caucasians, while heroin was the most common illicit drug among ED visits by Hispanics.

Similar results from the DAWN data suggest an increased trend in ED visits involving misuse or abuse of prescription opioids and benzodiazepines. The 2003 DAWN data indicated a significant increase in opiate misuse related deaths, especially among adults aged 35–54 [12]. Similar to benzodiazepine misuse in the TEDS, the majority (66–93% across states) of opiate-related deaths involved multiple substances. The DAWN findings also demonstrate that prescription opioids and benzodiazepines are the most commonly identified prescription-type psychoactive drugs of misuse among ED visits by both younger and older adults [13]. The majority of ED visits for these two drug classes also involved multiple substances, including alcohol [13]. The recent 2012 DAWN report further confirmed a significantly rising trend in ED visits for prescription drug misuse and abuse among adults aged 50 and older (115 798 ED visits in 2004 versus 300 084 ED visits in 2009) [14]. Increased numbers of ED visits involving prescription opioids (e.g. oxycodone) and anti-anxiety and insomnia drugs had also been reported. In 2009, a large proportion (44%) of these ED visits for prescription drug misuse and abuse occurred among patients aged 60 and older. These studies corroborate the increasing concern over prescription drug misuse and abuse alone or in combination with alcohol and/or other psychoactive drugs among older adults.

Co-morbidities among older substance misusers

Data from the subsample of adults aged 60 and older in the 2000-2001 National Epidemiologic Survey on Alcohol and Related Conditions (NESARC) suggested that major depression was the most common mental disorder experienced by adults with a severe alcohol use disorder, followed by anxiety disorder and antisocial personality disorder [15]. In the group of latent class analysis (LCA) defined high-risk alcohol users, 24.9% had a lifetime major depressive disorder, 8.9% had an anxiety disorder and 5.9% had an antisocial personality disorder. A community survey of older adults aged 65 and older in Canada showed that 31.3% of older adults with past-year benzodiazepine dependence also had either a mood or anxiety disorder in the past year [16]. Older drug users receiving addiction

treatment exhibit a pattern of severe comorbid conditions. In a sample of methadone maintenance patients, Lofwall *et al.* [17] found prevalent rates of lifetime
disorders among patients aged 50 and older, including: major depression, 34.1%;
alcohol use disorder, 75.6%; cocaine use disorder, 73.2%; opioid use disorder,
100%; cannabis use disorder, 41.5%; and sedative use disorder, 36.6%. In
another study of methadone maintenance patients, Rosen *et al.* [18] documented
high rates of past-year psychiatric and medical diagnoses among patients aged 50
and older that included: major depression, 32.9%; generalized anxiety disorder,
29.7%; post-traumatic stress disorder, 27.8%; any mood/anxiety disorder,
47.1%; arthritis, 54.3%; Hepatitis C, 49.3%; hypertension, 44.9%; heart condition, 17.9%; lung disease, 22.1%; alcoholic liver disease, 14.3%; and diabetes,
11.4%. More recently, Cicero *et al.* [19] found that opioid-dependent patients
aged 45 and older (n = 476) were more likely than younger opioid-dependent
patients (18–44 years) to have moderate to severe pain as well as anxiety/depres-
sive disorder or alcohol dependence. In summary, older drug abusers appear to
suffer psychiatric conditions that may further increase their likelihood for taking
medications and experiencing adverse drug interactions.

Psychopharmacology of alcohol and drug misuse in older people

Many age-related factors affect the pharmacokinetics and pharmacodynamics of
abused drugs [20, 21]. For example, older adults may have reduced kidney function
due to diminished renal blood flow and glomerular filtration rate, compromised
liver function because of reduced hepatic mass, a decrease in total body water due
to increased fat composition and reduced muscle mass, and a more permeable
blood–brain barrier. These age-related changes can result in alterations in absorption, distribution, metabolism and elimination of drugs, and consequently the systemic and brain exposure as well as the effects of these drugs. In addition, age-related
alterations in neurotransmitter function and receptor density can result in altered
pharmacodynamics of these drugs on the brain.

Neurocircuitry of abused substances

The reward or positive reinforcement derived from addictive drugs results from the
release of dopamine (DA) in the mesolimbic areas of the brain [22]. Alcohol, opiates, cannabinoids and benzodiazepines all accomplish this by reducing GABAgeric
inhibition of mesolimbic dopamine neurons, specifically the DA neurons that project from the ventral tegmental area (VTA) to basal forebrain areas, including the
nucleus accumbens (NAc), the medial prefrontal cortex (mPFC) and the bed nucleus
of the stria terminalis (BNST). This results in an increase in DA levels in these brain
areas demonstrated to be vital to reward [23–25]. In contrast, stimulants such as
amphetamine and cocaine increases DA levels by binding to dopamine transporters

[26] localized in presynaptic terminals in the substantia nigra and VTA, preventing reuptake of DA into pre-synaptic cells. Both mechanisms produce a sensation of euphoria, as a result of an increased level of DA in the brain's reward areas.

Alcohol

Alcohol affects a wide variety of neurotransmitter systems [25, 26]. It enhances actions at GABA-A receptors, inhibits N-methyl-D-aspartate (NMDA) and glutamate receptors and increases endogenous opioid, serotonin and dopamine release. Alcohol modulates the hypothalamic–pituitary–adrenal axis and chronic use leads to dysregulation of the normal stress response. Alcohol is a central nervous system (CNS) depressant and has a biphasic dose-response curve in that small doses (BAC <0.05) of alcohol stimulate pulse, motor activity and mood. Higher doses of ethanol impair cognitive and motor function, cause respiratory depression and, in severe cases, cause coma and death. Behavioural, psychomotor and cognitive changes begin to occur at a BAC of 0.02–0.03; this sensitivity may be altered, with larger changes seen in older individuals. Between 90–98% of ethanol is converted to acetaldehyde by alcohol dehydrogenase in the liver. Once converted, aldehyde dehydrogenase converts acetaldehyde to acetate and acetyl CoA. The other 2–10% is excreted through the lungs, sweat or urine.

There are only a few studies that have investigated age-related differences in alcohol pharmacokinetics (PK). Most of these studies have documented age-related changes in lean body mass and total body water, which results in decreased volumes of distribution and, therefore, higher alcohol levels [27, 28]. Age-related changes in first-pass metabolism and bioavailability of alcohol has also been observed [29, 30]. Studies that have examined sex- and age-related variations have used oral administration of alcohol, which prevents the effect of absorption from being separated from that of alcohol metabolism. This is additionally confounded by substantial variability in first-pass metabolism [31]. Furthermore, most of these studies have not examined the combined effects of age and sex on alcohol pharmacokinetics.

Additionally, older people are thought to be more sensitive to alcohol and show greater impairment than younger drinkers. However, it is unclear if these changes are due to pharmacokinetic or pharmacodynamic factors [32]. Pharmacokinetic changes, including a decrease in volume of distribution, can result in increased alcohol levels, and therefore increased impairment, in older participants following standard doses of alcohol. Pharmacodynamic factors may include a decrease in sensitivity to the initial impairing effects or a decreased ability to develop tolerance to the effects of alcohol [32–34]. Pre-existing medical conditions and even conditions associated with normal ageing can increase the risk of negative reactions to alcohol in older people. Alcohol can cause sleep problems, including impaired sleep and insomnia, as well as exacerbations of sleep apnoea by relaxing the muscles in the pharynx, resulting in snoring [35]. This effect becomes more prominent with advanced age, with reports of 75% of alcoholic men over age 60 showing symptoms of sleep apnoea [36]. Alcohol also impairs glycogenesis in the liver, which can cause fat accumulation in hepatic cells. It acutely lowers blood pressure and both causes and forces the heart to work harder. For drinkers with cardiac disease, this is particularly problematic. Chronic use of alcohol can cause hypertension. All of these effects have been shown to be exacerbated in older people.

A growing body of literature suggests that moderate drinking may have beneficial effects on coronary heart disease, dementia, mortality and bone metabolism [37–42]. Alcohol may play a role in psychosocial functioning, such as the consumption of alcoholic beverages during social gatherings or before dinner, which is becoming more common in retirement communities [37, 43]. While these association studies indicate emerging factors that encourage moderate alcohol consumption among older adults, the causal mechanisms underlying these effects remain unclear. Additionally, the regular intake of alcohol may slowly give way to craving and dependence, prompting higher consumption of alcohol.

Opioids/opiates

The effects of opiates are mediated primarily through the mu-opioid receptor (MOR). Opiates act as agonists at the mu-opioid receptors, which when activated result in the inhibition of gamma-aminobutyric acid (GABA) interneurons in the ventral tegmental area (VTA). This, is turn, causes hyperpolarization of dopaminergic neurons and release of dopamine (DA) in the nucleus accumbens [44, 45]. The primary route of elimination for opiates is via hepatic metabolism, with minor amounts excreted through urine or faeces. The duration of action varies greatly between different opiates. Morphine is short-lived with a half-life of about 2.5–3 hours in the general population, while methadone, the drug used most widely for heroin replacement in treatment clinics, has a half-life of about 22 hours. Opiates depress the CNS, resulting in analgesia, drowsiness, mood changes, euphoria, lethargy and depressed respiration. High doses can cause loss of consciousness.

Benzodiazepines and Sedative-Hypnotics (SH)

GABA is the primary inhibitory neurotransmitter in the CNS. Both sedatives and benzodiazepines operate through GABAgeric mechanisms. However, the mechanisms of action differ between benzodiazepines and SHs in which GABAA receptor subtype(s) the drug preferentially binds to. Benzodiazepines nonselectively target α1, α2, α3 or α5 GABAA receptor subunits [46]. This allosteric activation may result in both anxiolytic and sedative–hypnotic effects. Nonanxiolytic sedative–hypnotics also act through the GABAA receptors, but differ from benzodiazepines in that they specifically target α1 receptors [47]. These drugs depress the CNS at limbic and subcorticol levels. The half-life of SHs and benzodiazepines range from 1.5–5 h (triazolam) to 30–100 h (flurazepam) and vary in time to reach peak effect.

Older individuals demonstrate an increased sensitivity to the effects of anxiolytics and hypnotics [48, 49]. Even with α1 specific sedative–hypnotics (e.g. zolpidem), area under the plasma concentration–time curve values are higher in subjects aged 65 years and older than in younger individuals receiving the same dose [50]. Thus, the recommended dose of zolpidem in older patients,is 5 mg once daily, compared to the typical dose (10 mg) in younger adults. Decreased body water in older people can result in a prolonged duration of action for lipid soluble medications such as benzodiazepines. These drugs cause psychomotor and cognitive impairment [21, 51].

Cocaine

Cocaine exerts its effects primarily by binding to pre-synaptic dopamine transporters (DATs) to prevent the re-uptake of DA. Cocaine also prevents reuptake of serotonin (5-HT) and noradrenaline into post-synaptic cells [52, 53]. This leads to increased synaptic concentrations of DA, 5-HT and noradrenaline. Voluntary use of cocaine elicits long-lasting potentiation of glutamate function in the VTA and NAc that persist even after the person has stopped using cocaine. Cocaine also causes changes in glutamatergic transmission onto VTA DA neurons, thus altering DA release into terminal regions [54], altering reward learning and cue saliency [55]. Cocaine is metabolized by plasma esterase and cocaine metabolites are excreted in the urine. Effects of cocaine are short-lived, peaking 8–10 seconds (smoking) to 10–20 minutes (snorting) after administration and lasting less than an hour. The plasma half-life of cocaine is 45–60 minutes. There is a dose-dependent response of the CNS to cocaine – high doses enhance mood, raise body temperature, increase pulse and cause vasoconstriction. Due to cocaine's sympathomimetic properties, older people who use cocaine are at increased risk of serious adverse consequences, including cardiac arrhythmias, convulsions and stroke. Smoking crack has also been shown to cause liver damage; liver function is already depressed in the elderly.

Cannabis

Δ9-tetrahydrocannabinol (THC) is responsible for the main psychological effects of cannabis, though cannabis contains over 60 different cannabinoids [56]. THC is absorbed into the lungs and is quickly stored in many tissues. THC is metabolized in the liver and converted to the psychoactive compound 11-hydroxyl-THC and more than 20 other metabolites. CB1 and CB2 receptors are cannabinoid specific and are present in both the central and peripheral nervous systems.

There is virtually no research on the pharmacokinetics and pharmacological effects of cannabis or THC in older people. Given the increasing prevalence of marijuana use in this population, particularly as a result of increased prescription use of marijuana, there is a great need for increased research efforts to understand the pharmacokinetic and pharmacodynamic effects of marijuana in older individuals, as well as the potential for interactions with other prescribed and abused drugs and alcohol.

Alcohol–drug interactions in older adults

The use of prescription medications has escalated in recent years. Older adults use more medications than any other age group. The National Council on Patient Information and Education (NCPIE) report stated, 'this group comprises 13% of the population, but accounts for 34% of all prescription medication use and 30% of all *over-the-counter* (OTC) drug use' [57]. Polypharmacy is commonly seen in this population with two out of five patients taking five or more prescription medications [58]. The widespread prevalence of alcohol use and medication use indicates that the potential for interactions and consequences is significant.

Mechanisms of alcohol–medication interactions

Alcohol interacts with numerous medications through different mechanisms. The two most prevalent mechanisms are: (i) pharmacokinetic interactions (in which alcohol interferes with the metabolism of the medication) and (ii) pharmacodynamic interactions (in which alcohol influences the response to the medication) [59]. Age-related changes may further exacerbate the alcohol–medication interaction, rendering older adults more vulnerable to a variety of adverse events [60]. Alcohol is a CNS depressant like many other CNS-acting prescription medications [61]. The sedative effect of CNS-acting medications, including antidepressants, anxiolytics, anticonvulsants, opioid analgesics and certain antihistamines, is enhanced in the presence of alcohol, resulting in impaired psychomotor function, dizziness and increased risk of injury [60]. Alcohol, when combined with antihypertensive agents such as hydralazine, nitrates and α-blockers, potentiates orthostatic hypotension by impairing vasoconstriction [60]. Risk of gastrointestinal bleeding increases with concomitant use of alcohol and nonsteroidal anti-inflammatory drugs (NSAIDs). Alcohol affects the metabolism of various medications, mediated by the cytochrome P450 enzyme system, depending upon the type of drug and pattern of alcohol consumption. Chronic heavy drinkers have been shown to have amplified cytochrome P450 (CYP) 2E1 enzyme activity, which can enhance the metabolism of many drugs that are CYP 2E1 substrates, including warfarin, phenytoin, propranolol and isoniazid. However, during acute heavy drinking alcohol may compete with these drugs for liver enzymes, thereby decreasing the metabolism of the drugs. For example, acute alcohol consumption may increase anticoagulation by decreasing warfarin metabolism, whereas chronic alcohol intake decreases anticoagulation by increasing warfarin metabolism [59].

Significance of the problem

The ageing baby boomer generation faces an anticipated increase in alcohol-related problems as a result of higher alcohol consumption and relatively large size of the cohort. The rise in alcohol-related problems is likely to impose significant burden in health care resource use. A better understanding of adverse events resulting from alcohol and drug interaction among older adults will enable clinicians to focus on vulnerable older adults and to design measures that will mitigate adverse events attributable to hazardous drinking. Using baseline data from a randomized controlled trial, researchers found that 11.1% of the patients reported having had an alcohol-related discussion with a physician in the past two months, and drinking and driving and concerns raised by others were factors associated with alcohol-related discussion, whereas having co-morbidities or using medications that may interact with alcohol were not [62]. Awareness about alcohol-related risks, reading educational materials and physicians' advice may lead to a decline in alcohol intake by older at-risk drinkers [63]. These studies highlight the need to create awareness among healthcare professionals to address alcohol-related problems among older adults. Interventions such as preventive educational programmes and brief counselling have been useful in improving awareness among older adults regarding alcohol and drug interactions [64]. Providing educational materials to healthcare professionals as well as to older adults, and screening combined with counselling of older adults for hazardous drinking, are some ways to increase awareness among healthcare professionals and older adults.

Concurrent use of alcohol and potentially interacting medications

Several observational studies have been conducted to understand the prevalence and pattern of alcohol and medication use among older adults. A random sample of community-dwelling older adults was studied for concurrent use of alcohol and medications. One-quarter of this sample consumed one or more drugs with the potential to cause alcohol–drug interaction. Over-the-counter pain medications were the most commonly used medications [65]. A cross-sectional survey of older adults with low to moderate income found that 19% of the older adults taking an alcohol-interactive medication reported current drinking. This study also observed that NSAIDS were the most common alcohol-interactive medication being combined with alcohol followed by prescription anti-histamines and miscellaneous anti-hypertensives [66]. Analysis of the National Health and Nutrition Examination Survey (NHANES) data 1999–2002 indicated the absence of a significantly lower prevalence of alcohol use among older adults taking alcohol-interactive medications such as benzodiazepines, antidepressants and pain medications [67]. In a survey conducted in primary care clinics, a sampling of 549 current drinkers aged 65 years or older found that 11 and 35% were identified as harmful and hazardous drinkers, respectively, by the Alcohol-Related Problem Survey (ARPS). Use of arthritis and pain medications, histamine (H_2)-antagonists, antidepressants and antihypertensive medications conributed to hazardous drinking [68].

In a study involving a large, population-based sample of older adults, at-risk drinking was assessed using a validated measurement tool known as CARET (Comorbidity Alcohol Risk Evaluation Tool) [69]. This study reported that the prevalence of at-risk drinking in older adults between 1971 and 1974 was 10% (18% in men and 5% in women) and that 69% of these at-risk drinkers were identified as such solely because their amount of alcohol consumption was considered risky in the presence of certain co-morbidities and medication use. Pain medications were the most common medications used by at-risk drinkers, while ulcer disease and anxiety disorders were the most common disorders identifying at-risk drinking among women [69]. Another study evaluating at-risk drinking among older adults using CARET found that out of 3308 current drinkers, 1147 were at-risk drinkers. Among at-risk individuals, 61.9% had alcohol use in the context of high-risk comorbidities, 61.0% had high-risk medication use and 64.3% had high-risk alcohol behaviours [70].

The widespread use of CNS-acting medications has been well-documented in many settings, including community, assisted living facilities and nursing homes [71]. The prevalence of antidepressant use increased from 5.84% (95% CI: 5.47–6.23%) in 1996 to 10.12% (95% CI: 9.58–10.69%) in 2005 [72]. An emerging body of literature predicts a rise in the use of alcohol and psychotropic medications among older adults in the future. A study of the National Health Interview and Examination Survey showed previous-week prevalence of alcohol and psychotropic medications being 47.3 and 20.1%, respectively. The prevalence of combined use of alcohol and psychotropic medication was reported to be 7.6% [73]. A retrospective analysis of NHANES 2005–2008 data found the potential concomitant use of alcohol and CNS medication was 8.19% (95% CI: 6.33–10.05%) among older adults taking at least one prescription medication [74]. The study also indicated that antidepressants, opioid analgesics, anticonvulsants and anxiolytics were some of the most commonly use CNS-acting medications. Thus, studies have indicated that potential concomitant use of alcohol and CNS-acting medication is substantial among older adults, though lower in magnitude than their younger counterparts. Considering the vulnerability of this population, it is imperative to investigate and understand the impact of concurrent use of alcohol and medication in older adults.

Consequences of concurrent use of alcohol and medications

Alcohol has been implicated as a risk factor for various adverse health effects, including alcoholic liver disease, pancreatitis, cardiomyopathy, several different cancers, functional and cognitive impairment and accidental injuries. Many of these adverse effects may be confounded by the concurrent use of medications. A retrospective review of all zolpidem-related cases reported in the span of two years to the Illinois Poison Center showed co-ingestion of alcohol and zolpidem was associated with intensive care unit admissions [75]. The risk of acute upper gastrointestinal bleeding was further increased among aspirin and ibuprofen medication users, at all levels of alcohol consumption [76]. High alcohol consumption is associated with the risk of falls in older adults [77]. Very few studies have assessed the adverse health outcomes resulting from concomitant use of alcohol and medications among older adults, perhaps due to the difficulty in capturing the outcome at the appropriate time, underreporting of alcohol use, and lack of awareness of potentially harmful effects of alcohol.

Clinical presentation and evaluation of substance use disorders in the elderly

Unfortunately, because of lack of awareness, insufficient knowledge, limited research data, atypical presentations and hurried office visits, healthcare providers often fail to identify and treat substance abuse among elderly [78]. Diagnosis can be challenging because symptoms of substance abuse in the elderly can mimic symptoms of other medical and behavioural disorders common among this population, such as diabetes, dementia and depression. Patients are often reluctant or ashamed to seek professional help for what is traditionally considered to be a private matter; family disapproval or collusion may contribute to this reticence. Behaviour that would be considered a problem requiring immediate intervention in younger adults does not inspire the same urgency among older adults, although the elderly are likely to experience more adverse consequences from substance abuse than their younger counterparts. Ageing ushers in psychosocial transitions, plus biomedical changes that magnify the effects of alcohol and drugs on the body. Older substance abusers are also more likely to have psychiatric and medical co-morbidities. Epidemiological studies have found up to 30% of older alcohol abusers suffer from a primary mood disorder [79]. A comprehensive clinical evaluation is therefore essential when caring for the elderly. The following case vignettes describe some of the common clinical presentations of substance abuse among elderly patients.

Clinical presentations (case vignettes)

A. Alcohol dependence with medical problems

Harry has struggled with substance abuse since his late teens. Although drinking binges were often followed by periods of sobriety, he inevitably returned to his addiction. At 75 years old, he takes several prescription medications, including warfarin and metoprolol for atrial fibrillation and simvastatin for hyperlipidaemia. Harry has passed out after drinking alcohol and taking his medications, and woken up with bruises and abrasions. He has developed chronic headaches in the last couple of weeks and reports several recent falls. Although his children have been exhausted by previous futile pleas for their father to seek professional help, the family has hired an interventionist to confront Harry about his alcoholism and its negative consequences on his physical and mental health and its effect on his relationships with family and friends.

This case underscores that alcohol dependence is associated with the development of chronic medical conditions such as atrial fibrillation, cardiomyopathy and hyperlipidaemia. It also notes how medications used to treat atrial fibrillation can increase risk for bleeding and falls, especially with continuing misuse of alcohol. Increased head injuries have put the patient at increased risk for the development of subdural haematomas. Dehydration and muscle injury has also increased the patient's risk of rhabdomyolysis, especially if the patient is compliant with the statin.

B. Alcohol dependence with depression

In her early years, Eva would have been described as a 'teetotaller', because she detested the use of alcohol or other intoxicants. In her fifties, Eva began taking occasional sips of wine on special occasions or when she was feeling 'stressed out' and needed to 'relax'. But after her children moved away and her husband and many of her close friends died, Eva has turned to alcohol on a daily basis to cope with grief and loss. At the age of 82, Eva is an alcoholic struggling with depression, anxiety, and insomnia. She takes no medications and has not seen a doctor for 'years'. She has had passive thoughts of suicide, wishing that she could be with her husband. She is tired of living alone and being a burden to her children.

This case illustrates how a patient can develop alcoholism later in life. It also stresses how death, loss and loneliness can precipitate and perpetuate the cycle of addiction. Life changing events compounded with alcohol dependence have resulted in worsening depression, anxiety and insomnia. It is important to complete a safety assessment, especially since Eva is having suicidal ideation and lacks social support at home.

C. Prescription opioid dependence with chronic pain

Bob is 70 year old obese farmer who continues to work despite chronic back pain and arthritis of both knees. After injuring his back 10 years ago while lifting hay bales, Bob has remained on opioids for chronic pain management. Over the years, he has required increases in the dosage of opioids. His current regimen includes both long-acting and short-acting opioids. Bob also takes diazepam and cycloben-zaprine for muscle relaxation. Bob reports a 'boost of energy' when he takes his 'pain pills'. Over the last couple of months, he has consistently run out of his opi-oids prior to his next visit at the pain clinic. He has requested early refills more than once, prompting a warning from the pain clinic that he will be discharged from their practice if he continues these behaviours. He awakens each morning with 'chills, sweats and feeling nauseated'. His wife also notices that his speech is slurred and his gait is unsteady, particularly after his morning dose of medications. This is particularly worrisome since Bob continues to work on the family farm.

This case highlights the fact that a patient can potentially develop addiction from the chronic use of opioids for pain management. In addition to physiological depend-ence, the patient will experience symptoms of cravings, compulsion to obtain and use the substance, continued pattern of use despite negative consequences and loss of control. Opioids combined with benzodiazepines and muscle relaxants can increase risk for oversedation and falls. For chronic pain management, it is impor-tant to incorporate complementary and alternative methods to pain relief, for exam-ple meditation, mindfulness, chiropractic care and acupuncture.

D. Benzodiazepine dependence with anxiety

Alice is a 65 year old retired school teacher who has experienced anxiety since child-hood. As a young teenager, she was sexually abused by her uncle, who threatened to harm her and her parents if she reported the abuse. She developed nightmares and would often awaken in the middle of night screaming. At 16, her parents consulted a psychologist and psychiatrist who diagnosed her with post-traumatic stress disor-der and recommended psychotherapy with a trial of sertraline and clonazepam.

Alice said that the only treatment that 'worked' were the benzodiazepines. Throughout college and during her teaching career, she suffered worsening anxiety and developed increased tolerance to benzodiazepines. Since retiring in recent years, she awakens craving her next dose of clonazepam. She takes more clonazepam than prescribed throughout the day and has blacked out more than once. She has been treated at the emergency room and at urgent care clinics, seeking additional prescriptions for benzodiazepines.

This case underscores the fact that a patient predisposed to anxiety disorder, combined with a history of childhood sexual trauma and post-traumatic stress disorder is at increased risk of not only being prescribed benzodiazepines but also developing an addiction to benzodiazepines. Her symptoms of physiological withdrawal may be masked by her underlying anxiety and sleep disorders.

Medical co-morbidities

Co-morbid medical conditions, such as hypertension, heart disease, diabetes and gastro-oesophageal reflux disease (GERD), psychiatric disorders, including depression and anxiety, and cognitive disorders, such as mild cognitive impairment and Parkinson's disease, affect the presentation of substance use disorders in the elderly [80, 81]. Clinical evaluation should include a review of the multiple drug–drug interactions and an explanation of how poor nutrition (e.g. low albumin) might affect the protein-bound state of medications. Because of the potential social isolation of the elderly, it is recommended that the clinician consider patient medication compliance and follow up for multiple comorbid conditions.

Major alcohol- and drug-related health risks in the elderly may include:

- increased risk of falls;
- increased potential for drug interactions;
- sleep disturbances;
- memory problems, which could impair driving ability;
- worsening of existing medical conditions, such as GERD;
- increased prevalence of cancers (e.g. breast cancer due to longer exposure to alcohol);
- agitation or violent behaviours;
- increased risk of suicide.

Screening for substance use disorders

The co-morbidities described above can make it difficult to differentiate substance use disorders from the effects of ageing. Therefore, the clinician is advised to adopt a high index of suspicion while taking patient history. Every person age 60 or older should be screened for alcohol and other drug use, including prescription and over-the-counter medications as well as supplements [82]. It is recommended that screening for substance use disorders occur in community health and welfare settings, primary care offices, specialty clinics, urgent care, emergency departments

Table 12.1 Physical and psychiatric symptoms or signs that trigger evaluation for substance use disorders in the elderly

Physical Triggers	Psychiatric Triggers
• Seizures • Malnutrition and muscle wasting • Liver function abnormalities • Chronic pain or other unexplained somatic complaints • Incontinence, urinary retention, difficulty urinating • Poor hygiene and self-neglect • Complaints of dry mouth or dehydration • Unexplained nausea and vomiting or gastrointestinal distress • Motor incoordination and shuffling gait • Frequent falls and unexplained bruising and head injuries	• Sleep disturbances • Cognitive impairment with memory problems • Persistent irritability and/or anxiety • Change in mood with depression or elevated affect • Unusual restlessness and agitation • Unusual fatigue • Daytime sedation • Changes in eating habits • Difficulty with concentration • Difficulty with orientation

Source: Adapted from [78] Chapter 4, Figure 4.2.

and inpatient units with a validated tool, such as the AUDIT (Alcohol Use Disorders Identification Test) questionnaire. At-risk drinking patterns in elderly patients are a modifiable health risk and must be identified before treatment can be initiated. Elderly patients may not fit the profile of chronic drinkers. Patients commonly minimize the impact of their alcohol and drug use, and clinicians may overlook substance use assessment in the elderly patient. Physical and psychiatric symptoms/signs to trigger screening for substance use disorder in the elderly are summarized in Table 12.1. Clinicians should be familiar with signs and symptoms that arouse suspicion of possible substance abuse [78].

Evaluation of substance use disorders

A comprehensive evaluation of the elderly with substance use disorders should include assessment of the following conditions:

• physical;
• mental (psychological);
• cognitive capacity, which affects motivation, attention span, the ability to evaluate new situations and to acquire new skills;
• nutrition;
• chronic pain;
• social and environmental;
• overall general functioning;
• medication interactions.

Table 12.2 Clinical evaluation of substance use disorders in the elderly

- Alcohol and drug history
- Prescription drug history (e.g. confirm from pharmacy or prescription bottles and cross-check what patient takes with what is prescribed; confirm with prescription monitoring programme if database available)
- Psychiatric history and mental status with particular attention to depression, anxiety and insomnia
- Cognitive examination
- Collateral history from care giver and family for behavioural changes
- Physical and neurologic examination
- Laboratory tests, including alcohol levels, drug screens as necessary along with routine laboratory tests
- Additional studies if clinically indicated, such as brain MRI, liver ultrasound or upper endoscopy

These assessments (see also Table 12.2) should continually be updated to guide management, such as to monitor and treat withdrawal syndromes for when the elderly abstain from alcohol and/or drugs. Abstinence and sobriety may be associated with improvements in medical and/or psychiatric conditions. In the elderly, memory and executive skills may take weeks to months before significant improvements are observed on neuropsychological testing.

Cognitive impairment in the elderly with substance use disorders

Substance use may mask underlying conditions, such as cognitive impairment. It is important to determine whether cognitive impairment is acute, as in the case of delirium, or if it is chronic or an acute exacerbation of a chronic condition. The clinician should gather a thorough substance use history, especially for benzodiazepines and opioids; obtain collateral information; and order indicated laboratory tests, such as alcohol and drug levels.

Delirium may be secondary to drug intoxication or withdrawal (e.g. alcohol and/or benzodiazepines). Substances may worsen underlying medical conditions, such as liver cirrhosis, and lead to hepatic encephalopathy. Wernicke's encephalopathy due to thiamine deficiency should be considered in an alcoholic. Subdural hematoma following multiple head injuries while intoxicated can lead to acute confusion. Withdrawal seizures can also cause post-ictal confusion.

The following studies may be indicated depending on the clinical presentation:

- urinalysis;
- blood cultures;
- urine drug screen;
- blood alcohol concentration;
- routine blood tests (e.g. liver function, renal function, complete blood count (CBC) with differential, thyroid function, lipids);
- X-rays;

- electrocardiogram;
- electroencephalogram (EEG);
- computed tomography (CT) and/or magnetic resonance imageing (MRI) scans.

For nonacute or lingering cognitive impairment, differential diagnoses may include the following: alcohol-related frontal lobe impairment, alcoholic dementia, Korsakoff's syndrome, Alzheimer's dementia, neoplasm and/or cerebrovascular accident (CVA). Psychiatric disorders that may present with cognitive changes include major depressive disorder, mania, severe anxiety disorder and/or psychosis.

Safety assessment of the elderly with substance use disorders

A risk assessment can help determine whether it is safe for patient to live independently. Consulting a social worker along with occupational and physical therapists may be crucial in assessing safety and making recommendations for level of care. Whenever possible, it is important to involve the family in discussing the patient's limitations and requirements for daily living, including the possible need to move to a skilled nursing facility. If the patient suffers significant cognitive impairment, the treatment team should consider guardianship for the patient's safety. This may include involuntary treatment for life-threatening conditions.

Medications for individuals with substance use disorders

The US Food and Drug Administration (FDA)-approved medications for the treatment of alcohol dependence include the following [83–86]:

- *Disulfiram* causes an acutely toxic physical reaction when mixed with alcohol, which is considered to increase the patient's motivation to remain abstinent.
- *Acamprosate* helps modulate and normalize alcohol-related changes in brain activity, reducing symptoms of protracted withdrawal (e.g. disturbances in sleep or mood).
- *Oral naltrexone* reduces the rewarding effects of alcohol and the craving for it.
- *Extended-release injectable naltrexone* helps address patient nonadherence, which can limit the effectiveness of oral naltrexone.

In the United States, the Substance Abuse and Mental Health Services Administration (SAMHSA)'s Treatment Improvement Protocol (TIP) 49, 'Incorporating Alcohol Pharmacotherapies Into Medical Practice', gives a detailed description of clinical practice guidelines for using four medications in the medication-assisted treatment of alcoholism and alcohol abuse: acamprosate, disulfiram, oral naltrexone and extended-release injectable naltrexone [83]. In the United Kingdom, the National Institute for Health and Clinical Excellence (NICE) published, in 2011, Clinical Guidelines 'CG115 Alcohol-use disorders: diagnosis, assessment and management of harmful drinking and alcohol dependence' [87]. For harmful drinkers and people with mild alcohol dependence, NICE recommends offering a psychological intervention (such as cognitive behavioural therapies, behavioural therapies or social network and environment-based therapies) focused specifically on alcohol-related cognitions, behaviour, problems and social networks. Regarding interventions for moderate and severe alcohol dependence, NICE recommends offering acamprosate or oral naltrexone in combination with an individual psychological intervention (cognitive behavioural therapies, behavioural therapies or social network and environment-based therapies) focused specifically on alcohol misuse [87].

The FDA-approved medications for the treatment of opioid addiction include [88]:

- Naltrexone (oral and injectable depot Vivitrol®);
- Buprenorphine (Subutex®, Suboxone®; Zubsolv®);
- Methadone (Dolophine®).

SAMHSA's Treatment Improvement Protocol 40 (TIP 40), 'Clinical Guidelines for the Use of Buprenorphine', offers guidelines to physicians using buprenorphine for the medication-assisted treatment of opioid addiction, including the pharmacology of buprenorphine, patient assessment, treatment protocols, needs of special populations and policies and procedures [89]. Treatment Improvement Protocol 43 (TIP 43), 'Medication-Assisted Treatment for Opioid Addiction in Opioid Treatment Programs', provides updated information on effective treatment practices and care for individuals with opioid use disorders [88]. In July 2013, the FDA approved Zubsolv (buprenorphine/naloxone, Orexo AB) for maintenance treatment of opioid dependence (www.fda.gov/downloads/Drugs/DrugSafety/UCM362203.pdf).

In the United Kingdom, the National Institute for Health and Clinical Excellence published Technology Appraisal Guidance TA11, 'Naltrexone for the management of opioid dependence'. Naltrexone is recommended as a treatment option in detoxified formerly opioid-dependent people who are highly motivated to remain in an abstinence programme. According to NICE, naltrexone should only be administered under adequate supervision to people who have been fully informed of the potential adverse effects of treatment and it should be given as part of a programme of supportive care. The effectiveness of naltrexone in preventing opioid misuse in people being treated should be reviewed regularly and discontinuation of naltrexone treatment should be considered if there is evidence of such misuse [90].

Currently available FDA-approved pharmacotherapy for nicotine dependence includes [91, 92]:

- Nicotine Replacement Therapy: patch (NicoDerm CQ®), nasal spray (Nicotrol® NS), lozenge (Commit®), gum (Nicorette®) and oral inhaler (Nicotrol®).
- Bupropion sustained release formulation (Zyban®).
- Varenicline (Chantix®).

For additional reviews of treatments, refer to the following chapters: Tobacco Use Cessation (Chapter 15), Pharmacological and Integrated Treatments in Older Adults with Substance Use Disorders (Chapter 20) and Age-Sensitive Psychosocial Treatment for Older Adults with Substance Abuse (Chapter 22).

Conclusions

Substance abuse in the elderly is a significant and frequently unrecognized problem. Clinicians can help patients avoid potential health consequences through the use of screening tools and the development of an appropriate treatment strategy. Clinicians are advised to pay particular attention to co-morbid medical and psychiatric conditions and prescription medications with potential for drug interactions. Systematic screening of all patients reduces the chance that substance abuse will remain undetected. Once identified, at-risk individuals can benefit from brief interventions in clinic or community settings or a combination of pharmacotherapy and behavioural interventions.

References

1. Howden, L.M. and Meyer, A.J. (2011) *Age and Sex Composition: 2010*. 2010 Census Briefs, US Department of Commerce, Washington, DC.
2. Han, B., Gfroerer, J.C., Colliver, J.D. and Penne, M.A (2009) Substance use disorder among older adults in the United States in 2020. *Addiction*, **104**(1), 88–96.
3. Blazer, D.G. and Wu, L.-T. (2009) The epidemiology of substance use and disorders among middle aged and elderly community adults: national survey on drug use and health. *Am J Geriatr Psychiatry*, **17**(3), 237–245.
4. Blazer, D.G. and Wu, L.-T. (2009) The epidemiology of at-risk and binge drinking among middle-aged and elderly community adults: National Survey on Drug Use and Health. *Am J Psychiatry*, **166**(10), 1162–1169.
5. Merrick, E.S., Hodgkin, D., Garnick, D.W., *et al.*, (2011) Older adults' inpatient and emergency department utilization for ambulatory-care-sensitive conditions: relationship with alcohol consumption. *J Aging Health*, **23**(1), 86–111.
6. Wu, L.-T. and Blazer, D.G. (2011) Illicit and nonmedical drug use among older adults: a review. *J Aging Health*, **23**(3), 481–504.
7. Substance Abuse and Mental Health Services Administration (2011) *The NSDUH Report: Illicit Drug Use among Older Adults*. Substance Abuse and Mental Health Services Administration, Rockville, MD.
8. Blazer, D.G. and Wu, L.-T. (2009) Nonprescription use of pain relievers by middle-aged and elderly community-living adults: National Survey on Drug Use and Health. *J Am Geriatr Soc*, **57**(7), 1252–1257.
9. Substance Abuse and Mental Health Services Administration (2007) *The DASIS Report: Older Adults in Substance Abuse Treatment: 2005*. Substance Abuse and Mental Health Services Administration, Rockville, MD.
10. Substance Abuse and Mental Health Services Administration (2011) *The TEDS Report: Substance Abuse Treatment Admissions for Abuse of Benzodiazepines*. Substance Abuse and Mental Health Services Administration, Rockville, MD.
11. Substance Abuse and Mental Health Services Administration (2010) *The DAWN Report: Emergency Department Visits involving Illicit Drug Use by Older Adults: 2008*. Substance Abuse and Mental Health Services Administration, Rockville, MD.
12. Substance Abuse and Mental Health Services Administration (2006) *The DAWN Report: Opiate-related Drug Misuse Deaths in Six States: 2003*. Substance Abuse and Mental Health Services Administration, Rockville, MD.

13. Substance Abuse and Mental Health Services Administration (2009) *Emergency Department visits involving Nonmedical Use of Selected Pharmaceuticals*. Substance Abuse and Mental Health Services Administration, Rockville, MD.
14. Substance Abuse and Mental Health Services Administration (2012) *The DAWN Report: Drug-related Emergency Department Visits involving Pharmaceutical Misuse or Abuse by Older Adults: 2009*. Substance Abuse and Mental Health Services Administration, Rockville, MD.
15. Sacco, P., Bucholz, K.K. and Spitznagel, E.L. (2009) Alcohol use among older adults in the National Epidemiologic Survey on Alcohol and Related Conditions: a latent class analysis. *J Stud Alcohol Drugs*, **70**(6), 829–838.
16. Preville, M., Boyer, R., Grenier, S. *et al.* (2008) The epidemiology of psychiatric disorders in Quebec's older adult population. *Can J Psychiatry*, **53**(12), 822–832.
17. Lofwall, M.R., Brooner, R.K., Bigelow, G.E. *et al.* (2005) Characteristics of older opioid maintenance patients. *J Subst Abuse Treat*, **28**(3), 265–272.
18. Rosen, D., Smith, M.L. and Reynolds, C.F., 3rd (2008) The prevalence of mental and physical health disorders among older methadone patients. *Am J Geriatr Psychiatry*, **16**(6), 488–497.
19. Cicero, T.J., Surratt, H.L., Kurtz, S. *et al.* (2012) Patterns of prescription opioid abuse and comorbidity in an ageing treatment population. *J Subst Abuse Treat*, **42**(1), 87–94.
20. Shi, S. and Klotz, U. (2011) Age-related changes in pharmacokinetics. *Curr Drug Metab*, **12**(7), 601–610.
21. Bowie, M.W. and Slattum, P.W. (2007) Pharmacodynamics in older adults: a review. *Am J Geriatr Pharmacother*, **5**(3), 263–303.
22. Wise, R.A. and Bozarth, M.A. (1985) Brain mechanisms of drug reward and euphoria. *Psychiatr Med*, **3**(4), 445–460.
23. Koob, G.F. (1992) Drugs of abuse: anatomy, pharmacology and function of reward pathways. *Trends Pharmacol Sci*, **13**(5), 177–184.
24. Tzschentke, T.M. and Schmidt, W.J. (2000) Functional relationship among medial pre-frontal cortex, nucleus accumbens, and ventral tegmental area in locomotion and reward. *Crit Rev Neurobiol*, **14**(2), 131–142.
25. Koob, G.F. and Volkow, N.D. (2010) Neurocircuitry of addiction. *Neuropsychopharmacology*, **35**(1), 217–238.
26. Koob, G.F. and Nestler, E.J. (1997) The neurobiology of drug addiction. *J Neuropsychiatry Clin Neurosci*, **9**(3), 482–597.
27. Jones, A.W. and Neri, A. (1985) Age-related differences in blood ethanol parameters and subjective feelings of intoxication in healthy men. *Alcohol Alcohol*, **20**(1), 45–52.
28. Vestal, R.E., McGuire, E.A., Tobin, J.D. *et al.* (1977) Ageing and ethanol metabolism. *Clin Pharmacol Ther*, **21**(3), 343–354.
29. Pozzato, G., Moretti, M., Franzin, F. *et al.* (1995) Ethanol metabolism and ageing: the role of "first pass metabolism" and gastric alcohol dehydrogenase activity. *J Gerontol A Biol Sci Med Sci*, **50**(3), B135–141.
30. Oneta, C.M., Pedrosa, M., Rüttimann, S. *et al.* (2001) Age and bioavailability of alcohol. *Z Gastroenterol*, **39**(9), 783–788.
31. Ramchandani, V.A., W.F. Bosron, and T.K. Li, (2001) Research advances in ethanol metabolism. *Pathol Biol (Paris)*, **49**(9), 676–682.
32. Kalant, H. (1998) Pharmacological interactions of ageing and alcohol. In: *Alcohol Problems and Ageing* (eds E.S.L. Gomberg, A.M. Hegedus and R.A. Zucker). NIAAA Research Mongraph No. 33, NIH Publication No. 98-4163, NIAAA, Rockville, MD.
33. Lucey, M.R., Hill, E.M., Young, J.P. *et al.* (1999) The influences of age and gender on blood ethanol concentrations in healthy humans. *J Stud Alcohol*, **60**(1), 103–110.

34. Tupler, L.A., Hege, S. and Ellinwood, E.H., Jr. (1995) Alcohol pharmacodynamics in young-elderly adults contrasted with young and middle-aged subjects. *Psychopharmacology (Berl)*, **118**(4), 460–470.

35. Brower, K.J. (2001) Alcohol's effects on sleep in alcoholics. *Alcohol Res Health*, **25**(2), 110–125.

36. Schuckit, M.A. (2012) Alcohol and Alcoholism. In: *Harrison's Principles of Internal Medicine* (eds D.L. Longo, A. Fauci, D. Kasper *et al.*). McGraw-Hill Professional, New York, NY, pp. 3546–3551.

37. Ferreira, M.P. and Weems, M.K. (2008) Alcohol consumption by ageing adults in the United States: health benefits and detriments. *J Am Diet Assoc*, **108**(10), 1668–1676.

38. Mukamal, K.J., Chung, H., Jenny, N.S. *et al.* (2006) Alcohol consumption and risk of coronary heart disease in older adults: the Cardiovascular Health Study. *J Am Geriatr Soc*, **54**(1), 30–37.

39. Brien, S.E., Ronksley, P.E., Turner, B.J. *et al.* (2008) Effect of alcohol consumption on biological markers associated with risk of coronary heart disease: systematic review and meta-analysis of interventional studies. *BMJ*, 2011. **342**, d636.

40. Collins, M.A., Neafsey, E.J., Mukamal, K.J. *et al.* (2009) Alcohol in moderation, cardioprotection, and neuroprotection: epidemiological considerations and mechanistic studies. *Alcohol Clin Exp Res*, **33**(2), 206–219.

41. Ronksley, P.E., Brien, S.E., Turner, B.J. *et al.* (2011) Association of alcohol consumption with selected cardiovascular disease outcomes: a systematic review and meta-analysis. *BMJ*, **342**, d671.

42. Mukamal, K.J., Kuller, L.H., Fitzpatrick, A.L. *et al.* (2003) Prospective study of alcohol consumption and risk of dementia in older adults. *JAMA*, **289**(11), 1405–1413.

43. Resnick, B. (2003) Alcohol use in a continuing care retirement community. *J Gerontol Nurs*, **29**(10), 22–29.

44. Spanagel, R., Herz, A. and Shippenberg, T.S. (1992) Opposing tonically active endogenous opioid systems modulate the mesolimbic dopaminergic pathway. *Proc Natl Acad Sci USA*, **89**(6), 2046–2050.

45. Tanda, G. and Di Chiara, G. (1998) A dopamine-mu1 opioid link in the rat ventral tegmentum shared by palatable food (Fonzies) and non-psychostimulant drugs of abuse. *Eur J Neurosci*, **10**(3), 1179–1187.

46. Schoch, P., Richards, J.G., Häring, P. *et al.* (1985) Co-localization of GABA receptors and benzodiazepine receptors in the brain shown by monoclonal antibodies. *Nature*, **314**(6007), 168–171.

47. Sanger, D.J. (2004) The pharmacology and mechanisms of action of new generation, nonbenzodiazepine hypnotic agents. *CNS Drugs*, **18**(Suppl 1), 9–15 [discussion 41, 43–45].

48. Greenblatt, D.J., Harmatz, J.S. and Shader, R.I. (1991) Clinical pharmacokinetics of anxiolytics and hypnotics in the elderly. Therapeutic considerations (Part I). *Clin Pharmacokinet*, **21**(3), 165–177.

49. Greenblatt, D.J., Harmatz, J.S. and Shader, R.I. (1991) Clinical pharmacokinetics of anxiolytics and hypnotics in the elderly. Therapeutic considerations (Part II). *Clin Pharmacokinet*, **21**(4), 262–273.

50. Olubodun, J.O., Ochs, H.R., von Moltke, L.L. *et al.* (2003) Pharmacokinetic properties of zolpidem in elderly and young adults: possible modulation by testosterone in men. *Br J Clin Pharmacol*, **56**(3), 297–304.

51. Buffett-Jerrott, S.E. and Stewart, S.H. (2002) Cognitive and sedative effects of benzodiazepine use. *Curr Pharm Des*, **8**(1), 45–58.

52. Pifl, C., Drobny, H., Reither, H. *et al.* (1995) Mechanism of the dopamine-releasing actions of amphetamine and cocaine: plasmalemmal dopamine transporter versus vesicular monoamine transporter. *Mol Pharmacol*, **47**(2), 368–373.

53. White, F.J. and Kalivas, P.W. (1998) Neuroadaptations involved in amphetamine and cocaine addiction. *Drug Alcohol Depend*, 51(1–2), 141–153.
54. Bowers, M.S., Chen, B.T. and Bonci, A. (2010) AMPA receptor synaptic plasticity induced by psychostimulants: the past, present, and therapeutic future. *Neuron*, 67(1), 11–24.
55. Schultz, W. (1998) Predictive reward signal of dopamine neurons. *J Neurophysiol*, 80(1), 1–27.
56. Pertwee, R.G., Howlett, A.C., Abood, M.E. *et al.* (2010) International Union of Basic and Clinical Pharmacology. LXXIX. Cannabinoid receptors and their ligands: beyond CB(1) and CB(2). *Pharmacol Rev*, 62(4), 588–631.
57. NCPIE (National Council on Patient Information and Education) (2010) *Fact Sheet: Medicine Use and Older Adults. MUST (Medication Use Safety Training) for Seniors*, NCPIE, Rockville, MD. www.mustforseniors.org (last accessed 8 April 2014).
58. Wilson, I.B., Schoen, C., Neuman, P. *et al.* (2007) Physician–patient communication about prescription medication nonadherence: a 50-state study of America's seniors. *J Gen Intern Med*, 22(1), 6–12.
59. Weathermon, R. and Crabb, D.W. (1999) Alcohol and medication interactions. *Alcohol Res Health*, 23(1), 40–54.
60. Moore, A.A., Whiteman, E.J. and Ward, K.T. (2007) Risks of combined alcohol/medication use in older adults. *Am J Geriatr Pharmacother*, 5(1), 64–74.
61. Davies, M. (2003) The role of GABAA receptors in mediating the effects of alcohol in the central nervous system. *J Psychiatry Neurosci*, 28(4), 263–274.
62. Duru, O.K., Xu, H., Tseng, C.H. *et al.* (2010) Correlates of alcohol-related discussions between older adults and their physicians. *J Am Geriatr Soc*, 58(12), 2369–2374.
63. Lin, J.C., Karno, M.P., Barry, K.L. *et al.* (2010) Determinants of early reductions in drinking in older at-risk drinkers participating in the intervention arm of a trial to reduce at-risk drinking in primary care. *J Am Geriatr Soc*, 58(2), 227–233.
64. Benza, A.T., Calvert, S. and McQuown, C.B. (2010) Prevention BINGO: reducing medication and alcohol use risks for older adults. *Aging Ment Health*, 14(8), 1008–1014.
65. Forster, L.E., Pollow, R. and Stoller, E.P. (1993) Alcohol use and potential risk for alcohol-related adverse drug reactions among community-based elderly. *J Community Health*, 18(4), 225–239.
66. Pringle, K.E., Ahern, F.M., Heller, D.A. *et al.* (2005) Potential for alcohol and prescription drug interactions in older people. *J Am Geriatr Soc*, 53(11), 1930–1936.
67. Jalbert, J.J. and Lapane, K.L. (2008) Unhealthy alcohol consumption among older adults. *J Am Geriatr Soc*, 56(9), 1769–1770.
68. Fink, A., Morton, S.C., Beck, J.C. *et al.* (2002) The alcohol-related problems survey: identifying hazardous and harmful drinking in older primary care patients. *J Am Geriatr Soc*, 50(10), 1717–1722.
69. Moore, A.A., Giuli, L., Gould, R. *et al.* (2006) Alcohol use, comorbidity, and mortality. *J Am Geriatr Soc*, 54(5), 757–762.
70. Barnes, A.J., Moore, A.A., Xu, H. *et al.* (2010) Prevalence and correlates of at-risk drinking among older adults: the project SHARE study. *J Gen Intern Med*, 25(8), 840–846.
71. Lindsey, P.L. (2009) Psychotropic medication use among older adults: what all nurses need to know. *J Gerontol Nurs*, 35(9), 28–38.
72. Olfson, M. and Marcus, S.C. (2009) National patterns in antidepressant medication treatment. *Arch Gen Psychiatry*, 66(8), 848–856.
73. Du, Y., Scheidt-Nave, C. and Knopf, H. (2008) Use of psychotropic drugs and alcohol among non-institutionalised elderly adults in Germany. *Pharmacopsychiatry*, 41(6), 242–251.
74. Mohanty, M., Harpe, S.E. and Slattum, P.W. (2012) Concurrent use of alcohol and central nervous system (CNS)-acting medications among older adults. *Clin Pharmacol Ther*, 91(Suppl), S134.

75. Zosel, A., Osterberg, E.C. and Mycyk, M.B. (2011) Zolpidem misuse with other medications or alcohol frequently results in intensive care unit admission. *Am J Ther*, **18**(4), 305–308.

76. Kaufman, D.W., Kelly, J.P., Wiholm, B.E. *et al.* (1999) The risk of acute major upper gastrointestinal bleeding among users of aspirin and ibuprofen at various levels of alcohol consumption. *Am J Gastroenterol*, **94**(11), 3189–3196.

77. Mukamal, K.J., Mittleman, M.A., Longstreth, W.T. Jr *et al.* (2004) Self-reported alcohol consumption and falls in older adults: cross-sectional and longitudinal analyses of the cardiovascular health study. *J Am Geriatr Soc*, **52**(7), 1174–1179.

78. Substance Abuse and Mental Health Services Administration (1998) *Substance Abuse among Older Adults*. Treatment Improvement Protocol (TIP) Series No. 26, Substance Abuse and Mental Health Services Administration, Rockville, MD.

79. Lin, J.C., Karno, M.P., Grella, C.E. *et al.* (2011) Alcohol, tobacco, and nonmedical drug use disorders in U.S. Adults aged 65 years and older: data from the 2001–2002 National Epidemiologic Survey of Alcohol and Related Conditions. *Am J Geriatr Psychiatry*, **19**(3), 292–299.

80. Ryan, M., Merrick, E.L., Hodgkin, D. *et al.* (2013) Drinking patterns of older adults with chronic medical conditions. *J Gen Intern Med*, **28**(10), 1326–1332.

81. Blow, F.C., Serras, A.M. and Barry, K.L. (2007) Late-life depression and alcoholism. *Curr Psychiatry Rep*, **9**(1), 14–19.

82. Haber, P., Lintzeris, N., Proude, E. and Lopatko, O. (2009) *Guidelines for the Treatment of Alcohol Problems*. Department of Health and Ageing, Australia.

83. Substance Abuse and Mental Health Services Administration (2009) *Incorporating Alcohol Pharmacotherapies Into Medical Practice*. Treatment Improvement Protocol (TIP) Series 49, Substance Abuse and Mental Health Services Administration, Rockville, MD.

84. Ooteman, W., Naassila, M., Koeter, M.W. *et al.* (2009) Predicting the effect of naltrexone and acamprosate in alcohol-dependent patients using genetic indicators. *Addict Biol*, **14**(3), 328–337.

85. Lee, J.D., Grossman, E., DiRocco, D. *et al.* (2010) Extended-release naltrexone for treatment of alcohol dependence in primary care. *J Subst Abuse Treat*, **39**(1), 14–21.

86. Pettinati, H.M., Oslin, D.W., Kampman, K.M. *et al.* (2010) A double-blind, placebo-controlled trial combining sertraline and naltrexone for treating co-occurring depression and alcohol dependence. *Am J Psychiatry*, **167**(6), 668–675.

87. NICE (2011) *Alcohol-Use Disorders: Diagnosis, Assessment and Management of Harmful Drinking and Alcohol Dependence*. Clinical Guidelines CG115, NICE (National Institute for Health and Care Excellence), UK.

88. Substance Abuse and Mental Health Services Administration (2008) *Medication-Assisted Treatment for Opioid Addiction in Opioid Treatment Programs*. Treatment Improvement Protocol (TIP) Series 43, Substance Abuse and Mental Health Services Administration, Rockville, MD.

89. Substance Abuse and Mental Health Services Administration (2005) *Clinical Guidelines for the Use of Buprenorphine in the Treatment of Opioid Addiction*. Treatment Improvement Protocol (TIP) Series 40, Substance Abuse and Mental Health Services Administration, Rockville, MD.

90. NICE (2007) Naltrexone for the Management of Opioid Dependence. Technology Appraisal Guidance TA11, NICE (National Institute for Health and Care Excellence), UK.

91. FDA (Food and Drug Administration) (2012) *FDA 101: Smoking Cessation Products*. Food and Drug Administration, Silver Spring, MD.

92. Update Panel, Liaisons and Staff (2008) A clinical practice guideline for treating tobacco use and dependence: 2008 update. A US Public Health Service report. *Am J Prev Med*, **35**(2), 158–176.

Section 4

COMPREHENSIVE GERIATRIC ASSESSMENT AND SPECIAL NEEDS OF OLDER PEOPLE

Chapter 13

COMPREHENSIVE GERIATRIC ASSESSMENT AND THE SPECIAL NEEDS OF OLDER PEOPLE

Dan Wilson[1], Stephen Jackson[1], Ilana B. Crome[2,3,4,5], Rahul (Tony) Rao[6] and Peter Crome[7]

[1] King's College Hospital NHS Foundation Trust, UK
[2] Keele University, UK
[3] Queen Mary University of London, UK
[4] Imperial College University of London, UK
[5] South Staffordshire and Shropshire Healthcare NHS Foundation Trust, UK
[6] Institute of Psychiatry/South London and Maudsley NHS Foundation Trust, UK
[7] University College London, UK

Background

Older people continue to form a progressively larger proportion of the general population. This, in turn, is compounded by changes in attitudes towards substance use for the so-called *baby boomer* population, the oldest of whom are now in their seventh decade [1]. There is some evidence to suggest that those older people who drink alcohol in later life continue to do so into their ninth and tenth decades, with the emergence of an increasing 'oldest old' population [2]. The number of people aged 90+ in England and Wales accounted for 1% of the population in 2011. This population has increased by 26% since 2002 [3] and will continue to rise.

With growing numbers of older people requiring care for substance misuse, it is imperative that their needs are addressed and met within clinical services [4, 5]. Such service provision should take into account not only the special considerations inherent in the ageing process but also sociocultural influences, such as the effects of previous occupation [6] and ethnicity [7, 8]. Some geographical areas, such as those covering inner city populations offer additional challenges through a combination of both these risk factors as well as that of socioeconomic deprivation [9]

In the United Kingdom, some progress has been made in providing an evidence base, the findings of which have been used to influence policy through the implementation of national frameworks, particularly in the screening of alcohol misuse in primary care, review of safe drinking limits for older people and service provision for alcohol-related brain injury [10, 11].

Substance Use and Older People, First Edition.
Edited by Ilana B. Crome, Li-Tzy Wu, Rahul (Tony) Rao and Peter Crome.
© 2015 John Wiley & Sons, Ltd. Published 2015 by John Wiley & Sons, Ltd.

Clinical services, such as those found within geriatric inpatient units and community old age psychiatry settings, are still ill-equipped to provide the knowledge, skills and attitudes needed for the comprehensive assessment, treatment and care of older people with substance misuse [12, 13].

Integrated service models that combine expertise in care of the elderly medicine, old age psychiatry and substance misuse remain in their infancy but the development of dual diagnosis training within these services is a positive step and may pave the way for a wider programme to improve competencies in professionals who come into contact with older substance misusers in their everyday clinical practice [14].

For the purposes of this chapter, the terms substance use, misuse, abuse, dependence and addiction are used interchangeably.

For the purposes of diagnosis two classification systems can be used: DSM-5 [15] and ICD-10 [16]. However, older people may not fulfil the criteria required to come to a diagnosis of substance use disorder according DSM-5 or dependence syndrome in ICD-10. This is illustrated in Table 13.1. For example, older people: may not develop withdrawal symptoms; may not be able to discern whether they are taking larger amounts over a longer period than was intended because cognitive impairment may affect self-monitoring; might not have tried to cut down on use because there may be reduced social pressure to do so; may not have had to spend increased time obtaining substances because of lower levels of use than younger people; might not have had to give up activities because of use because activities are

Table 13.1 Diagnostic and statistical manual criteria for substance use disorder (SUD)

The presence of at least two of these symptoms indicates a Substance Use Disorder (SUD). The severity of SUD is defined as Mild (the presence of 2–3 symptoms); Moderate (presence of 4–5 symptoms) or Severe (the presence of 6 or more symptoms). However, this is based on an adult population, rather than older adults.

	Criteria	Special considerations for older adults
1	Substance taken in larger amounts or over a longer period than intended	Cognitive impairment may interfere with self-monitoring
2	There is a persistent desire or unsuccessful efforts to cut down or control substance use	There may be reduced social pressures to decrease harmful use
3	A great of time is spent in activities necessary to obtain substances, or recover from effects	Negative effects may occur at relatively low levels of use
4 New criterion	Craving or a strong desire or urge to use substances	Older people may not recognize the urges as cravings, or may attribute it to something else

Table 13.1 (*continued*)

	Criteria	Special considerations for older adults
5	Recurrent substance use resulting in failure to fulfil major role obligations of work, school or home	The roles and expectations of older people and their families might have changed so that this is not acknowledged as a problem
6	Continued use despite having persistent or recurrent social or interpersonal problems caused or exacerbated by substance use	Older people may not realize that the problems are associated with substance use
7	Important social occupational or recreational activities are given up or reduced due to substance use	Older people may have decreased activities due to physical and psychiatric co-morbidities or 'slowing down'
		Social isolation and disabilities may detection more difficult
8	Recurrent use in situations in which it is physically hazardous	Older people may not realize that a situation that was once safe, has become physically hazardous
9	Substance use is continued despite knowledge of having a persistent or recurrent physical or psychological problem that is likely to have been caused or exacerbated by substances	Older people may not realise that these symptoms are substance related Practitioners may not attribute some or all problems as substance related

Adapted from DSM-5 [15], Blow [17] and Crome [1]

reduced due to co-morbid disorders, social isolation and disability; might continue use despite being made aware of the relationship of substance use to physical and psychological problems because of lack of understanding or poor memory.

Assessment

The components of the assessment process will be determined by the setting in which this initially takes place, the culture of the environment in relation to older people and substance misuse, particularly barriers to assessment and high risk features in the presenting situation and clinical presentation, opportunities to engage with colleagues and carers in obtaining additional information and the general principles of physical and psychiatric assessment of older people.

Setting

The initial setting for the assessment of older people with substance misuse will also determine the nature and depth of assessment carried out. This will, in turn, be influenced by the training received. At the very least, all staff should be equipped with the core skills in the detection of substance misuse, so that brief intervention and further assessment may offered in a timely manner.

In hospital settings, it is essential that frontline clinical staff have the competencies to be able to detect the acute and chronic effects of substances, including intoxication, overdose, withdrawal and dependence. This is particularly important for the assessment of alcohol misuse, with extra vigilance over accompanying physical disorders such as hypertension, diabetes mellitus and disorders affecting mobility. Interactions with prescribed and over-the-counter medication should also not be overlooked.

It is important that patient management does not stop at assessment and treatment of the acute phase of substance misuse, so that further assessment can offer the chance for extended brief interventions, referral to specialist services and developing an integrated care plan that includes harm reduction and social integration.

In the community, there is a wealth of untapped expertise for primary care, old age psychiatry and addiction psychiatry services to work together. There currently exists both sequential and parallel service delivery for older people with substance misuse. For example, old age psychiatrists are most likely to see older people with alcohol misuse and dual diagnosis; addiction services provide care for the majority of older people with illicit opiate misuse and primary care professionals are most likely to see a wide variety of substance misuse problems, mainly alcohol but also misuse of sedative/hypnotics, over-the-counter medication and prescribed opiate-containing analgesics. Geriatric medicine services are likely to see a combination of the above.

It should also be borne in mind that nonmedical professionals are likely to encounter older substance misusers. This group of professionals includes those working in voluntary sector and third party service provider organizations, social workers, liaison nurses and those working in supported housing and long-term care settings.

Barriers to assessment

Barriers to assessment in the detection of substance misuse remain considerable. Ageism is problematic and frequently encountered, particularly from carers and relatives (more so than from health professionals), with perceptions ranging from 'it is all that (s)he has left in life' to '(s)he has always been a poor sleeper' and '(s)he has always been fussy with food'. It is acknowledged that geriatricians are less likely than general physicians to screen for alcohol use [18]. Older people are known to under-report their substance misuse, with up to a fourfold difference when compared to their younger counterparts [19]. Self-underreporting may be associated with self-perceived moral weakness and the stigma associated with substance misuse. In a busy clinical setting, the clinical signs of substance misuse, such as lack of energy and changes in mood, may be misattributed to depression or physical illness. Lastly, a lower level of detection may be attributable to stereotyping, such as not asking about substance misuse in older women [20]. Time constraints and lack of sufficient training may also impact on carrying out a complete assessment that can fully inform referral and treatment [21, 22].

There are also several other barriers to screening. Transport is problematic in rural communities [23]. The effect of reduced social support networks [24] will mean a reduced likelihood that carers and other sources of support will be able to provide collateral information. Financial constraints may also apply where the structure of insurance policies can be a barrier to initial assessment.

High-risk groups

There are some similarities between older and younger people in their risk profile for substance misuse. These risk factors include homelessness [25], a past history of substance misuse [26] and depression [27]. However, other risk factors have greater relevance for older people, such as recent bereavement [28], retirement [29], social isolation [30] and immobility [31].

Presenting problems

The clinical presentation will be affected by the pharmacology of the drug or combination of drugs, the quantity, frequency, route of use, contaminants and purity. A recent publication by the British Medical Association [32] has presented detailed up-to-date information on the effects, acute adverse reactions, intoxication and chronic use of illicit drugs. The following is a brief summary of the impact of the use of such drugs.

In acute hospital settings, older people may present with acute intoxication, rendering further assessment problematic, particularly for alcohol intoxication. Alcohol intoxication increases the risk of other pathologies, for example trauma from head injury. There is no absolute threshold below which there are no effects. At a blood alcohol concentration (BAC) of 25 mg% the person may feel euphoric. Disinhibition, aggression, lability of mood may be associated. Between a BAC of 50 and 100 mg% there is lack of coordination, and between a BAC of 100 and 200 mg% there is unsteadiness, ataxia and poor judgment. Amnesic periods ensue at a BAC of 200–400 mg%. Slurred speech, nystagmus, flushed facies and conjunctival injection may accompany other symptoms. High tolerance may be associated with high alcohol levels but low levels of impairment. A low alcohol dose in the elderly is associated with greater subjective perception of intoxication than an adult and the effects last longer. The impact of alcohol on psychomotor ability is more detrimental in older people than adults.

Alcohol withdrawal is on a continuum from mild to severe where delirium comprising disorientation, seizures and hallucinations is the main feature. This can follow low volume drinking in the older person.

In some cases patients may present with the care triad of symptoms of Wernicke's Encephalopathy – nystagmus, ophthalmoplegia and ataxia, accompanied by disorientation and memory impairment as a result of thiamine deficiency. This must be distinguished from delirium with which it can be easily confused. This can progress to Korsakoff's Syndrome which presents with lack of insight, apathy and amnesia. Correct diagnosis is vital to prevent fatality or deterioration into Korsakoff's Syndrome.

There may also be acute local and systemic complications from intravenous drug use and a withdrawal syndrome from opiate misuse. The possibility of opiate and benzodiazepine overdose should also be recognized. Benzodiezapine intoxication can present with dizziness, tiredness and unsteadiness, and combined with alcohol and opiates can present with an overdose and can be fatal. Even low doses can lead to dependence. Convulsions and a confusional state are common on withdrawal.

As mentioned above, opiate intoxication can lead to sedation, decreased level of consciousness and depressed respiration, and result in death, especially if the patient is using other substances. Craving, sweatiness, shivering and muscle aches are withdrawal symptoms.

Cannabis intoxication produces euphoria, disinhibition, anxiety, agitation, paranoid ideation, hallucinations, depersonalization and derealization, increased appetite, conjunctival injection, tachycardia, impaired reaction time and poor judgement. Withdrawal leads to irritability, craving, sweating and muscle aches.

Stimulant intoxication leads to euphoria, increased energy, agitation and weight loss, paranoid states with hallucinations, aggressive behaviour and convulsions. Withdrawal may lead to lethargy, craving, increased appetite, depression and suicide. Intravenous use may results in fits, stroke and cardiac pain.

The other acute and long-term systemic effects of substances on the gastrointestinal, respiratory, cardiovascular and musculoskeletal systems should be considered. Presentations include alcoholic hepatitis, Mallory Weiss tears and acute pancreatitis from alcohol misuse or acute and chronic respiratory symptoms from tobacco, cannabis and cocaine. Cardiac symptoms, such as syncope, arrhythmia, tachycardia and cardiac arrest, may also be sequelae of stimulant use. Common presentations where substance misuse may be overlooked include stroke and falls.

The presentation to mental health services may occur both in hospital and community settings and includes self-harm, depression, psychotic symptoms and personality disorder [5, 13, 33–37]. See also Chapters 5, 14 and 18.

Collateral information

Given the stigma and associated underreporting of substance use in older people, supplementing clinical information from a variety of sources can be invaluable. This is also especially informative in patients with cognitive impairment or who have problems with communication.

Valuable information may be obtained from a variety of sources; these include:

- relatives, friends and informal carers (taking account of information sharing and confidentiality);
- GP consultations;
- hospital discharge summaries;
- social care assessments;
- home carer observations;
- day centre observations;
- reports from housing officers/wardens of supported housing;
- criminal justice agencies;
- results from previous investigations (including cognitive testing and neuro-imaging).

General principles of assessment

History

When taking a history as part of comprehensive assessment, it may be difficult to focus on one particular set of symptoms or a single disease process. In part this may be because patients have multiple interacting problems. Another challenge arises because many problems in older people present atypically compared with younger adults [5, 38, 39]. This is particularly the case with delirium, which may be a sign of the (sometimes incorrectly diagnosed) urinary infection but can equally well be the presenting feature in intoxication and withdrawal from substances, typically in delirium tremens. In patients with pre-existing dementia, symptoms such as pain, thirst or hunger may present only with changes in behaviour, such as restlessness or social withdrawal.

It is particularly important to ask specifically about those physical and psychological problems that are more frequently encountered in older people, since these could be related to substance misuse. Asking about the geriatric giants of immobility, instability and falls, incontinence and impairment of intellect is essential, as is a nutritional history. Objective testing for impaired function in these areas may also be required as part of the examination prompted by the relevant history.

Time and an appropriate environment will be needed to take into account potential problems with sight, hearing and language deficits, which are known to accumulate with older age and particularly frailty [40].

Reductions in the clearance of drugs in older age and increased risk of drug interactions with complex regimens are well recognized [41]. The drug history must include not only the details of the regular prescriptions but the actual consumption, which often includes over-the-counter medicines as well as alternative medicines such as homeopathic and herbal remedies and food supplements.

Drug use histories, which should (but may not) include prescribed medications, non-prescribed medications and illicit drugs, are commonly taken by ward pharmacists, which is very useful but sources of history or of supplier of prescribed as well as nonprescribed medications should be noted. If the history or information was only taken from the patient's General Practice, nonprescribed medicines will be missing. The drug history will, as the assessment progresses, lead to a medication review when the antecedent problems have been clarified. The medication review seeks to identify the indications for all the medicines, including those indications no longer active, and to re-evaluate them. There is a potential role for pharmacists in this undertaking.

Examination

Frailty may appear obvious at a glance, though out of context (such as in a gown in a hospital bed) appearances can sometimes be deceiving. How well kempt a patient is, or how clean they or their clothes are, can give clues to their physical or cognitive abilities or may suggest that there are deficiencies in support networks. Gait and balance may reveal obvious diagnoses such as Parkinson's disease with tremor and festination or the spastic hemiplegia of a previous stroke. Use of walking aids can give clues about rheumatological and neurological diagnoses.

Complete examination should include a thorough inspection of all the skin, including the genital areas, looking for evidence of injury (accidental or not), pressure area breakdown, evidence of damage from incontinence and ulceration.

Risk for future skin damage (for instance dry or papery thin skin or areas that have been sun-damaged) should be noted and appropriate advice given about protecting from pressure damage, sun exposure or use of emollients.

With regard to the older person who may be misusing drugs or alcohol, any organ system may be involved. Tar staining of the fingers and hair will give clues about tobacco use and nicotine addiction. Urine screening for drugs may be clinically appropriate in order not to miss commonly misused substances whether prescribed, illicit or over-the-counter.

There may be evidence of liver cirrhosis, such as palmar erythema, spider naevi and caput medusae or jaundice, which can give clues to previous alcohol misuse or might point to exposure to hepatitis C virus transmitted from needle sharing [42, 43]. Alcohol misuse is associated with psoriasis, increased risk of skin carcinomata and porphyria cutanea tarda (also prevalent in hepatitis C).

Injected drugs of abuse are associated with thrombosed superficial and deep veins, ulceration and sinus formation. In bacterial endocarditis, which can be as a result of injecting drugs, immune complex deposits can lead to nail fold infarcts, splinter haemorrhages and Osler's nodes in the pulps of the digits. Janeway lesions (tender nodules in the palms or soles) are due to septic emboli.

HIV is increasingly recognized in older people as both survival increases and also with increased numbers of cases arising de novo over the age of 50. Rosen *et al.* [37], in a literature review of older heroin addicts, demonstrated that between 14.6 and 29.2% of older heroin users reported HIV/AIDS. Cutaneous manifestations are diverse and include a macular rash in seroconversion, increased rates of bacterial, viral and fungal infections, higher rates of skin cancers, higher rates of drug reactions and specific reactions to antiretroviral therapy. Psoriasis and sebhorrhoeic dermatitis are also seen more commonly. Poor nutrition, which often accompanies substance misuse, may be evident from gum disease and dental caries, or the cork-screw shaped body hair seen in scurvy (Vitamin C deficiency). Methamphetamine use is particularly associated with dental problems.

When examining cardiovascular and respiratory systems, particular attention should be given to looking for complications of drug and alcohol misuse. Patients with COPD (chronic obstructive pulmonary disease), for example, may have purse-lipped breathing, a barrel-shaped chest or signs of pulmonary hypertension. Hypertension may co-exist with smoking; alcohol may cause hypertension and both increase the likelihood of ischaemic heart disease, vascular disease, heart failure and stroke. Some stimulant drugs, particularly cocaine, can induce myocardial infarction and also stroke [32].

Stigmata of liver disease mentioned earlier may be accompanied by specific abdominal findings of a macronodular liver, a liver tumour or ascites. Rectal examination may reveal the pale stools of malabsorption associated with pancreatic insufficiency.

Neurological manifestations of alcohol, drugs and associated complications such as HIV and hepatitis C are also common and diverse [32]. Cognitive impairment and dementia are caused by alcohol. Delirium may present due to intoxication or withdrawal states. Recognizing delirium tremens in acute hospital settings is especially important, as it has a high morbidity and mortality and is treatable. More important is to recognize those at risk before or in the earliest stages of withdrawal to ensure they are given appropriate detoxification plans and nutritional support. Other neurological complications of alcohol include cerebellar syndromes and peripheral neuropathies. These may result in injuries (as can intoxication), so examination will need to look for these, including altered mental status or focal neurology that might accompany traumatic intracerebral bleeding sometimes without evidence of external injury.

Functional status

The impact of ill health on both acute and chronic functional ability has long been recognized. An approach is needed that covers a wide range of daily activities, is sensitive to the individual's own objectives, but also aims to challenge limitations that might have arisen from both ill health and prejudice. Most assessment scales are very systematic, covering a variety of set functions, such as in the Barthel Index [44].

The Barthel Index rates an individual's ability to perform a number of activities of daily living (ADLs), such as feeding, toilet use, mobility and transfers. It has good reliability and has practical uses both in research and clinical settings [45].

An alternative way to take a functional history is to ask patients to describe a typical day or week and establish where they and their relatives or carers perceive or experience difficulties. This has the advantage of being more person-centred and focusing on areas of need important to the patient. It has limitations if patients are cognitively impaired or have low expectations of their ability.

In most geriatric ward settings, assessment of activities of daily living (ADL) commonly falls to occupational therapists, with contributions from physiotherapists (gait, balance, endurance) and sometimes speech and language therapists (swallowing as well as communication). It is essential to recognize the role of assessment from nursing staff who have specific skills, for example in assessment of continence or medication management, and also are often best placed to inform the rest of the team on daily ADL activity; for inpatients they are usually uniquely placed to assess function at night time. The benefits of this multiprofessional approach are clear but there can also be a risk of overreliance on assessment, especially in hospitals or clinics where it is all too often out of context. Recognizing the context and limitations of an assessment or how to balance risk after an assessment has taken place is one of the most important roles of the multidisciplinary team.

Whilst the vast majority of investigations should be triggered by clinical questions arising from the history, examination and functional assessment, a small number of screening tests have value. These include the standard biochemistry screen covering renal, liver and bone function, the full blood count and thyroid function tests – there being an age-related increased prevalence of hypothyroidism. As mentioned previously drug screening may be appropriate.

Screening

Screening is a portal to a more thorough clinical assessment, by identifying patients at highest risk. Most of the literature around screening for probable substance use disorders in older people concerns alcohol misuse, with most instruments developed for use in younger populations. This requires certain adaptions and considerations to be taken into account to ensure that these are age appropriate. The CAGE questionnaire [46] is quick to administer and detects the core features of alcohol dependence but is relatively insensitive to harmful/ hazardous drinking. Although validated in older people, one study showed that up to 60% of older people at risk of alcohol dependence in a community sample were CAGE-negative [47].

The most widely used age-specific screening tool, the Short Michigan Alcoholism Screening Test – Geriatric version [48] has been validated for use in older hospital inpatients [49]. It asks questions that tap into problems more commonly seen in older people such as 'drinking after a significant loss' or to 'take your mind off problems'. Various adaptations of the Alcohol Use Disorders Identification Test (AUDIT) tool [50] have been validated in older populations. These include the AUDIT-5, a five-item version of the full AUDIT [51] and the AUDIT-C, which asks only the three alcohol consumption questions of the full AUDIT [52]. Given the lack of specific screening tools for alcohol problems in older people, such tools need to be combined with quantity/frequency measures and a comprehensive assessment that covers substance use, misuse and dependence. While the DAST (Drug Abuse Screening Tool) [53] has been developed, this is not validated in an older population. Furthermore, Lam and Cheung [54] have suggested a tool for prevention of inappropriate prescribing which could be used for screening. A recent review identified and described 13 instruments that could be useful in general hospital wards for screening of illicit drug use, including the DAST [55]. There is, however, lack of evaluation of illicit drug use screening instruments in general hospital wards. Currently, clinicians or researchers searching for a simple, reliable, general screening instrument for current drug use to guide practice or research in general hospital wards do not have enough comparative evidence to choose between the available measures [55].

Psychiatric assessment

As detailed in Chapter 23, the prevalence of substance misuse and co-morbid mental disorders (also referred to as 'dual diagnosis') ranges from 21 to 66% [56].

26% of people aged 65 and over have a mental disorder; this includes 16% with a primary mental disorder, 3% with dementia complicated by significant psychiatric symptoms and 7% with uncomplicated dementia [57]. In community settings, the highest level of co-morbidity in older people is most common in the 75–84 age group and largely attributable to benzodiazepine use.

The commonest presentations when assessing mental health problems in the context of substance misuse in older people are mood disorders and cognitive impairment. Depression and anxiety are commonly associated with both substances, with evidence to suggest that the direction of causality is for alcohol misuse to increase the likelihood of depression [58]. It is not uncommon to find an atypical presentation of symptoms suggestive of a mood disorder. These include being 'masked' by cognitive impairment or else being 'somatized' by presenting as physical symptoms such as lack of energy or physical discomfort.

The presence of multiple physical co-morbidities may make the detection of depression and anxiety all the more problematic, particularly somatic symptoms of depression such as anergia, poor appetite, weight loss and sleep disturbance, which are also associated with many physical disorders such as rheumatological and neurological disease. The skill in detecting mood disorders then relies on the presence of cognitive and behavioural symptoms, such as poor concentration, pessimism, suicidal ideation and irritability. The assessment of depression is particularly important in older people at highest risk of completed suicide, where alcohol misuse often accompanies the worsening of depressive symptoms and the actual act of suicide itself.

Cognitive impairment associated with alcohol misuse may present with alcohol-related brain injury in the form of amnestic disorders confined to memory impairment, or with alcohol-related dementia where there is a more global loss of cognitive function. In either case, screening cognitive function using a tool covering a range of cognitive domains, such as the mini mental state examination (MMSE) [59], is required.

However, it should be borne in mind that this screening tool does not assess frontal lobe function, which is known to be more sensitive than other brain areas to the initial effects of alcohol toxicity [60]. If a more comprehensive assessment of cognitive function is required, the Addenbrookes Cognitive Examination offers such a screen [61].

Psychotic symptoms can be also associated with the acute effects of a variety of substances such as cannabinoids, stimulants and hallucinogens. Withdrawal states accompanying alcohol and/or sedatives/hypnotics are also commonly associated with transient psychotic symptoms.

Case presentations

The following case presentations cover six clinical scenarios that include clinical encounters likely to be seen by health and social care professionals involved in the assessment and treatment of older people with substance misuse.

Driving and substance misuse

CT is a 70 year old man who was found wandering around his local area picking up cigarette stubs, looking dishevelled. He insisted on driving even though he had recently had a drink driving conviction for which he was supposed to attend a community-based course to enable him to reduce his drinking. He had lost his job at the age of 69 because he had been drinking heavily. He had had chest pains and asthma and had been noted to have hypertension. CT had not taken the treatment for his cardiovascular problems for several months, was not eating properly and was neglecting himself.

He had experienced a period of heavy drinking years ago but had managed to cut down. His wife died suddenly and his social network seemed to have contracted to such an extent that he was isolated and bored, especially at the weekends. On admission to a geriatric unit, he was diagnosed as having alcohol-induced dementia. He was encouraged to inform the DVLA (Driver and Vehicle Licensing Agency) and to stop driving; he was also referred to a specialist addiction unit. It proved possible to reduce his alcohol intake substantially, but memory deficits persisted, though he did engage with treatment and agreed to write to the DVLA.

Older women and alcohol misuse

AB is a 78 year old lady referred by her family doctor for an assessment of mood. She has attended the surgery every week for the past two months with a variety of nonspecific symptoms, such as poor sleep, appetite loss, falls, lack of energy and episodes of incontinence. She is noted to have started neglecting her hygiene. A collateral history from her daughter reveals no problems with memory, mood or activities of daily living, but she has noticed her mother to be unusually tired when she visits every week.

At interview, AB appears defensive and irritable and denies any problems with her mood, memory or level of function. Only when a tactful and nonjudgemental approach is taken to enquiring into her alcohol intake, does she reveal that she sometimes likes a 'drop of gin' but does not divulge any further information. At a follow-up visit, she talks about her sleep problems and how alcohol helps her to get a good night's sleep, also stating her life has changed since she lost her husband and has become more socially isolated. A more detailed account of quantity/frequency of alcohol intake emerges when questions are built around current and past problems and difficulties, with a typical drinking day providing a complete picture that now involves purchasing a bottle of gin three times a week. Only when speaking to home carers is it discovered that they are commonly asked to buy alcohol for AB and they are also asked to throw away empty bottles.

Further blood investigations reveal a high mean corpuscular volume (MCV) and raised gamma glutamyl transferase. Following further assessment and brief intervention, a care plan is developed to address social isolation and harm reduction from alcohol misuse.

Polysubstance misuse

PS is a 62 year old man presented to the emergency clinic for detoxification. He has a long-standing history of substance misuse, with his first taste of alcohol at the age of five years and he started drinking regularly at 12 years. PS had tried almost every substance, including solvents, amphetamines, ecstasy, magic mushrooms and heroin. He had been in custody for three periods because of theft, burglary and shoplifting offences, committed to fund drugs or to maintain basic living needs. At the time of presentation, he was drinking more than the 'safe recommended limits' for alcohol (for adults) using benzodiazepines and topping up his methadone prescription with street opiates.

PS lived with his partner and had a central role in the care of his two grandchildren. He was encouraged to attend the substance misuse service for a full initial assessment after the prescribing GP was contacted.

After a thorough assessment, it was concluded that he probably suffered from harmful use of alcohol, opiate dependence and harmful use of stimulants and benzodiazepine dependence. The care of his grandchildren was rearranged so that his daughter provided support to them and to him. The decision was made to admit him for detoxification from alcohol and benzodiazepines and stabilization of opiates. His mental state on cessation of stimulants would be monitored in case he became depressed. Following admission, and after detoxification, he became depressed.

He was seen and treated with antidepressants and psychosocial interventions by an old age psychiatrist. Follow-up continues by both services; although abstinent from opiates and stimulants, he has become dependent again on benzodiazepines, as well as showing harmful use of alcohol.

The frequent attender

LJ is an 80 year old man living in supported accommodation. He lives alone and has problems with mobility secondary to shortness of breath and osteoarthritis. Over the past month, he has been seen at the Accident and Emergency Department on five separate occasions, in each case having been brought in by ambulance after pulling the emergency cord in his room. Each presentation has been slightly different, ranging from being unable to get up after a fall, to breathlessness and to feeling that he wants to 'end it all'. During the first three presentations, he was admitted to an acute medical ward, with several investigations having been carried out.

Apart from discovering an incidental hiatus hernia and an MCV of 98 fl, no other abnormalities were detected. LJ then started being sent home directly from the emergency department, eventually being referred to the community mental health team.

At initial assessment on a home visit, his flat is cluttered with little furniture and no food in the refrigerator. Although he maintains an independent lifestyle, he has clearly neglected his self-care and food intake, mostly eating take-away food and buying other food from the local shop. At interview, he is irritable and suspicious and appears to be responding to external stimuli. He has sealed his letterbox and keeps the curtains permanently closed. On mental state examination, he is restless and distractible and talks about the council and the police being involved in a 'plot' to get him out of his flat. He also hears second and third person auditory hallucinations. After careful exploration, he reports that these had been present for three months, since he started 'hitting the bottle' following the death of a close friend who had lived next door to him and that alcohol helped to 'drown out the voices'. LJ was admitted voluntarily to a mental health unit, where he underwent detoxification and an antipsychotic was started. He returned to his supported accommodation, is compliant with medication, received a care package and has started attending a day centre, also engaging in motivational interviewing to address his alcohol misuse.

Alcohol and cognitive impairment

AX is a 68 year old single gentleman who was referred by the housing department for failure to pay his rent for the past six months and is being threatened with eviction. He refused to see his family doctor but information from his social worker suggests problems with 'forgetfulness'. He had locked himself out of the flat on two occasions, as well as forgetting to take his medication regularly.

AX was not expecting you when you visit, stating that he had not received the appointment letter. His flat was cluttered and unclean. There were boxes of medication that were out of date; with the same applying to the food in his refrigerator. He denied any problems with memory, stating that he was independent with all activities of daily living, but you noticed reminders for payment of rent and his telephone line had been disconnected. There was a one litre bottle of whiskey on the cupboard which was two-thirds empty and a glass on the floor containing the same. AX was dishevelled and there were food stains on his clothes. His affect was irritable but there was no evidence of depression. Further assessment revealed that AX started drinking 50 units of alcohol per week six months previously, when he was diagnosed with prostate cancer.

On the Mini Mental State Examination, he scored 25/30, losing points for orientation to day and date, losing 1 point for object recall and losing a further 2 points for concentration. On a screen of frontal lobe testing, there were deficits in abstract thinking, as well as cognitive estimates and set-shifting.

The Addenbrookes Cognitive Assessment Revised (ACE-R) showed global deficits in memory and verbal fluency that are more severely affected than visuospatial function and language. There was also evidence of a decline in functional activities of daily living, such as management of finances.

A diagnosis of alcohol-related dementia was made, with the successful implementation of harm reductions measures resulting in complete abstinence from alcohol. After a further 12 months, repeat neuropsychological testing shows some improvement in verbal fluency and memory.

Pain and substance misuse

RS is a 66 year old man who presented to the drug service with a positive urine test for opiates. He was shocked, as were the staff, as he had been stable on a dose of 50 mg/ml methadone for one year. RS had begun a prescription for methadone when he had become dependent on heroin following the need for pain relief for back ache. When probed as to whether he had taken any new medications for any reason he volunteered that he had taken what he thought was some aspirin that he had found in his brother's flat. His brother had recently died and RS felt low and 'lost'.

The urine sample was sent for toxicological analysis where codeine was found, after which he brought in some of the tablets, which were analysed and were a combination of codeine and aspirin.

RS stopped using these and he was advised to take them to a pharmacy for disposal. His mood was monitored for evidence of clinical depression, but he appeared to respond to cognitive behavioural therapy.

Discussion

The assessment of older people with substance misuse is complex, largely owing to the wide variety of presentations, many of which are either masked by other co-morbidities or else atypical in their presentation. Given the multiple needs that require assessment of both physical and mental health as well as an assessment of functional abilities and social support, an integrated approach is required. Such approach will need to involve joint assessment from professionals with skills in assessing both older people and substance misuse [62], in order to offer a seamless approach to care to improve both health and social outcomes in older people.

Conclusion

The field of substance misuse in older people will continue to grow over the coming decades, with the likely emergence of higher levels of illicit drug misuse and of prescription drugs [63] in addition to the already growing burden of alcohol misuse.

There remains immense scope for the provision of skills to meet this need within mainstream services, while at the same time, drawing upon the expertise of substance misuse services in more complex cases. The wide variation in presentation, as illustrated by the case vignettes above, mandates that practitioners must have awareness that older people may have a substance misuse problem as a principal or subsidiary factor in their illness.

This requires that staff treating older people should be adequately trained so that they are comfortable screening patients and asking them about substance issues, as well as having knowledge about the relationship between signs and symptoms of disease and the range of substances people might take. This should be more than just asking whether people smoke, drink and what pharmaceutical drugs they take. Specific validated tools for older people would be a great help and there should also be help readily available from appropriate specialists for mental and physical health needs. Patients should be encouraged to engage with continuing treatment and follow-up is required.

References

1. Crome, I., Dar, K., Janikiewicz, S. *et al.* (2011) *Our Invisible Addicts*. Report of the Older Persons' Substance Misuse Working Group of the Royal College of Psychiatrists, College Report 165, Royal College of Psychiatrists, London.
2. Cherry, K.E., Walker, E.J. and Brown, J.S. (2013) Social Engagement and Health in Younger, Older, and Oldest-Old Adults in the Louisiana Healthy Aging Study. *Journal of Applied Gerontology*, **32**, 51–75.
3. Office of National Statistics (2013) Estimates of the Very Old (including Centenarians), 2002–2011, England and Wales. Office of National Statistics, London.
4. Crome, I. and Bloor, R. (2005) Older substance misusers still deserve better services – an update (Part 1). *Reviews in Clinical Gerontology*, **15**, 125.
5. Crome, I. and Bloor, R. (2005) Older substance misusers still deserve better diagnosis – an update (Part 2). *Reviews in Clinical Gerontology*, 2005; **15**, 255.
6. Rao, R. and Shanks, A. (2011) Development and implementation of a dual diagnosis strategy for older people in south east London. *Advances in Dual Diagnosis*, **4**, 28–35.
7. Rao, R. (2006) Alcohol misuse and ethnicity – Hidden populations need specific services – and more research. *British Medical Journal*, **332**, 682-A.
8. Rao, R., Wolff, K. and Marshall, E.J. (2008) Alcohol use and misuse in older people: a local prevalence study comparing English and Irish inner-city residents living in the UK. *Journal of Substance Use*, **13**, 17–26.
9. Bardsley, M., Hamm, J., Lowdell, C. *et al.* (2000) *Developing Health Assessment for Black and Ethnic Minority Groups: Analysing Routine Health Information*. The Health of Londoners Project, NHS Executive, London.
10. Alcohol Concern (2009) *All Party Parliamentary on Alcohol. The Future of Alcohol Treatment*. Alcohol Concern, London.
11. HM Government (2012) *The Government's Alcohol Strategy*. HMSO, London.
12. Crome, I.B., Crome, P. and Rao, R. (2011) Addiction and ageing – awareness, assessment and action. *Age and Ageing*, **40**, 657–658.
13. Rao, R.T. (2011) Older people and dual diagnosis – out of sight, but not out of mind. *Advances in Dual Diagnosis*, **4**, 1.

14. Saxton, L., Lancashire, S. and Kipping, C. (2011) Meeting the training needs of staff working with older people with dual diagnosis. *Advances in Dual Diagnosis*, 4, 36–46.
15. American Psychiatric Association (2013) *Diagnostic and Statistical Manual of Mental Disorders*, 5th edn (DSM-5). American Psychiatric Association, Arlington, VA.
16. World Health Organization (1992) *The ICD-10 Classification of Mental and Behavioural Disorders: Clinical Descriptions and Diagnostic Guidelines*. World Health Organization, Geneva, Switzerland.
17. Blow, F.C. (1998) *Substance Abuse Amongst Older Adults*. Treatment Improvement Protocol (TIP) Series 26, DHSS Publication Number (SMA) 98-3179, Substance Abuse and Mental Health Services Administration, Centre for Substance Abuse Treatment, US Department of Health and Human Services, Rockville, MD.
18. Carrington Reid, M., Tinetti, M.E., Brown, C.J. and Concato, J. (1998) Physician awareness of alcohol use disorders among older patients. *Journal of General Internal Medicine*, 13, 729–734.
19. Rockett, I.R.H., Putnam, S.L., Jia, H. and Smith, G.S. (2006) Declared and undeclared substance use among emergency department patients: a population-based study. *Addiction*, 101, 706–712.
20. Arnd, S., Schultz, S.K., Turvey, C. and Petersen, A. (2002) Screening for alcoholism in the primary care setting. *Journal of Family Practice*, 51, 41–50.
21. Friedmann, P.D., McCullough, D., Chin, M.H. and Saitz, R. (2000) Screening and intervention for alcohol problems. *Journal of General Internal Medicine*, 15(2), 84–91.
22. Anderson, D., Cattell, H. and Bentley, E. (2008) Nurse-led liaison psychiatry service for older adults: service evaluation. *Psychiatric Bulletin*, 32(8), 298–302.
23. Norfolk Drug and Alcohol Partnership (2012) *Adult Substance Misuse Related Needs Assessment*. Norfolk DAAT Research and Information Team, Norwich, UK.
24. Zunzunegui, M.V., Koné, A., Johri, M. *et al.* (2008) Social networks and self-rated health in two French-speaking Canadian community dwelling populations over 65. *Social Science and Medicine*, 58(10), 2069–2081.
25. Crane, M. (2001) *Our Forgotten Elders: Older People on the Streets and in Hostels*. St Mungo's, London.
26. Welte, J.W. and Mirand, A.L. (1995) Drinking, problem drinking and life stressors in the elderly general population. *Journal of Studies on Alcohol*, 56, 67–73.
27. Saunders, P.A., Copeland, J.R., Dewey, M.E. *et al.* (1991) Heavy drinking as a risk factor for depression and dementia in elderly men: Findings from the Liverpool Longitudinal Community Study. *British Journal of Psychiatry*, 159, 213–216.
28. Byrne, G.J., Raphael, B. and Arnold, E. (1999) Alcohol consumption and psychological distress in recently widowed older men. *Australia and New Zealand Journal of Psychiatry*, 33, 740–747.
29. Carstensen, L.L., Rychtarik, R.G. and Prue, D.M. (1985) Behavioral treatment of the geriatric alcohol abuser: A long term follow-up study. *Addictive Behaviors*, 10, 307–311.
30. Hanson, B.S. (1994) Social network, social support and heavy drinking in elderly men – a population study of men born in 1914, Malmö, Sweden. *Addiction*, 89, 725–732.
31. Fink, A., Hays, R.D., Moore, A.A. and Beck, J.C. (1996) Alcohol-related problems in older persons: determinants, consequences, and screening. *Archives of Internal Medicine*, 156, 1150–1156.
32. British Medical Association (2013) *Drugs of Dependence: The Role of Medical Professionals*. British Medical Association, London.
33. Rao, R., Buxey, R. and Jalloh, K. (2011) Alcohol and dual diagnosis in older people. In: *Mental Health and Later Life: Delivering an Holistic Model for Practice* (eds J. Keady and S. Watts). Routledge, Abingdon.

34. Crome, P. (1984) ABC of poisoning the elderly. *British Medical Journal*, **289**, 546–548.
35. Lin, J.C., Karno, M.P., Grella, C.E. *et al.* (2011) Alcohol, tobacco and nonmedical drug use disorders in US adults age 65 years and older: data from 2001–2002. National Epidemiologic Survey of Alcohol and Related Conditions. *American Journal of Geriatric Psychiatry*, **19**, 292–299.
36. Cicero, T.J., Surratt, H.L., Kurtz, S., *et al.* (2012) Patterns of prescription opioid abuse and comorbidity in an aging treatment population. *Journal of Substance Abuse Treatment*, **42**, 87–94.
37. Rosen, D., Hunsaker, A., Albert, S.M. *et al.* (2011) Characteristics and consequences of heroin use among older adults in the US: a review of the literature, treatment implications and recommendations for further research. *Addictive Behaviours*, **36**, 279–285.
38. O'Connell, H., Chin, A., Cunningham, C. *et al.* (2003) Alcohol use disorders in elderly people: refining an age old problem in old age. *British Medical Journal*, **327**, 664–667.
39. McInnes, E. and Powell, J. (1994) Drug and alcohol referrals: are elderly substance abuse diagnoses and referrals being missed? *British Medical Journal*, **308**, 444–446.
40. Cummings, N.M.C. and Kidd, S. (1988) Forgetting falls. The limited accuracy of recall of falls in the elderly. *Journal of the American Geriatric Society*, **36**, 613–616.
41. Mangoni, A.A. and Jackson, S.H.D. (2004) Age-related changes in pharmacokinetics and pharmacodynamics: basic principles and practical applications. *British Journal of Clinical Pharmacology*, **57**, 6–14.
42. Hser, Y.I., Hoffman, V., Grella, C.E. and Anglin, M.D. (2001) A 33-year follow-up of narcotics addicts. *Archives of General Psychiatry*, **58**(5), 503–508.
43. Rosen, D., Smith, M.L. and Reynolds, C.F., 3rd. (2008) The prevalence of mental and physical health disorders among older methadone patients. *American Journal of Geriatric Psychiatry*, **16**, 488–497.
44. Mahoney, F.I. and Barthel, D.W. (1965) Functional evaluation: the Barthel index. *Maryland State Medical Journal*, **14**, 61–65.
45. Wade, D.T. and Collin, C. (1988) The Barthel ADL Index: a standard measure of physical disability? *International Disability Studies*, **10**, 64–67.
46. Ewing, J.A. (1984) Detecting alcoholism: the CAGE questionnaire. *Journal of the American Medical Association*, **252**, 1905–1907.
47. Adams, W.L., Barry, K.L. and Fleming, M.F. (1996) Screening for problem drinking in older primary care patients. *Journal of the American Medical Association*, **276**, 1964–1967.
48. Blow, F.C., Gillespie, B.W. and Barry, K.L. (1998) Brief screening for alcohol problems in elderly populations using the Short Michigan Alcoholism Screening Test – Geriatric Version (SMAST-G). *Alcoholism: Clinical and Experimental Research*, **22**(Suppl), 131A.
49. Joseph, C.L., Ganzini, L. and Atkinson, R.M. (1995) Screening for alcohol use disorders in the nursing home. *Journal of the American Geriatrics Society*, **43**, 368–373.
50. Saunders, J.B., Aasland, O.G. and Babor, T.F. (1993) Development of the Alcohol Use Disorders Identification Test (AUDIT): WHO Collaborative Project on Early Detection of Persons with Harmful Alcohol Consumption – II. *Addiction*, **88**, 791–804.
51. Piccinelli, M., Tessari, E. and Bortolomasi, M. (1997) Efficacy of the Alcohol Use Disorders Identification Test as a screening tool for hazardous alcohol intake and related disorders in primary care: a validity study. *British Medical Journal*, **314**, 420–424.
52. Bush, K., Kivlahan, D.R. and McDonnell, M.B. (1998) The AUDIT Alcohol Consumption Questions (AUDIT-C): an effective, brief screening test for problem drinking. *Archives of Internal Medicine*, **158**, 1789–1795.
53. Skinner, H.A. (1982) The drug abuse screening test. *Addictive Behaviors*, 7(4), 363–371.
54. Lam, M.P. and Cheung, B.M. (2012) The use of the STOPP/START criteria as a screening tool for assessing the appropriateness of medications in the elderly population. *Expert Review of Clinical Pharmacology*, **5**, 187–197.

55. Mdege, N.D. and Lang, J. (2011) Screening instruments for detecting illicit drug use/abuse that could be useful in general hospital wards: a systematic review. *Addictive Behaviors*, **36**(12), 1111–1119. doi: 10.1016/j.addbeh.2011.07.007.
56. Bartels, S.J., Blow, F.C., van Citters, A.D. *et al.* (2006) Dual diagnosis among older adults: co-occurring substance abuse and psychiatric illness. *Journal of Dual Diagnosis*, **2**, 9–30.
57. Bartels, S.J., Blow, F.C., Brockmann, L.M. and Van Citters, A.D. (2005) Substance abuse and mental health among older Americans: The state of the knowledge and future directions. WESTAT, Rockville, MD.
58. Boden, J.M. and Fergusson, D.M. (2001) Alcohol and depression. *Addiction*, **106**(5), 906–914.
59. Folstein, M.F., Folstein, S.E. and McHugh, P.R. (1975) 'Mini Mental State". A practical method for grading the cognitive state of patients for the clinician. *Journal of Psychiatric Research*, **12**, 189–198.
60. Zahr, N.M., Kaufman, K.L. and Harper, C.G. (2011) Clinical and pathological features of alcohol-related brain damage. *Nature Reviews Neurology*, **7**, 284–294.
61. Mioshi, E., Dawson, K., Mitchell, J. *et al.* (2006) The Addenbrooke's Cognitive Examination Revised (ACE-R): a brief cognitive test battery for dementia screening. *International Journal of Geriatric Psychiatry*, **21**, 1078–1085.
62. Rao, R. (2013) Outcomes from liaison psychiatry referrals for older people with alcohol use disorders in the UK. *Mental Health and Substance Use*, **6**(4), 1–7.
63. Finlayson, R.E. (1995) Misuse of prescription drugs. *Substance Use and Misuse*, **30**, 1871–1901.

SCREENING AND INTERVENTION IN HEALTH CARE SETTINGS

Chapter 14

SCREENING AND BRIEF INTERVENTION IN THE PSYCHIATRIC SETTING

M. Shafi Siddiqui[1] and Michael Fleming[2]

[1] Linden Oaks Medical Group, USA
[2] Department of Psychiatry and Family Medicine, Northwestern University, USA

Overview

This chapter focuses on substance abuse screening and brief intervention in the context of routine psychiatric care [1]. Although tobacco addiction remains an important clinical and public health concern, substances discussed in this chapter are limited to alcohol, illegal drugs and prescription medications. The goal of the chapter is to present evidence-based clinical guidelines on how to screen and conduct brief counselling for people with substance use disorder. Screening is different from assessment and is designed to identify patients at risk and is generally limited to 1–2 questions for each substance. Screening can be conducted by a self-administered screening tool or face-to-face in a few minutes. A substance use disorder assessment on the other hand is usually conducted to determine Diagnostic and Statistical Manual of Mental Disorders (DSM)-IV criteria for a particular substance [2] and can take up to an hour to conduct.

The chapter is divided into five sections. The first section provides an overview on screening and brief intervention for older adults. The second discusses a number of alcohol screening tests. The third reviews screening tests for illegal drugs, including specific questions and toxicology testing. The fourth presents the limited information available on screening for prescription drug abuse – primarily opioids, benzodiazepines and amphetamines. The final section reviews what is known about brief intervention for alcohol, illegal drugs and prescription drugs. While there is limited evidence-based information on screening and brief intervention as a component of routine psychiatric care for older adults, there is a wealth of evidence-based research that may be applicable to this setting. Most of the research presented in this chapter was conducted in primary care settings.

Screening and assessment are separate processes, with the former implying the routine administration of a series of questions by interview, pencil and paper questionnaire or electronic device (office computer, online web sites, text messaging). Screening is generally conducted on all new and continuing care patients at regular

Substance Use and Older People, First Edition.
Edited by Ilana B. Crome, Li-Tzy Wu, Rahul (Tony) Rao and Peter Crome.
© 2015 John Wiley & Sons, Ltd. Published 2015 by John Wiley & Sons, Ltd.

intervals. The frequency of the screening depends on the substance, the age of the patient and co-morbid factors. Alcohol use screening for older adults is generally recommended once a year. Recommendations for screening of illicit or nonmedical prescription drug use vary by professional organization but, in general, there is less enthusiasm for routine screening, since there is limited evidence to support this activity. Screening implies the use of a single or limited number of questions. The goal of most substance abuse screening procedures is to document 'use' as opposed to an 'assessment', the goal of which is to make a diagnosis of substance abuse or dependence.

While most clinicians report routine screening of older adults for substances at the initial visit and/or before starting pharmacotherapy, there is limited consensus on how to screen, which questions to ask and how often to do so. For example, is it adequate to ask an older adult:

'Have you had any alcohol to drink or used any illegal drugs in the past month?'

If the answer is 'yes', what then? Should a psychiatrist administer a questionnaire such as CAGE (an acronym for cut down, annoyed by criticism, guilty about drinking, eye-opener drinks), the 10 question Alcohol Use Disorder Inventory Test (AUDIT) or the eight-question National Institute of Drug Abuse (NIDA) drug screen? [3]. Should they conduct a full DSM-IV diagnostic interview schedule? Should they obtain a urine drug test or alcohol biomarker test on all new patients or people going on medication? Should screening be limited to patients with whom there is a clinical concern about potential substance problems as in other fields of medicine most of the psychiatrist's time is spent on medication management with limited time for counselling?

While referral to an alcohol and drug counsellor is standard practice for people who meet diagnostic criteria for '*dependence or addiction*', there may be more uncertainty about patients who screen positive for heavy alcohol use, illicit drug or prescription drug use but who are not dependent. Screening procedures for older adults in the psychiatric setting will identify many more risky drinkers and infrequent (low-level) drug users than they will people who are addicted. How much alcohol or marijuana or opioids is too much in the context of medication management for depression or anxiety or bipolar disorders? When does a psychiatrist use brief intervention, motivational interviewing, psychotherapy or other counselling methods? What is the goal in the context of the nondependent user where limited use may have no direct effect on the patient's mental health problem?

One of the principles of screening for any health issue, whether for high blood pressure, diabetes, depression, suicidal thoughts or substance use disorders, is the need to have evidenced-based guidelines on what to do about a positive screen. Another principle used by the US Preventive Services Task Force is the need for evidence that screening can improve the health of the people who are screened (i.e. older adults in the context of this book chapter). For example, the controversy about the benefit of screening all women for breast cancer under the age of 50 continues despite billions of dollars and hundreds of trials trying to address this question. Making a decision to screen or not screen for substance abuse in the psychiatric setting is a complicated process since the evidence is insufficient.

The current recommendations, by most professional societies and the US Preventative Task Force, for alcohol screening include asking about current alcohol use once a year for adults ≥8 years of age, including older adults [4]. Most groups do not recommend routine screening for illicit or prescription drugs due to the lack of evidence that screening makes a difference in the lives of the patients screened. However, patients in the mental health care setting often have co-morbid problems that place them at greater risk for substance abuse and substance-related harm [5]. So it may be possible to justify routine screening for alcohol, illicit drugs and prescription drug abuse in this setting.

Many patients coming into a psychiatrist's office have depression, anxiety or Post-traumatic Stress Disorder (PTSD) that may be exacerbated by alcohol, illicit or prescription drugs. In addition, most medications used in the mental health setting directly interact with alcohol and drugs, may affect the efficacy of the medication and can be associated serious adverse effects – that is drug overdoses. This is especially an issue in older adults who do not metabolize drugs or medication in the same way as younger adults.

One of the important aspects of screening is to be able to identify patients who are at varying levels of risk for substance related mental health issues and to provide appropriate counselling and treatment [6]. This could vary from a single session of brief advice to cut down their use, to multiple sessions using motivational interviewing or cognitive behavioural therapy, to anticraving medication, to referral to a specialized alcohol and drug treatment programme. For example, a patient who is drinking 5–6 drinks on weekends and is being treated for depression may respond to a single session of brief advice. Daily heavy drinkers who are drinking in the morning to prevent shaking and tremors generally require more intensive treatment than can be provided in the context of general psychiatric care. An attempt is made here to address many of the clinical questions raised during this brief overview.

Screening and assessment for alcohol use disorders

Screening for alcohol use disorders includes asking about the quantity and frequency of use, frequency of heavy drinking, symptoms of abuse or dependence and indirect proxy questions [7]. There are also an increasing number of biomarkers to detect recent or chronic use. Screening can also be accomplished by direct interview, pencil and paper and electronic methods.

Single question screen for an alcohol use disorder

If a psychiatrist has time for a single question, the best question, which enquires about the frequency of heavy drinking, is:

'How many times in the last 30 days did you have 4 or more drinks?'

Research suggests that this single question will detect >90% of patients who use alcohol above recommended limits [8]. It is less specific than other tests but it can identify patients who require more extensive assessment.

In general, any older adult who reports four or more times per month would be considered a positive screen. In some high risk older adults on medication, any heavy drinking episodes should be a considered a positive screen. A positive screen would be followed up by additional questions on the quantity and frequency of use as well as symptoms of abuse and dependence.

Quantity and frequency questions

There are two primary alcohol use questions. The first inquires about the frequency of use and the second about quantity [9, 10]. The time frame is generally limited to the last year:

'In the last year about how many times per week do you have a drink containing alcohol?'
'In the last year about how many drinks do you have on a day when you have alcohol?'

Using the US National Institute on Alcohol Abuse and Alcoholism (NIAAA) criteria, men under the age of 65, who drink >2 drinks per day or >14 drinks per week and women who drink >1 drink per day or >7 drinks a week are considered at risk for alcohol-related problems or alcohol dependent [11]. NIAAA recommends that men and women 65 years or older do not drink more seven drinks a week and no more than one drink per day. The NIAAA also suggests no alcohol use in older adults with certain co-morbid disorders (e.g. hypertension, severe depression, diabetes, elevated lipids) and taking medication that interacts with alcohol (e.g. sedatives, regular doses of acetaminophen).

Proxy questions such as CAGE

One of the most frequently used set of alcohol screening questions is CAGE (the acronym for cut down, annoyed by criticism, guilty about drinking, eye-opener drinks). While these four questions do not inquire about current alcohol use, specific DSM-IV dependence criteria or a specific time period, a positive response to one or more questions suggests a lifetime history of an alcohol use disorder. While the CAGE has a low sensitivity and specificity in the detection of heavy alcohol use it does correlate alcohol abuse and dependence [12]. The CAGE questions are as follows.

'Have you ever felt a need to cut down or control your drinking?'
'Have you felt annoyed when someone criticizes your drinking?'
'Have you ever felt guilty about your drinking?'
'Do you ever have an eye opener in the morning to get going?'

A positive CAGE should be followed up by an assessment of current alcohol use and symptoms of alcohol dependence.

Symptoms of abuse or dependence

There are two screening/assessment pencil and paper questionnaires commonly used in general clinical settings. These include the Alcohol Use Disorders Identification Test (AUDIT) and the geriatric version of the Michigan Alcohol Screening Test. The AUDIT is probably the most widely used pencil and paper test used in the United States and many other countries [13]. It was originally developed and tested in 10 countries by a working group of the World Health Organization. The AUDIT consists of three questions on alcohol use, three questions related to alcohol dependence (unable to control, failure to complete expectations, alcohol withdrawal) two questions on morbidity (injury and blackouts) and family member concern Box 14.1. For adults a score of six or less is considered low-risk drinking. A score of 7–12 is considered risky or at-risk drinking, 12–15 correlates with a DSM diagnosis of alcohol abuse and >15 alcohol dependence [7]. There are no specific data on AUDIT scores in older adults.

The short geriatric version of the Michigan Alcohol Screening Test (MAST) – Short Michigan Alcoholism Screening Test-Geriatric Version (SMAST-G) – is a 10-question screening questionnaire that can be administered as part of the initial patient vision or during medication therapy [14]. A positive response to three or more questions suggests an alcohol use disorder. Like the original MAST, the questions are based on lifetime use, there are no alcohol use questions and it contains proxy questions related to DSM dependence criteria [15]. While not as widely used as the CAGE or the AUDIT, it can provide additional information and may be more sensitive in the older adult population. The 10 questions have dichotomous yes/no responses (Box 14.2). Three or more positive responses are considered a positive test and should be followed up with brief intervention and possible referral to a substance abuse program.

Alcohol biomarkers

There is increasing interest in the use of biomarkers to detect recent alcohol use [16]. While traditional liver function tests such as gamma-glutamyl transferase (GGT) are neither sensitive nor specific, a number of new markers offer promise. Blood alcohol levels can be useful to assess tolerance and risk of withdrawal. However, since most people metabolize at the rate of one drink per hour, the blood alcohol level has limited value as a screening test. Recently developed alcohol biomarkers include carbohydrate deficient transferase (CDT), ethyl glucuronide (EtG), ethyl sulfate (EtS) and phosphatidyl ethanol (PET) [16]

CDT measures the percentage of asialo, monoasialo and disialo isoforms of transferrin in serum. These isoforms are elevated in the presence of sustained heavy alcohol use. The test is able to detect daily heavy drinking >4 drinks/day over the previous four weeks. The test has the highest sensitivity in men, daily heavy drinkers and patients with normal liver function tests and is less useful in binge drinkers, women and young adults (<25 years of age). False positives are

Box 14.1 Alcohol Use Disorders Identification Test (AUDIT)

The Alcohol Use Disorders Identification Test: Interview Version

Read questions as written. Record answers carefully. Begin the AUDIT by saying "Now I am going to ask you some questions about your use of alcoholic beverages during this past year." Explain what is meant by "alcoholic beverages" by using local examples of beer, wine, vodka, etc. Code answers in terms of "standard drinks". Place the correct answer number in the box at the right.

1. How often do you have a drink containing alcohol?
   (0) Never [Skip to Qs 9-10]
   (1) Monthly or less
   (2) 2 to 4 times a month
   (3) 2 to 3 times a week
   (4) 4 or more times a week

2. How many drinks containing alcohol do you have on a typical day when you are drinking?
   (0) 1 or 2
   (1) 3 or 4
   (2) 5 or 6
   (3) 7, 8, or 9
   (4) 10 or more

3. How often do you have six or more drinks on one occasion?
   (0) Never
   (1) Less than monthly
   (2) Monthly
   (3) Weekly
   (4) Daily or almost daily
   Skip to Questions 9 and 10 if Total Score for Questions 2 and 3 = 0

4. How often during the last year have you found that you were not able to stop drinking once you had started?
   (0) Never
   (1) Less than monthly
   (2) Monthly
   (3) Weekly
   (4) Daily or almost daily

5. How often during the last year have you failed to do what was normally expected from you because of drinking?
   (0) Never
   (1) Less than monthly
   (2) Monthly
   (3) Weekly
   (4) Daily or almost daily

6. How often during the last year have you needed a first drink in the morning to get yourself going after a heavy drinking session?
   (0) Never
   (1) Less than monthly
   (2) Monthly
   (3) Weekly
   (4) Daily or almost daily

7. How often during the last year have you had a feeling of guilt or remorse after drinking?
   (0) Never
   (1) Less than monthly
   (2) Monthly
   (3) Weekly
   (4) Daily or almost daily

8. How often during the last year have you been unable to remember what happened the night before because you had been drinking?
   (0) Never
   (1) Less than monthly
   (2) Monthly
   (3) Weekly
   (4) Daily or almost daily

9. Have you or someone else been injured as a result of your drinking?
   (0) No
   (2) Yes, but not in the last year
   (4) Yes, during the last year

10. Has a relative or friend or a doctor or another health worker been concerned about your drinking or suggested you cut down?
   (0) No
   (2) Yes, but not in the last year
   (4) Yes, during the last year

Record total of specific items here

If total is greater than recommended cut-off, consult User's Manual.

Box 14.2   SMAST-G [14]

1. *When talking with others do you ever underestimate how much you actually drink?*
2. *After a few drinks, have you sometimes not eaten, or skipped a meal because you didn't feel hungry?*
3. *Does having a few drinks help decrease your shakiness or tremors?*
4. *Does alcohol sometimes make it hard for you to remember parts of the day or night?*
5. *Do you usually take a drink to relax or calm your nerves?*
6. *Do you drink to take your mind off of your problems?*
7. *Have you ever increased your drinking after experiencing a loss in your life?*
8. *Has a doctor or nurse ever said they were worried or concerned about your drinking?*
9. *Have you ever made rules to manage your drinking?*
10. *When you feel lonely does having a drink help?*

---

common in patients with liver disease and chronic immunological diseases. CDT levels >2.5% are considered a positive test [17].

Phosphatidyl ethanol (PET) is a new test that is able to detect heavy drinking (>4–5 drinks) in the previous four weeks [18]. PET is produced by phospholipase D, which converts phosphatidyl choline to PET in the presence of alcohol. The assay requires whole blood and intact red blood cells. The test is highly sensitive and specific in patients who drink four or more drinks per occasion in the previous 3–4 weeks. PET can also be detected in nails. There are no known false positives. While the assay is not widely available in most clinical laboratories it offers great promise and is being tested to monitor persons under court sanctions for drunk driving, persons who have received liver transplants and in cord blood to detect foetal alcohol exposure in the third trimester. Its use in high-risk psychiatric populations is a new area of research.

Ethyl sulfate and ethyl glucuronide are direct metabolites of alcohol and can be useful biomarkers. They can be detected in urine, blood, nails and hair samples. They are not as sensitive or specific as PET but can offer additional information on alcohol use in the previous 2–3 weeks.

In summary, screening for alcohol use and alcohol abuse/dependence is an important component of routine psychiatric care. Positive screens need to be followed up with a more intensive assessment, brief intervention and potential referral. The prevalence of clinically important alcohol use and disorders may exceed one out of every 10 older adults seen by psychiatrists. Alcohol interacts with a number of psychiatric medications and impairs effective treatment for many mental health disorders.

Illicit drugs

Rationale for screening older adults for marijuana, cocaine and other illicit drugs

Illicit drug use typically declines as individuals move through young adulthood and into maturity. Recent evidence, however, suggests the baby boomer generation (persons born between 1946 and 1964) has relatively higher drug use rates than previous generations [19]. An estimated 4.8 million adults aged 50 or older, or 5.2% of adults in that range, have used an illicit drug in the past year [19]. Although the use of illicit drugs is problematic for individuals of all ages, it may be of particular concern for older adults because they experience physiological, psychological and social changes that place them at greater risk of harm from illicit drug use [20, 21].

Screening for illegal drugs in the psychiatric setting

There are number of methods that can be used for screening, including simple screening questions that can be administered by a psychiatrist as part of a routine care, pencil and paper or computer administered assessment tools and toxicology testing. To assess current use patterns, it is important to ask about the frequency, quantity and ingestion method [3, 11]. There is a clear dose-response effect with the greater the frequency and dose, the greater the likelihood of a clinical problem such as depression, suicide ideation, hallucinations, mania and drug interactions with psychiatric medication. As with tobacco use, inhalation of marijuana, cocaine and opioids through smoking can be toxic to the pulmonary and cardiac system as well as the brain.

Recommended screening questions to detect drug use

Routine questions to screen for drug use include:

- *Have you used any marijuana in the past year? If yes, about how many times a month? When you used marijuana, how much do you use? (If patient is sure how to respond ask about the number of joints.)*
- *Have you used any cocaine in the past year? If yes, did you use by nasal inhalation, smoking crack? IV injection? If yes, about how many times a month? If yes, how much did you use?*
- *Have you used any illegally obtained narcotics in the past month? If yes, what kind did you use? (e.g. include morphine, heroin, oxycontin, methadone, vicodin) If yes, did you take it orally? Smoke it? Inject IV? If yes, about how many times a month? If yes, how much do you use?*
- *The same questions can be used to assess for other drugs that may be more common in some communities and older adult populations; these include methamphetamine, hallucinogens and benzodiazepines.*

Screening for drug abuse/dependence

If interested in screening for abuse or dependence by direct interview, the following set of questions are useful with reasonable sensitivity and specificity:

- *Have you ever felt the need to cut down or control your drug use?*
- *Have you been annoyed when someone criticized your drug use?*
- *Have you felt guilty about your drug use?*
- *Has your drug use interfered with your job? Your finances? Your relationships with your family or friends? Your health?*
- *Do you experience symptoms of drug withdrawal after prolonged daily use?*

Another method that can be used for screening and assessment is to simply ask:

'Have you used marijuana in the past year?'

Those patients who report 'yes' can be asked to complete the NIDA-Modified ASSIST questionnaire, called NM-ASSIST, available as an interactive web-based (www.drugabuse.gov/nmassist) or 'full text' survey (www.drugabuse.gov/sites/default/files/pdf/nmassist.pdf) [3].

The eight-question NM-ASSIST (http://www.drugabuse.gov/publications/resource-guide/nida-quick-screen) inquires about the type of drugs, frequency of their use and symptoms suggestive of abuse or dependence. Its total score, the so-called *Substance Involvement Score,* determines the level of risk associated with illicit or nonmedical prescription drug use (0–3 points: low, 4–26 points: moderate and 27+ points: high risk) [3]. If more than one drug is reported, the patient receives a score for *each* substance endorsed, rather than a single cumulative score. Therefore, the patient's risk level may differ from drug to drug. In addition to its 'scored' questions, the NM-ASSIST also includes a question about intravenous (IV) drug use. Clinicians should use clinical judgment when deciding whether to deliver an intervention for drug use (especially if the risk level is low). The screen is only one indicator of a patient's potential drug use problem. In case of an elevated 'risk level' identified for more than one drug (substance), a decision about which substance to address first needs to be clinically driven; in general, focusing intervention on the substance with the 'highest risk' or the patient's expressed greatest 'motivation to change' may produce best results. There are also a number of computer administered drug assessment tests based on DSM-IV criteria that can be used in the office setting to minimize psychiatrist time, such as the CIDI (Composite International Diagnostic Interview) [22].

Screening for illicit drug use with toxicology screening

Urine toxicology testing [23–25] as part of an office-based screening system is underused by most clinicians and can detect illicit drug use in up to 5% of patients seen for routine older adult care. Rates in psychiatric populations are probably higher. There are a number of reasons to consider routine toxicology testing, including the frequent association of drug use and psychiatric disorders, interaction of illegal drugs with psychiatric medication and detection of an important treatable, clinical problem. Older adults minimize their drug use with their physician. Reasons for this minimization include shame and embarrassment, fear of being judged and treated differently, concern about legal prosecution and, in patients who are drug dependent, unwillingness stop or to give up 'their best friend'.

The use of routine drug testing as part of a new patient visit or prior to starting medication is controversial. Most physicians reserve drug testing for patients at highest risk, such as patients who have a past history of dependence or extensive use, those in whom medication is not working and patients who avoid talking about prior drug use. When ordering a urine toxicology test, it is important to tell the patient why you are ordering the test and what drugs you are testing for. Use the following approach:

'As part of my initial patient assessment, I always obtain a urine test for drugs on all of my new patients. We test for marijuana, stimulants, opioids and sedatives. I want to be sure the medication we are going to use is safe and effective. Is that OK?'

While most patients understand the importance of screening of drug testing as a routine part of psychiatric care, some patients are resistant, especially those who are minimizing their drug use. It is not uncommon for patients to reveal the extent of their drug use when asked to give a urine test for drugs. In addition, if a patient refuses the test or leaves the office/laboratory without giving a urine sample, current use has to be assumed. It is important to check with the laboratory to understand what illegal drugs are tested, the assay procedure, the metabolites detected, cut-off values, duration of detection, substances that may alter the sensitivity of the assay as well as the cost to the patient. It is also important to write the drug on the laboratory request if a specific drug is being looked for. While common drugs, such as marijuana, cocaine and benzodiazepines, are included in standard drug panels, designer drugs, hallucinogens and synthetic opioids (e.g. methadone, oxycodone, oxycontin, fentanyl) are not. Some drugs, such as marijuana, can also be detected in the urine for months depending on the cut-off used to report a positive test.

In summary, there are many reasons why a psychiatrist may want to include routine urine drug testing in older adults for new patients, especially those being placed on psychotropic medication. A test result, positive or negative, can inform decisions made by the clinician regarding treatment and prescription management. Illicit drug use can have important clinical implications in vulnerable older adults, false positive tests are rare and a drug test can identify patients who may not otherwise receive addiction treatment. Addiction remains an important cause of mortality in psychiatric patients.

Prescription drug abuse

Rationale for screening older adults

There are number of medical and mental health disorders that are managed with mood altering drugs that have a high potential for abuse. These drugs include opioids for chronic pain, amphetamines for adult attention deficit disorders, muscle relaxants for leg spasms and sedatives for anxiety and sleep [26, 27].

Chronic pain in the elderly is being increasingly treated with opioids for benign clinical problems such as osteoarthritis, chronic neck pain and chronic back pain. It is no longer unusual for patients to be placed on long acting morphine, oxycodone and methadone by their primary care clinician or pain clinic provider. Co-management of these patients by a psychiatrist, geriatricians and primary care physician complicates the use and monitoring of potentially abusive medications.

The use of amphetamines in older adults to treat adult attention deficit disorders is uncommon. However, as the current adult population that has received prescription amphetamines becomes older, an increasing frequency of abuse of this drug can be expected in older adult populations. Muscle relaxants such as cyclobenzaprine and carisoprodol are other prescription medications with high abuse potential when used to treat chronic pain, for example leg cramps.

Screening for prescription drug abuse

The development and testing of screening for alcohol and illicit drugs use disorders has been an active of research since the 1970s. Screening for prescription drug abuse is a more recent endeavour. The strongest predictors of prescription drug abuse include recent diagnosis of addiction, lifetime history of a psychiatric hospitalization, a positive toxicology screen for cocaine or marijuana and aberrant drug behaviours. As a result of these observations, researchers have approached screening by developing questions and procedures that inquire about aberrant drug behaviours, prior history of addiction, illegal drug activities, urine toxicology screens, escalating doses and presence of psychiatric treatment.

Screening by asking about aberrant drug behaviours

A recent study conducted on a sample of 1000 patients receiving opioids from a primary care physician found that a history of four or more aberrant behaviours was associated with prescription drug abuse [28]. Aberrant behaviours most strongly associated with medication abuse include requests for early refills, felt intoxicated, increased dose on own, purposely oversedating themselves. Other aberrant drug behaviours included seeking medication from more than one physician, hoarding medication, using opioids for other reasons, lost medication or prescriptions.

Screening using urine toxicology testing

While the issue of routine toxicology testing remains controversial, including its use with older adults, most clinicians who work in the area of chronic pain recommend a urine toxicology testing prior to the initiation of opioid therapy. This not only protects the prescriber from potential legal action but gives a measure of credibility to an elderly patient's denial of illicit drug use. While illicit drugs are less commonly used in older adults, drugs generally included in routine toxicology screens include marijuana, cocaine and its metabolites, benzodiazepines, amphetamines and naturally occurring opioids such as morphine. If a physician has concerns about synthetic opioids or wants to confirm current prescription use, a specific assay for oxycodone, hydrocodone, methadone and fentanyl has to be ordered.

Costs can be a consideration and the laboratory fees and potential cost to the patient should be checked. When ordering a toxicology screening, it is important to tell the patient why the test is being ordered, how the information will be recorded in the medical record and how patient confidentiality is safeguarded. Drug addicts who are requesting prescriptions for opioids or other drugs will often leave the medical setting without complying with the request for a urine drug test.

Brief intervention for alcohol, prescription drug abuse and illegal drug use

Brief intervention (BI) is one of many treatment methods available to help patients with excessive alcohol use, illegal and prescription drug abuse [11, 29]. BI has been shown to decrease alcohol use and morbidity when administered in primary care settings [30–36]. While there have been a limited number of trials conducted in older adults that show a similar positive effect as those conducted in other populations [37], the efficacy of brief intervention in primary care settings is well accepted for college students, pregnant and post-partum women, adults and older adults. There is less information on the efficacy of BI in the emergency department, inpatient care and psychiatric setting. While there is more information on reducing alcohol use, recent research suggests BI can be effective for illicit drug and prescription drug abuse [38]. BI is less useful in people who are dependent but may be effective in motivating dependent patients to seek treatment in a traditional substance abuse treatment programme [39].

Brief intervention is a time-limited brief counselling session that can be delivered in the context of routine medical or mental health care. BI is based on the concepts and techniques of motivational interviewing (MI), cognitive behavioural therapy (CBT) and the clinician–client relationship. While the terms BI and MI are used often used interchangeably by researchers and clinicians, they are not equivalent. BI may be a simple statement by a provider such as:

> '*I am concerned about your alcohol use and how it is affecting your depression and the medication I have prescribed? I would like you to stop drinking for a while to see how things go.*'
> '*The urine toxicology test we conducted last week contained cocaine and marijuana. In order for us to continue to work together you need stop using drugs. I also need you to see an alcohol and drug counsellor.*'

This is a traditional clinician directed statement and prescriptive advice. These kinds of statements are the core of what physicians say to patients, whether it is focused on pharmacotherapy, behavioural change or reducing substance use. These statements take <20 seconds to deliver and can begin the process of change. There is nothing in the statement that is client centred or MI based. It simply states the clinical evidence and the physician's recommendation. The patient may or may be not be ready to accept the physician's treatment recommendation.

Motivational interviewing, on the other hand, is a technique that explores what the patients think about their alcohol or drug use and if they are ready to change. The clinician tries to develop discrepancy, accepts patient ambiguity and rolls with the patient's resistance to change. The clinician goes along with the patient perspectives and tries to move them in direction that will help them reduce substance use and harm.

To effectively use these techniques, it is very difficult for an MI session to be less than 30 minutes. While physicians practicing medicine in today's practice model have limited time to practice traditional MI methods, BI may include elements of MI such:

'Would you be willing to reduce your alcohol use for a while to help the medicine be more effective?'
'What do you think about cutting back to no more than 1–2 drinks a day to allow your medication to work.'
'It seems like you have been having a hard time cutting back. What do you think about going to talk with a colleague of mine to help you with your drinking?'

The 5As has been recommended to guide screening and brief intervention – ASK, ADVISE, ASSESS, ASSIST and ARRANGE [11]:

- ASK – Screening for substance use and abuse is the first step to determine the level of use and presence or absence of substance-related problems and symptoms of abuse and/or dependence. This can be conducted by a clinical staff person, questionnaire completed in the waiting, computer or the physician.
- *ADVISE* – Patients who screen positive for at-risk substance use or substance abuse/dependence may respond to brief physician ADVICE. The brief intervention should include a summary of what was learned from the screening/assessment process, feedback on health/family/social related effects and recommendations on reducing substance use. It is important to relate the health/family/social adverse consequences to something the patient cares about:

'I am concerned about your alcohol/marijuana use.'
'I think your depression may be related to your alcohol or drug use. The medication I would like to prescribe will be more effective if you cut down to a few drinks a week and no more than 2–3 per occasion.'

In patients who have symptoms of dependence the following series of statements is suggested:

'I am concerned that you may have a serious alcohol/drug problem.'
'It will be difficult for me to work with you on treating your depression unless you completely stop drinking.'

- *ASSESS* – The next step in the process is to assess the patient's willingness ('readiness') to change the unhealthy behaviour (reduction of use or quitting). If the patient is not willing to change his or her substance use, the clinician should restate the substance use-related health concerns, reaffirm a willingness to help when the patient is ready and encourage the patient to reflect about perceived 'benefits' of continued use versus decreasing or stopping use, and barriers to change:

'Let's talk about setting a specific amount of alcohol you should drink per week.'
'It sounds like you are not ready to cut down your use. Why don't you think about what we discussed and come back in a week. I am glad to help you with your depression but first I need you to think about cutting down on your drinking.'

- *ASSIST* – involves helping the agreeable patient develop a treatment plan that follows the patient's personal goals. Using behaviour change techniques (e.g. motivational interviewing), the clinician should aid the patient in achieving agreed-upon goals and acquiring the appropriate skills, confidence and social/environmental support. It is helpful if the plan describes in concrete terms the specific steps the patient elects to take to reduce/quit drinking. For example, a maximum number of drinks per day or week, how to prevent and manage high-risk situations or establish a support network. Starting with 'small steps' while working toward a larger goal (abstinence or safe use) may be most reasonable and achievable for many patients.

    There are a number of tools physicians may want to recommend to patients, such as tracking cards, online education and intervention programmes, seeing a substance abuse counsellor or self-help groups.
- Finally, *ARRANGE* – refers to the consideration of a follow-up visit and specialty referrals. A follow-up appointment should be *arranged* for all patients who screened positive to provide continuing assistance and adjust the treatment plan as needed. Optimally, all patients should also receive educational materials.

Summary

Screening and brief intervention for substance abuse disorders in older adults is an important component of routine clinical care for all physicians, including psychiatrists and geriatricians. While substance misuse is less common in older adults, alcohol, opioid or marijuana use disorders impact the treatment of mental health problems and pharmacotherapy. The clinical importance of varying levels of substance use in older adults is less defined due individual differences in drug metabolism, severity of the mental health issues and interactions with other medications, such as cardiac drugs and hypertensive medication. In many patients, abstinence from all mood altering substances is the safest approach. Toxicology testing is underused and offers opportunities to detect substances that directly affect treatment. Another issue is linking screening and brief intervention to specialty addiction treatment and counselling and more affective referral strategies, as many patients are reluctant to be participate in alcohol and drug treatment programmes or self-help groups such as Alcoholics Anonymous.

References

1. Coulton, S., Watson, J., Bland, M. *et al.* (2008) The effectiveness and cost-effectiveness of opportunistic screening and stepped care interventions for older hazardous alcohol users in primary care (AESOPS) – a randomized control trial protocol. *BMC Health Serv Res*, **8**, 129.
2. American Psychiatric Association (2000) *Diagnostic and Statistical Manual*, 4th edn, text revision. American Psychiatric Association Press, Washington, DC.
3. National Institute on Drug Abuse (2012) Screening for Drug Use in General Medical Settings: Resource Guide. http://www.drugabuse.gov/sites/default/files/resource_guide.pdf (last accessed 10 April 2014).
4. Moyer, V.A. (2013) Screening and Behavioral Counseling Interventions in Primary Care to Reduce Alcohol Misuse: U.S. Preventive Services Task Force Recommendation Statement. *Ann Intern Med*, **159**(3), 210–218. doi: 10.7326/0003-4819-159-3-201308060-00652.
5. Moore, A.A., Whiteman, E.J. and Ward, K.T. (2007) Risks of combined alcohol/medication use in older adults. *Am J of Geriatr Pharmacother*, **5**(1), 64–74.
6. Lee, H.S., Mericle, A.A., Ayalon, L. and Areán, P.A. (2009) Harm reduction among at-risk elderly drinkers: a site-specific analysis from the multi-site Primary Care Research in Substance Abuse and Mental Health for Elderly (PRISM-E) study. *Int J Geriatr Psychiatry*, **24**(1), 54–60.
7. Berks, J. and McCormick, R. (2008) Screening for alcohol misuse in elderly primary care patients: a systematic literature review. *Int Psychogeriatr*, **20**(6), 1090–1103.
8. Smith, P.C., Schmidt, S.M., Allensworth-Davies, D. and Saitz, R. (2009) Primary care validation of a single-question alcohol screening test. *J Gen Intern Med*, **24**(7), 783–788.
9. Bradley, K.A., McDonell, M.B., Bush, K. *et al.* (1998) The AUDIT Alcohol Consumption Questions: reliability, validity, and responsiveness to change in older male primary care patients. *Alcohol Clin Exp Res*, **22**(8), 1842–1849.
10. Bradley, K.A., DeBenedetti, A.F., Volk, R.J. *et al.* (2007) AUDIT-C as a brief screen for alcohol misuse in primary care. *Alcohol Clin Exp Res*, **31**(7), 1208–1217.
11. National Institute on Alcohol Abuse and Alcoholism (2007) *Helping Patients Who Drink Too Much: A Clinician's Guide* (updated 2005 edition). NIH publication no. 07-3769. US Department of Health and Human Services, National Institutes of Health, National Institute on Alcohol Abuse and Alcoholism, Bethesda, MD.
12. Adams, W.L., Barry, K.L. and Fleming, M.F. (1996) Screening for problem drinking in older primary care patients. *JAMA*, **276**, 1964–1967.
13. Aalto, M., Alho, H., Halme, J. and Seppa, K. (2011) The Alcohol Use Disorders Identification Test (AUDIT) and its derivatives in screening for heavy drinking among the elderly. *Int J Geriatr Psychiatry*, **26**, 881–885.
14. Blow, F.C., Gillespie, B.W., Barry, K.L. *et al.* (1998) Brief screening for alcohol problems in elderly populations using the Short Michigan Alcoholism Screening Test-Geriatric Version (SMAST-G). *Alcoholism Clin Exp Res*, **22**(Suppl), 131A.
15. Beullens, J. and Aertgeerts, B. (2004) Screening for alcohol abuse and dependence in older people using DSM criteria: a review. *Aging Ment Health*, **8**(1), 76–82.
16. Peterson, K. (2004–2005) Biomarkers for alcohol use and abuse–a summary. *Alcohol Res Health*, **28**(1), 30–37.
17. Fleming, M.F., Spies, C. and Anton, R. (2004) A review of genetic, biological, pharmacological and clinical that affect CDT levels. *Alcohol Clin Exp Res*, **28**(9), 1347–1355.
18. Nalesso, A., Viel, G., Cecchetto, G. *et al.* (2010) Analysis of the alcohol biomarker phosphatidylethanol by NACE with on-line ESI-MS. *Electrophoresis*, **31**(7), 1227–1233.

19. Substance Abuse and Mental Health Services Administration (2011) *The NSDUH Report: Illicit Drug Use among Older Adults.* Center for Behavioral Health Statistics and Quality, Substance Abuse and Mental Health Services Administration, Rockville, MD.

20. American Society of Addiction Medicine (2012) State-Level Proposals to Legalize Marijuana. American Society of Addiction Medicine, Chevy Chase, MD. http://www.asam.org/policies/state-level-proposals-to-legalize-marijuana (last accessed 10 April 2014).

21. Wu, L.-T. and Blazer, D.G. (2011) Illicit and nonmedical drug use among older adults: a review. *J Aging Health,* **23**(3), 481–504.

22. World Health Organization (1990) *Composite International Diagnostic Interview.* World Health Organization, Geneva, Switzerland.

23. Bottros, M. and Christo, P.J. (2011) Urine Drug Testing: An Underused Tool. *Pain Management Today,* **1**(7). http://newsletter.qhc.com/JFP/JFP_pain022311.htm (last accessed 10 April 2014).

24. Owen, G.T., Burton, A.W., Schade, C.M. and Passik, S. (2012) Urine drug testing: current recommendations and best practices. *Pain Physician,* **15**(3 Suppl), ES119–133.

25. Heller, J.L. (2011) *Toxicology screen: MedlinePlus Medical Encyclopedia.* Medline Plus, US National Library of Medicine, National Institutes of Health. http://www.nlm.nih.gov/medlineplus/ency/article/003578.htm (last accessed 10 April 2014).

26. Substance Abuse and Mental Health Services Administration (2012) *The DAWN Report: Drug-Related Emergency Department Visits Involving Pharmaceutical Misuse or Abuse by Older Adults: 2009.* Center for Behavioral Health Statistics and Quality, Substance Abuse and Mental Health Services Administration, Rockville, MD.

27. Substance Abuse and Mental Health Services Administration (2011) *The TEDS Report: Substance Abuse Treatment Admissions for Abuse of Benzodiazepines.* Center for Behavioral Health Statistics and Quality, Substance Abuse and Mental Health Services Administration, Rockville, MD.

28. Fleming, M.F., Balousek, S.L., Klessig, C.L. *et al.* (2007) Substance use disorders in a primary care sample receiving daily opioid therapy. *J Pain,* **8**(7), 573–582.

29. Fink, A., Elliott, M.N., Tsai, M. and Beck, J.C. (2005) An evaluation of an intervention to assist primary care physicians in screening and educating older patients who use alcohol. *J Am Geriatr Soc,* **53**(11), 1937–1943.

30. Fleming, M.F., Barry, K.L., Manwell, L.B. *et al.* (1997) Brief physician advice for problem alcohol drinkers. A randomized controlled trial in community-based primary care practices. *JAMA,* **277**(13), 1039–1045.

31. Fleming, M.F., Manwell L.B., Barry, K.L. *et al.* (1999) Brief physician advice for alcohol problems in older adults: a randomized community-based trial. *J Fam Pract,* **148**(5), 378–384.

32. Fleming, M.F., Mundt, M.P., French, M.T. *et al.* (2002) Brief physician advice for problem drinkers: Long-term efficacy and benefit-cost analysis. *Alcohol Clin Exp Res,* **26**(1), 36–43.

33. Fleming, M.F., Balousek, S.L., Grossberg, P.M. *et al.* (2010) Brief physician advice for heavy drinking college students: a randomized controlled trial in college health clinics. *J Stud Alcohol Drugs,* **71**(1), 23–31.

34. Fleming, M.F., Lund, M.R., Wilton, G. *et al.* (2008) The healthy moms study: the efficacy of brief alcohol intervention in postpartum women. *Alcohol Clin Exp Res,* **32**(9), 1–7.

35. Cuijpers, P., Riper, H. and Lemmers, L. (2004) The effects of mortality of brief interventions for problem drinkers: a meta-analysis. *Addiction,* **99**, 839–845.

36. Bertholet, N., Daeppen, J.B., Wietlisbach, V. *et al.* (2005) Reduction of alcohol consumption by brief alcohol intervention in primary care: systematic review and meta-analysis. *Arch Intern Med*, **165**(9), 986–995.

37. Anderson, P., Scafato, E. and Gauzzo, L. (VINTAGE Project Working Group) (2012) Alcohol and older people from a public health perspective. *Ann Ist Super Sanita*, **48**(3), 232–247.

38. Bernstein, J., Bernstein, E., Tassiopoulos, K. *et al.* (2005) Brief motivational intervention at a clinic visit reduces cocaine and heroin use. *Drug Alcohol Depend*, **77**(1), 49–59.

39. Copeland, J., Swift, W., Roffman, R. and Stephens, R. (2001) A randomized controlled trial of brief cognitive-behavioral interventions for cannabis use disorder. *J Subst Abuse Treat*, **21**(2), 55–64; discussion 65–56.

Chapter 15

TOBACCO USE CESSATION

Daniel J. Pilowsky[1] and Li-Tzy Wu[2]

[1] Department of Epidemiology, Mailman School of Public Health/Department of Psychiatry, Columbia College of Physicians and Surgeons, USA
[2] Department of Psychiatry and Behavioral Sciences, Duke University School of Medicine, USA

Introduction

Tobacco smoking is less prevalent among older than younger adults but it remains common in the older population. A study using a large community sample of American adults (N = 5691) found self-reported prevalences of current smoking of 29.1 and 19.5 % among younger (18–50 years) and older (≥50 years) adults, respectively. Both age groups had similar prevalences of past 12-month nicotine dependence as defined in the fourth edition of the Diagnostic and Statistical Manual of Mental Disorders (DSM-IV), that is 4.6 and 3.1% in younger and older adults, respectively, as well as lifetime dependence, that is 8.6 and 8.2%, respectively [1]. Data from the 2000–2001 National Epidemiologic Survey on Alcohol and Related Conditions (NESARC) showed similar nicotine dependence prevalences in adults aged ≥65 years, that is 8.7% lifetime dependence (vs 8.2%) and 4.0% past-year dependence (vs 3.1%) [2]. A study of a Brazilian sample of individuals aged 60 years and older revealed that nearly one in five elderly individuals surveyed were current tobacco smokers [3]. A review of worldwide tobacco use surveys targeting older adults found that the prevalence of elderly tobacco use was higher in richer countries than prevalences in low and middle income countries [4]. This finding contrasts with reports indicating that low socioeconomic status is associated with tobacco use at the individual level. Thus, it appears that tobacco control programmes in developed countries usually focus on young adults, leaving the elderly unexposed to prevention efforts [4]. Given the increasing use of tobacco in low income countries [5], seen by some as part of the globalization of risk factors [6], the prevalence of elderly tobacco use in these countries may increase over time.

Extant research suggests a low rate of smoking cessation among older adults. Older adults are less likely to attempt to quit smoking, and less likely to quit, compared to younger adults. In the United States, 53.8% of adults aged 65 and older surveyed in 2010 were interested in quitting smoking, compared to 69.0% among those aged 45–64 years; quitting attempts were reported by 43.5 and 45.5% in the these age groups, respectively [7]. During the period 2001–2010, the prevalence of

Substance Use and Older People, First Edition.
Edited by Ilana B. Crome, Li-Tzy Wu, Rahul (Tony) Rao and Peter Crome.
© 2015 John Wiley & Sons, Ltd. Published 2015 by John Wiley & Sons, Ltd.

quit attempts remained stable among smokers aged 65 and older [7]. In the same report, recent cessation (former smokers who quit smoking in the past year for six months or more) was somewhat similar among elders aged 65 and older (5.3%) and adults aged 45–64 (4.7%) but was much higher among younger adults (8.2% among adults aged 18–24; 7.1% among adults aged 25–44).

Because of the deterioration of health status with ageing, tobacco use (cigarettes, cigars, smokeless tobacco products) among older adults is associated with heightened health risks and increasing mortality [8, 9]. Health risks include heart disease and stroke [10], increased mortality and overall ill health [11]. A study of older adults (aged 60–70 years) showed that the crude mortality rate (deaths per 1000 population per year) was higher among current (40.9) and former (40.7) compared to never smokers (34.1). Heavy smokers were also about two times more likely to experience difficulty walking several blocks, more likely to be dependent in at least one activity of daily living, to be hospitalized in the last year and to self-report fair or poor health compared to those that never smoke [11]. Despite the elevated health risks, correlates of tobacco use among older adults have received less attention than among adolescents or young adults. Blazer and Wu examined correlates of tobacco use among adults aged 50–64 and ≥65 using data from the 2008–2009 National Survey on Drug Use and Health (NSDUH) [8]. In their sample, about a quarter (24%) of adults aged ≥50 years reported tobacco use in the past year. In the 50–64 age group, past-year cigarette smoking was associated with being male, less educated, not currently married, having a low income and being White or African American (compared to Hispanic). Elders aged ≥65 followed a similar pattern, except that there were no statistically significant differences by income or ethnicity. A possible interpretation of these differences between middle aged and senior smokers is that those aged 50–64 became adults when smoking began to be considered deviant and those 65+ when smoking was socially acceptable. In the same study, past-year cigarette smoking was associated with increased odds of binge drinking (alcohol), illicit drug use and nonmedical use of prescription drugs in middle aged and older individuals. Past-year cigarette smoking was not associated with depression in either age group and was associated with self-reported anxiety only in the middle aged cohort. This finding concurs with an often reported association between anxiety-related symptoms and smoking in the general adult population [1].

Another study found that American smokers aged ≥50 years without nicotine dependence had significantly higher rates of 12-month psychiatric disorders than their nonsmoking same-age peers, including affective disorders (0.9 vs 0.1%), dysthymia (4.1 vs 1.6%), major depressive disorder (6.4 vs 3.9%) and alcohol abuse (1.5 vs 0.1%) [1]. Similar findings have been reported for alcohol, the nonmedical use of prescription drugs and illicit substances in community and clinical samples [12–16], with a higher prevalence of depressive disorders in particular and of psychiatric disorders in general among individuals with substance use disorders compared to those without these disorders and to nonusers. Older smokers with nicotine dependence differed from non-nicotine-dependent same-age smokers in several respects, including a higher prevalence of past 12-month generalized anxiety disorder (13.6 vs 2.6%) and other anxiety disorders, as well as alcohol abuse (3.0 vs 1.5%) [1]. A limitation of these estimates is that the sample size of older adults was not sufficiently large to generate reliable estimates for some DSM-IV psychiatric disorders (e.g. panic disorder, drug abuse/dependence). Nevertheless, these data suggest that a higher prevalence of co-morbid DSM-IV disorders, and most prominently anxiety disorders, distinguished nicotine-dependent older smokers from nondependent same-age smokers. The high prevalence of most anxiety disorders among nicotine-dependent older smokers stands in sharp contrast to the low prevalence of most DSM-IV anxiety/depressive disorders among older adults [17], but it is not saliently different from prevalences reported in younger adult smokers [18]. Research suggests that co-morbid psychopathology makes it difficult to quit smoking with or without smoking cessation interventions [18]. These findings support the 'selection hypothesis of smoking', which posits that smokers with co-morbid psychiatric disorders or distress are less likely to successfully complete quitting attempts than those without such comorbid profiles [1].

Smoking cessation interventions among older adults

There are few studies examining smoking cessation interventions among older adults. A recent review found only 13 randomized controlled trials that provide findings about the effectiveness of smoking cessation interventions among older adults (ages 50 and older), including 10 American studies [19]. Nine of thirteen studies reported a significant intervention effect at one or more follow-up assessments, suggesting that successful interventions with older adults are available and feasible, although the best results are obtained with interventions of longer duration. Most studies included counselling of varying intensity and eight provided medication for smoking cessation, including bupropion, nicotine patches, nicotine gum or varenicline. The relevant findings are summarized here.

Multimodal interventions

According to a recent review [19], eight studies tested multimodal interventions that combined counselling, psychoeducation or one of the smoking cessation medications listed above [20–27]. The proportion of participants who quit smoking varied widely across these studies, from 7 to 66%. Overall, studies with the longest intervention length have shown the highest quit rates. These studies included three studies that reported results separately for elderly participants [20, 21, 25] and five studies that targeted exclusively older adults [22–24, 26, 27]. Table 15.1 summarizes the results of these studies.

A British study assessed smoking cessation following an intervention that provided individual or group-based behavioural treatment combined with nicotine replacement therapy (NRT) (78.6%) or bupropion (15.7%). Most received weekly treatment for eight weeks. The sample was large (N = 2546 at baseline); of these, 386 individuals aged 61 years and over completed the 52-week follow-up [28].

Table 15.1 Multimodal interventions for older smokers: A review of randomized trials

Reference	N/Age (years)	Intervention/duration	Results
Hall et al. [22]	402/50+	Compared extended NRT, extended CBT, and both administered concurrently to UC	Only extended CBT was significantly more effective than UC with 55% abstinence[a] at the 2-year F/U
Hill et al. [23]	82/50+	Compared behavioural training alone and combined with NRT or physical exercise to physical exercise only	No difference in abstinence[a] rates at the 12-month F/U
Joyce et al. [24]	7354/65+	Compared provider counselling (with and without pharmacotherapy) and telephone counselling with NRT to UC	At the 12-month F/U, all active treatments (14.1–19.3% abstinence[a]) were significantly more effective than UC (10.2% abstinence[a])
Morgan et al. [26]	659/50–74	Compared brief physician-delivered counselling to UC	At the 6-month F/U, 9.3% of UC and 17.8% of active group participants, respectively, were abstinent[a] (p < 0.005)
Orleans et al. [27]	470/65+	Compared providing a smoking guide and seven personalized computer-generated messages to UC	At the 6-month F/U, 40% in the active and 33% in the UC conditions, respectively, were abstinent[a] (p < 0.05) but there were no statistically significant differences at the 12-month F/U

Abbreviations: CBT = Cognitive-behavioural therapy; F/U = Follow-up; NRT = Nicotine replacement therapy; UC = Usual care
[a] Refers to abstinence from tobacco as defined in each study.

Assuming that loss to follow-up is equivalent to relapse, the cessation rate at 52 weeks (21.5%) was greater for older smokers (61 and over) than for other age groups. This rate compares to 7.8% among those aged 16–30; 11.7% (aged 31–40); 15.2% (aged 41–50); and 17.3% (aged 51–60). The investigators speculated that older individuals have a greater probability of adhering to a treatment programme and smaller risk of relapse, compared to their younger counterparts. A similar age effect was noted in a smoking cessation programme in Spain. Excluding those receiving only advice to stop smoking (n = 992), 211 primary care patients received advice, psychoeducation, follow-up and nicotine patches (63%), with the remaining 37% (n = 79) refusing the patches [29]. Older age was associated with a decreased likelihood of a biochemically validated relapse between 12 and

24 months post-intervention (adjusted odds ratio of validated abstinence = 1.32 [95% confidence interval: 1.13–0.44] for every additional 10 years of age).

Medication-based interventions

Four studies tested medication-based interventions among older adults. Joyce *et al.* [24] completed a study with a large sample of Medicare beneficiaries (n = 7354). This study appears to include the largest sample size of seniors studied as part of a smoking cessation randomized controlled trial [24]. Abstinence from tobacco was defined as self-reported smoking cessation in the past seven days. At the 12 month follow-up, as shown in Table 15.1, all active interventions were significantly more effective than usual care, with 12-month tobacco-abstinence rates of 14.1–19.3% for these interventions versus 10.2% for usual care. Another study that combined bupropion with brief counselling found that bupropion was effective in increasing the quitting rate [20]. Although all doses included in that trial (100 mg, 150 mg and 300 mg per day) were significantly more effective than placebo, the quit rate increased with higher bupropion doses. Hill *et al.* studied 82 chronic smokers aged 50 and older in a randomized trial with four arms, including three intervention groups (behavioural training; behavioural training and nicotine gum; behavioural training and physical exercise) and a control condition (physical exercise only) [23]. At the one-year follow-up, quitting rates were higher in the three intervention groups (27.8–31.8%) compared to the 10% rate in the control condition. However, differences in quitting rates at the one-year follow-up were not statistically significant (Table 15.1). The study might not have had enough statistical power to demonstrate differences in quitting rates across the arms.

Hall *et al.* studied 402 smokers aged 50 and older who smoked ten or more cigarettes per day [22]. Their randomized controlled trial was a unique and particularly interesting study for two reasons: (i) while most tobacco cessation interventions are brief, Hall *et al.* provided treatment of longer duration; and (ii) the main outcome was past seven-day smoking abstinence biochemically verified. Study participants were randomized into four arms, usual care and three extended treatment conditions, each having a one-year duration. The three extended treatments were: (i) extended nicotine replacement therapy (E-NRT); (ii) extended cognitive behavioural therapy (E-CBT); and (iii) extended combined treatment (e-combined), consisting of E-NRT and E-CBT. Usual care consisted of 12 weeks of bupropion and 10 weeks of nicotine gum as well as counselling. Participants in the four arms were followed up at week 104 (i.e. one year after completion of the extended treatments). As shown in Table 15.1, the only treatment condition that differed significantly from usual care one year after completion of the extended treatments was E-CBT. Neither E-NRT nor e-combined achieved significantly higher rates of abstinence than usual care. E-CBT was associated with over 50% abstinence at week 104, compared to over 30% in the usual care arm. The two most important findings were the long-term efficacy of E-CBT and, contrary to expectations, the failure to increase tobacco abstinence rates as a result of adding nicotine replacement therapy to E-CBT. The investigators speculated that, while those in the combined intervention may have attributed abstinence to nicotine replacement therapy, E-CBT participants may have gained a sense of self-efficacy, as a result of attributing their success in abstaining to the skills they gained during the E-CBT intervention.

Counselling and behavioural interventions

In this section, we focus on counselling/behavioural interventions often without co-occurring treatment with medication. Most studies offered brief interventions. Interventions that included a limited number of sessions, typically 3–10 sessions, uniformly found a significant short-term impact on smoking cessation but long-term effects varied and were often nonsignificant. These interventions, which are described in detail elsewhere [19], often comprise educational materials and may include booster sessions or treatment of co-morbid psychiatric conditions when applicable. For example, McFall *et al.* investigated a smoking cessation intervention combined with treatment of post-traumatic stress disorder among veterans [25]. The intervention effect was compared to standard treatment, and the difference remained significant at the 18 month follow-up. More typically, brief interventions are not effective, or do not have a lasting impact. For example, Doolan *et al.* studied the effectiveness of a smoking-cessation intervention for female smokers with cardiovascular disease [21]. They compared cessation rates among those aged 62 and older to their younger counterparts, that is participants younger than 62 years. At six-month follow-up, the counselling intervention was effective among older female smokers but not at 12 months (compared to a control condition consisting of being advised to quit smoking). It is noteworthy that older women did better than their younger counterparts, as evidenced by 52.0% and 38.1% quitting rates at the 12-month follow-up among older and younger female smokers, respectively, a significant difference (OR [odds ratio] = 1.77; 95% confidence interval: 1.02–3.06).

Overall, interventions of longer duration show more consistent results but very few trials have been conducted using this intensive approach. The aforementioned extended cognitive behavioural intervention (E-CBT) was more effective than a standard intervention over multiple follow-up intervals [22].

Physician-delivered interventions

Physician-delivered interventions, typically very brief, are associated with low-to-modest quitting rates (12–16%) [19]. For example, Vetter and Ford reported that a personally delivered physician advice followed by brief counselling by a nurse resulted in a six-month quitting rate of 15% compared to 9% among controls [30]. In his study of Medicare beneficiaries, Joyce *et al.* found that provider counselling alone (i.e. without pharmacotherapy) was more effective, as evidenced by 12-month quitting rates, than usual care (14.1 vs 10.2% for counselling and usual care, respectively; p ≤ 0.05) [24]. Twelve-month quitting rates were also higher for provider counselling with pharmacotherapy compared to usual care (15.8 and 10.2%, respectively; p ≤ 0.05).

Other interventions

Self-help guides targeting older tobacco users have been used either as a single intervention or in combination with calls, mailings or transdermal nicotine [27, 31, 32]. Telephone quit-lines typically provide counselling over the phone to individuals who wish to quit smoking. This is the most commonly used service to quit smoking and there is abundant evidence of its effectiveness [33]. Abstinence rates among quit-line users are modest overall but these interventions have a lower cost than most other interventions and have the potential to serve a large number of smokers. For example, a large randomized controlled trial assigned callers to a treatment group (N = 1973) or a control condition (N = 1309). All participants received self-help materials. The active intervention included up to seven counselling sessions. Those in the control group received counselling only if they called back after randomization [34]. Rates of abstinence at the 12-month follow-up were 9.1 and 6.9% in the active and control condition, respectively (p < 0.001). Unfortunately, little information is available regarding the comparative effectiveness of this approach in older versus younger adults. Older adults seem to be less likely to know about quit-lines than their younger counterparts. For example, a study of the awareness and use of tobacco quit-lines revealed that younger individuals (aged 18–34) were more than twice as likely to be aware of quit-lines than their older counterparts, aged 65 and older (OR = 2.10; 95% CI [confidence interval]: 1.65–2.66) [35]. Although data on quit-lines (used as the only intervention) in the elderly do not seem to be available, the aforementioned study of Medicare beneficiaries investigated the use of quit-line combined with nicotine replacement [24]. At the 12-month follow-up, quit rates were 19.3%, among those using a quit-line in combination with nicotine replacement, a rate higher than those receiving usual care as well as those receiving other active interventions. This finding is suggestive of a potential effectiveness of quit-lines in this age group. Clearly, this area deserves further attention from investigators.

Conclusions

About one fifth of older adults aged ≥50 years are current tobacco smokers [1]. Given that the health consequences of smoking in old age are serious, including increased health care use and mortality, this is an important public health problem. There is evidence that older smokers are interested in quitting. For example, a study of smokers invited to participate in a smoking cessation trial showed that older smokers were more likely to enrol than their younger counterparts, with a 4% increased likelihood of enrolling for every year increase in age [36]. Studies have demonstrated that older adults can quit. Nevertheless, the rate of smoking cessation among older adults is relatively low. A recent review indicates that most treatment approaches targeting this population have short-term effectiveness, and only few have reported statistically significant lasting treatment effects (12 months or longer) [19]. Intensive and multimodal interventions are more likely to be associated with tobacco cessation than short and single modality interventions. Unfortunately, little is known about types of interventions or aspects of intervention design that older adults may find preferable and convenient. Similarly, relatively little is known about the effectiveness of quit-lines among older, compared to younger adults. Thus, additional research focusing on aspects of intervention design that are acceptable to older adults and effective in this age group, including quit-lines, are needed.

References

1. Sachs-Ericsson, N., Collins, N., Schmidt, B. and Zvolensky, M. (2011) Older adults and smoking: Characteristics, nicotine dependence and prevalence of DSM-IV 12-month disorders. *Aging and Mental Health*, **15**(1), 132–141.
2. Lin, J.C., Karno, M.P., Grella, C.E. *et al.* (2011) Alcohol, tobacco, and nonmedical drug use disorders in U.S. Adults aged 65 years and older: data from the 2001–2002 National Epidemiologic Survey of Alcohol and Related Conditions. *American Journal of Geriatric Psychiatry*, **19**(3), 292–299.
3. Madruga, C., Ferri, C., Pinsky, I. *et al.* (2010) Tobacco use among the elderly: The first Brazilian National Survey (BNAS). *Aging and Mental Health*, **14**(6), 720–724.
4. Marinho, V., Laks, J., Coutinho, E.S.F. and Blay, S.L. (2010) Tobacco use among the elderly: a systematic review and meta-analysis. *Cadernos de Saude Publica*, **26**(12), 2213–2233.
5. Strong, K., Mathers, C., Leeder, S. and Beaglehole, R. (2005) Preventing chronic diseases: how many lives can we save? *Lancet*, **366**(9496), 1578–1582.
6. Samb, B., Desai, N., Nishtar, S. *et al.* (2010) Prevention and management of chronic disease: a litmus test for health-systems strengthening in low-income and middle-income countries. *Lancet*, **376**(9754), 1785–1797.
7. Centers for Disease Control and Prevention (2011) Quitting smoking among adults – United States, 2001–2010. *MMWR – Morbidity & Mortality Weekly Report*, **60**, 1513–1519.
8. Blazer, D.G. and Wu, L.-T. (2012) Patterns of tobacco use and tobacco-related psychiatric morbidity and substance use among middle-aged and older adults in the United States. *Aging and Mental Health*, **16**(3), 296–304.
9. Tice, J.A., Kanaya, A., Hue, T. *et al.* (2006) Risk factors for mortality in middle-aged women. *Archives of Internal Medicine*, **166**(22), 2469–2477.
10. Go, A.S., Mozaffarian, D., Roger, V.L. *et al.* (2013) Executive summary: heart disease and stroke statistics – 2013 update: a report from the American Heart Association. *Circulation*, **127**(1), 143–152.
11. Ostbye, T., Taylor, D.H. and Jung, S.-H. (2002) A longitudinal study of the effects of tobacco smoking and other modifiable risk factors on ill health in middle-aged and old Americans: results from the Health and Retirement Study and Asset and Health Dynamics among the Oldest Old survey. *Preventive Medicine*, **34**(3), 334–345.
12. Hasin, D., Samet, S., Nunes, E. *et al.* (2006) Diagnosis of comorbid psychiatric disorders in substance users assessed with the Psychiatric Research Interview for Substance and Mental Disorders for DSM-IV. *American Journal of Psychiatry*, **163**(4), 689–696.

13. Hasin, D.S. and Grant, B.F. (2004) The co-occurrence of DSM-IV alcohol abuse in DSM-IV alcohol dependence: Results of the National Epidemiologic Survey on Alcohol and Related Conditions on heterogeneity that differ by population subgroup. *Archives of General Psychiatry*, **61**(9), 891–896.
14. Hasin, D.S. and Grant, B.F. (2002) Major depression in 6050 former drinkers: association with past alcohol dependence. *Archives of General Psychiatry*, **59**(9), 794–800.
15. Hasin, D.S., Stinson, F.S., Ogburn, E. and Grant, B.F. (2007) Prevalence, correlates, disability, and comorbidity of DSM-IV alcohol abuse and dependence in the United States: Results from the National Epidemiologic Survey on Alcohol and Related Conditions. *Archives of General Psychiatry*, **64**(7), 830–842.
16. Becker, W.C., Sullivan, L.E., Tetrault, J.M. *et al.* (2008) Non-medical use, abuse and dependence on prescription opioids among U.S. adults: psychiatric, medical and substance use correlates. *Drug and Alcohol Dependence*, **94**(1–3), 38–47.
17. Scott, K.M., Von Korff, M., Alonso, J. *et al.* (2008) Age patterns in the prevalence of DSM-IV depressive/anxiety disorders with and without physical co-morbidity. *Psychological Medicine*, **38**(11), 1659–1669.
18. Piper, M.E., Smith, S.S., Schlam, T.R. *et al.* (2010) Psychiatric disorders in smokers seeking treatment for tobacco dependence: relations with tobacco dependence and cessation. *Journal of Consulting and Clinical Psychology*, **78**(1), 13–23.
19. Zbikowski, S.M., Magnusson, B., Pockey, J.R. *et al.* (2012) A review of smoking cessation interventions for smokers aged 50 and older. *Maturitas*, **71**(2), 131–141.
20. Dale, L.C., Glover, E.D., Sachs, D.P. *et al.* (2001) Bupropion for smoking cessation: predictors of successful outcome. *Chest*, **119**(5), 1357–1364.
21. Doolan, D.M., Stotts, N.A., Benowitz, N.L. *et al.* (2008) The Women's Initiative for Nonsmoking (WINS) XI: age-related differences in smoking cessation responses among women with cardiovascular disease. *American Journal of Geriatric Cardiology*, **17**(1), 37–47.
22. Hall, S.M., Humfleet, G.L., Munoz, R.F. *et al.* (2009) Extended treatment of older cigarette smokers. *Addiction*, **104**(6), 1043–1052. [Erratum appears in *Addiction*, 2011; **106**(6), 1204].
23. Hill, R.D., Rigdon, M. and Johnson, S. (1993) Behavioral smoking cessation treatment for older chronic smokers. *Behavior Therapy*, **24**(2), 321–329.
24. Joyce, G.F., Niaura, R., Maglione, M. *et al.* (2008) The effectiveness of covering smoking cessation services for medicare beneficiaries. *Health Services Research*, **43**(6), 2106–2123.
25. McFall, M., Saxon, A.J., Malte, C.A. *et al.* (2010) Integrating tobacco cessation into mental health care for posttraumatic stress disorder: a randomized controlled trial. *JAMA*, **304**(22), 2485–2493.
26. Morgan, G.D., Noll, E.L., Orleans, C.T. *et al.* (1996) Reaching midlife and older smokers: tailored interventions for routine medical care. *Preventive Medicine*, **25**(3), 346–354.
27. Orleans, C.T., Boyd, N.R., Noll, E. *et al.* (2000) Computer tailored intervention for older smokers using transdermal nicotine. *Tobacco Control*, **9**(Suppl 1), I53.
28. Ferguson, J., Bauld, L., Chesterman, J. and Judge, K. (2005) The English smoking treatment services: one-year outcomes. *Addiction*, **100**(Suppl 2), 59–69.
29. Grandes, G., Cortada, J.M., Arrazola, A. and Laka, J.P. (2003) Predictors of long-term outcome of a smoking cessation programme in primary care. *British Journal of General Practice*, **53**(487), 101–107.
30. Vetter, N.J. and Ford, D. (1990) Smoking prevention among people aged 60 and over: a randomized controlled trial. *Age and Ageing*, **19**(3), 164–168.
31. Ossip-Klein, D.J., Carosella, A.M. and Krusch, D.A. (1997) Self-help interventions for older smokers. *Tobacco Control*, **6**(3), 188–193.

32. Rimer, B.K., Orleans, C.T., Fleisher, L. *et al.* (1994) Does tailoring matter? The impact of a tailored guide on ratings and short-term smoking-related outcomes for older smokers. *Health Education Research*, **9**(1), 69–84.

33. Hopkins, D.P., Briss, P.A., Ricard, C.J. *et al.* (2001) Reviews of evidence regarding interventions to reduce tobacco use and exposure to environmental tobacco smoke. *American Journal of Preventive Medicine*, **20**(2 Suppl), 16–66.

34. Zhu, S.-H., Anderson, C.M., Tedeschi, G.J. *et al.* (2002) Evidence of real-world effectiveness of a telephone quitline for smokers. *New England Journal of Medicine*, **347**(14), 1087–1093.

35. Kaufman, A., Augustson, E., Davis, K. and Finney Rutten, L.J. (2010) Awareness and use of tobacco quitlines: evidence from the Health Information National Trends Survey. *Journal of Health Communication*, **15**(Suppl 3), 264–278.

36. Dahm, J.L., Cook, E., Baugh, K. *et al.* (2009) Predictors of enrollment in a smoking cessation clinical trial after eligibility screening. *Journal of the National Medical Association*, **101**(5), 450–455.

USE OF SUBSTANCE ABUSE TREATMENT SERVICES AMONG OLDER ADULTS

Chapter 16

EPIDEMIOLOGY OF USE OF TREATMENT SERVICES FOR SUBSTANCE USE PROBLEMS

Shawna L. Carroll Chapman and Li-Tzy Wu

Department of Psychiatry and Behavioral Sciences, School of Medicine, Duke University Medical Center, USA

Introduction

Due to the ageing baby boomer population (people born 1946–1964), the number of older adults (aged ≥65 years) in the United States is projected to grow rapidly (13–19% from 2010–2030) [1]. This growth will present challenges to policy makers and healthcare providers [1], particularly in the area of substance abuse treatment [2]. Because baby boomers came of age when substance use was popular, they may be at risk for drug use problems throughout their lives [3]. Gfroerer *et al.* [2] estimated that the number of people with a substance use disorder (alcohol or drug) aged ≥50 years would double from 1999–2020 (1.7–4.4 million). Because 2020 is only the midpoint of when baby boomers will reach age 65, this prediction may underrepresent the scope of the problem [4]. To understand the context of substance abuse treatment service use and characteristics associated with service use, studies on the epidemiology of substance abuse treatment utilization among individuals aged ≥50 years have been reviewed and summarized. To provide context, substance use and abuse prevalences are presented in Table 16.1 [5], [6]. Summaries of tobacco, alcohol and illicit or nonmedical prescription drug abuse treatment literature follow. The chapter concludes with a discussion of findings, making suggestions for next steps in future research.

Tobacco cessation service use and characteristics

Six studies on use of tobacco cessation interventions among older adults aged ≥55 years are summarized in Table 16.2. All focused on cigarette cessation treatment. Studies included men and women, with sample sizes ranging from 115 to 58 000.

Substance Use and Older People, First Edition.
Edited by Ilana B. Crome, Li-Tzy Wu, Rahul (Tony) Rao and Peter Crome.
© 2015 John Wiley & Sons, Ltd. Published 2015 by John Wiley & Sons, Ltd.

Table 16.1 Prevalences of substance use among older adults in the United States

	Prevalence in the past year (%)	Prevalence in the past month (%)
Tobacco use[a]		
Aged 65+	14.5	12.6
Aged 60–64	21.9	19.3
Aged 55–59	26.7	23.1
General population (aged 12 or older)	31.8	26.5
Alcohol use[a]		
Any use		
Aged 65+	51.5	40.3
Aged 60–64	65.6	50.9
Aged 55–59	67.6	52.8
General population (aged 12 or older)	66.2	51.8
Binge drinking[a]		
Aged 65+	N/A	8.3
Aged 60–64	N/A	14.5
Aged 55–59	N/A	18.0
General population (aged 12 or older)	N/A	22.6
Heavy drinking[a]		
Aged 65+	N/A	1.7
Aged 60–64	N/A	4.4
Aged 55–59	N/A	4.5
General population (aged 12 or older)	N/A	6.2
Alcohol use disorder[b,c]		
Aged 65+	1.5	N/A
Aged 50–64	4.2	N/A
Illicit or nonmedical drug use[a,d]		
Aged 65+	1.6	1.0
Aged 60–64	5.9	2.7
Aged 55–59	9.5	6.0
General population (aged 12 or older)	14.9	8.7

[a]SAMHSA, 2012 [5]
[b]Blazer and Wu, 2011 [6]
[c]2005–2007 Data
[d]Marijuana/hashish, cocaine and crack cocaine, heroin, hallucinogens, inhalants and nonmedical use of prescription-type psychotherapeutics

Table 16.2 Studies of tobacco treatment among older adults

Citation	Sample and location	Design and data	Findings
Ossip-Klein et al. [8]	• 1454 smokers (>10 cigarettes per day for 10 years) aged 50+ planning to quit. • 15 counties around Rochester, NY. • 92.48% White, 62.10% female, 48.83% married, 88.53% graduated high school, 49.56% employed.	• Cross-sectional; • Survey	• 81.43% received physician advice to quit in the past year; 57.26% welcomed advice, 31.68% said it improved their confidence in quitting ability, 50.90% said it influenced their decision to quit. • Having fair (OR 2.30, CI 1.18–4.44) or poor (OR 6.91, CI 2.08–31.71) health, number of past-year hospital stays (OR 1.71, CI 1.09, 2.79) and married (OR 1.50, CI 1.09, 2.09) predicted cessation advice.
Brown et al. [9]	• 788 cigarette smoking Medicare enrollees aged 65+. • Admitted to acute care in North Carolina with acute myocardial infarction and discharged alive. • 86% White, 60% male.	• Retrospective cohort. • Medical records.	• 60% of smokers did not receive smoking cessation counselling at index hospitalization. • No counselling correlated with being female, Black, older, and having a high prevalence of hypertension (p = 0.01), heart failure (p = 0.01) and stroke (p = 0.01). • Counselling correlated with a history of COPD and being less likely to be discharged to a skilled nursing facility. • Age-adjusted mortality decreased among those who received counselling.
Watt et al. [10]	• 115 Nurses and nurses assistants. • Long term care facility in Rochester, NY.	• Cross-sectional; • Survey.	• 45.6% of participants reported providing cessation information, and this was more common among licensed nurses compared to assistants (54.8% and 34.6%, respectively), x^2 (1, N = 114) = 4.662, p = 0.05. • 24.7% of participants consistently advised residents to quit, with smokers less likely to consistently advise than nonsmoking staff (t (78.21) = 2.05, p = 0.05). • 64.5% did not think the smoking policy at their facility should be changed, and whether staff indicated a desire to change smoking policy at their facility depended on their smoking status $F_{(8, 77)}$ = 8.725, p < 0.001; whether they gave cessation advice, $F_{(8, 76)}$ = 4.318, p < 0.001; and their job classification $F_{(8, 77)}$ = 2.138, p < 0.050.

(continued)

Table 16.2 (continued)

Citation	Sample and location	Design and data	Findings
Steinberg et al. [7]	• 58 000 individuals seeking health care. • United States.	• Cross-sectional. • NAMCS[a].	• Those aged 65+ (21.6%) were least likely to receive cessation counselling (18–24 = 22.7%, 25–44 = 22.8%, 45–64 = 22.6%) but the difference was not significant. • Those aged 65+ (0.9%) were least likely to receive tobacco cessation medication (OR = 0.14, CI = 0.03–0.63).
Whitson et al. [12]	• 573. • North Carolina (NC). • 43% Black; 57% female, 41% married, 26% some college.	• Prospective cohort; • NC EPESE[b]	• Quitters were more likely to be female (OR = 1.70, CI = 1.04–2.77).
Hall et al. [11]	• 810. • Western United States. • Aged <50 = 70.3% White, 37.5% female, 36.7% married, 16.6% high school or less. • Aged 50+ = 75.7% White, 41.2% female, 42.6% married, 12.1% high school or less.	• Randomized trial. • Survey.	• Smokers aged 50+ had better mental health scores and lower stress than those <50. • 66.2% of smokers aged 50+ had a goal of complete abstinence, compared to 40.5% of those aged <50. • Younger smokers were more likely to be abuse alcohol (38.7%) or be alcohol dependent (24.6%) compared to older smokers (32.0 and 17.0%, respectively). • Men aged 50+ were more likely to use marijuana than women aged 50+ (past week 21.4 vs 11.6%). • Men aged 50+ were more likely to abuse alcohol than women 50+ (41.6 vs 18.5%).

[a]National Ambulatory Medical Care Survey
[b]Established Populations for the Study of the Elderly

Tobacco users often seek cessation services from a primary health provider or receive related information when providers encourage them to improve their health behaviours. Steinberg *et al.* [7] examined 2001–2102 National Ambulatory Medical Care Survey data and found that 11.4% of physician/patient encounters (N > 58 000) involved a cigarette smoking patient. While proportions of smokers were not provided for specific age groups, Steinberg *et al.* [7] found that only about 22% of those aged ≥65 years received cigarette cessation counselling from providers (age: 18–24 = 22.7%, 25–44 = 22.8%, 45–64 = 22.6%, 65+ years = 21.6%). Of patients who received cessation counselling, about 1% of adults aged ≥65 years received tobacco cessation medications (18–24 = 1.3%, 25–44 = 3.4%, 45–64 = 2.3%, 65+ years = 0.9%) [7]. Ossip-Klein *et al.* (2000) [8] surveyed 1454 predominantly White, female, New York cigarette smokers aged ≥50 years drawn from participants (N = 1975) in a smoking cessation trial. They found that 81.43% were advised to quit at a past-year physician visit. The high percentage found by Ossip-Klein (2000) may reflect that women were motivated to make a quit attempt and thus likely to recall physician advice. In addition, 15% of participants were referred to the study by their physician or brochure in their physician's office [8].

Cigarette smokers with related health conditions need cessation information regardless of whether or not they ask for it. To examine the frequency with which health providers offer such information to individuals aged ≥65 years with smoking related conditions, Brown *et al.* [9] analysed data from medical records of 788 patients aged ≥65 years, predominantly White, male, cigarette smoking Medicare beneficiaries admitted to a North Carolina care facility with acute myocardial infarction. They found that 60% did not receive quit advice at first hospitalization [9].

Providers at senior care facilities also have opportunities for providing behavioural intervention with elders whose health is at risk. Watt *et al.* [10] surveyed 115 nursing staff at a New York senior care facility and found that only 45.6% had ever provided smoking cessation information to patients. Only 24.7% did so consistently. Members of the nursing staff were more likely to provide quit information when licensed (54.8%) compared with unlicensed assistants (34.6%). Additionally, identified barriers to providing quit information included: considering it was a physician's responsibility, residents' lack of interest and the institution's lenient cigarette smoking policy.

Similarly, Ossip-Klein *et al.* [8] found that health providers were likely to offer cigarette smoking cessation information to patients in fair or poor health, those with a high number of past-year hospital stays and those who were married. In terms of health status, individuals aged ≥65 years with a history of heart attack, hypertension, stroke, emphysema, asthma or chronic bronchitis were the most likely to receive advice to quit cigarettes. Steinberg *et al.* [7] found the strongest determinant of receiving cessation medication was presenting to providers with quit intent (34.9%). The second determinant was a tobacco-related diagnosis (6%). Brown *et al.* [9] found correlates of receiving cessation information among patients with myocardial infarction included a history of chronic obstructive pulmonary disorder and not being discharged to a skilled nursing facility. Brown *et al.* [9] also identified factors related to not receiving quit information, which were being female, Black, older aged and diagnosed with hypertension, heart failure or stroke. Therefore, these findings suggest that poor health, particularly having a smoking-related diagnosis or condition, is a primary correlate of receiving smoking cessation information.

Cigarette smokers wanting to quit may also seek assistance from smoking cessation programmes. Hall *et al.* [11] examined survey responses of 810 (56.9% aged ≥50 years) predominantly White, male, cigarette smokers seeking treatment for tobacco dependence through two clinical trials at a treatment facility in an urban area of the Western United States. They found that elder treatment seekers aged ≥50 years more often desired complete abstinence, had better mental health scores and lower stress scores and worse physical health scores than treatment seekers aged <50 years. Elder treatment seekers were the least likely to report alcohol abuse or dependence or marijuana use. In both age groups (aged <50 and ≥50 years), male treatment seekers were more likely than women to use marijuana and abuse alcohol, but this pattern was more pronounced among treatment seekers aged ≥50 years.

Few studies reported cessation outcomes for aged ≥50 years cigarette smokers seeking treatment. Whitson *et al.* [12] analysed Established Populations for Epidemiologic Studies of the Elderly (aged ≥65 years) data and found that 17% of respondents (n = 4162) smoked cigarettes in 1986–1987. By 1989–1990, 17.5% of follow-up respondents (n = 573) had quit. Information on how they quit was not provided. However, quitters were more likely to be female (57%) than male and nonblack (57%) than Black. Ossip-Klein *et al.* [8] did not report cessation outcomes but did report that 57.26% of patients who received cigarette cessation advice from their care provider welcomed it, 50.90% said it influenced their decision to quit and 31.68% said it improved their self-efficacy in quitting. Brown *et al.* [9] also found that patients who received counselling had reduced mortality at 30 days, six month, and one and five years.

In summary, studies showed that older adult cigarette smokers wanted to, attempted to and successfully quit smoking cigarettes. However, healthcare providers inconsistently offered intervention to older adult cigarette smokers. Only poor health was a consistent correlate of receiving cessation advice.

Alcohol treatment use and characteristics

Ten studies that include information on treatment use for alcohol abuse or dependence among elders are summarized in Table 16.3. Topics that studies covered included treatment in the general population and subpopulations (four on veterans and one on women), characteristics associated with seeking alcohol treatment or in treatment. Presenting for alcohol withdrawal was also described. Finally, six studies reported treatment outcomes.

There are limited data about the prevalences of older adults seeking or using treatment for alcohol use problems. In an analysis of 2001–2002 data from the National Epidemiologic Survey on Alcohol and Related Conditions (NESARC) for

Table 16.3 Studies of alcohol treatment use among older adults

Citation	Sample and location	Design and data	Findings
Christie et al. [14]	• 585. • Aged 55+. • 94% White, 61.5% male, 57% married, 57% retired. • United Kingdom.	• Prospective cohort. • United Kingdom National Health Service Trust Community Alcohol Team problem drinking assessments.	• While older adult assessments increased, the percentage for those aged 60+ remained consistent. • The increase was greater for men than for women. • The mean amount of alcohol consumed per week decreased from 1988–1989 to 1998–1999 but increased each year from 2003–2008. • Women tended to drink because of anxiety or loneliness/depression, while men tended to drink because of habit/dependency or anxiety.
Al-Otaiba et al. [18]	• 181. • 100% Women, 96% White, 85% married, 58% employed. • 50% of women were aged <45, 35% were aged 45–55, and 17% were aged 55+. • United States.	• Randomized trial. • Survey/interview.	**The older group:** • Drank more often, reported greater heavy drinking and had later age of alcohol initiation and onset of alcohol abuse or dependence. • Used fewer types of drugs, had fewer Axis I mental disorders, and smaller percentages of heavy drinkers in their social networks than the middle or younger groups. • Reduced their percentage of drinking and heavy drinking days more than younger women.
Sacco et al. [13]	• 4646; • Aged 60+. • United States.	• Cross-sectional. • National Epidemiologic Survey on Alcohol and Related Conditions (NESARC).	• 3.9% reported past-year alcohol abuse or dependence. • 0.34% of older adults reported past-year alcohol related service use, 1.24% of all age drinkers (n = 26,946) reported such service use, and 1.40% of the NESARC sample (n = 43 093) reported such service use. • 1.48% of elder adults contemplated seeking help for drinking, 3.48% of all age drinkers did so, and 3.33% of the NESARC sample did so. • Among elders, 0.10% low-risk drinkers sought alcohol-related services, 1.67% of moderate-risk drinkers sought services, and 7.46% of high-risk drinkers did so. • 0.85% of elder low-risk drinkers contemplated treatment, 2.51% of moderate-risk drinkers did so, and 28.59% of high-risk drinkers did so.

(continued)

Table 16.3 (continued)

Citation	Sample and location	Design and data	Findings
Oslin et al. [19]	• 1358 first time admits for alcohol but not drug dependence. • 97.5% white, 56% male, and 60.6% married. • Minnesota.	• Prospective cohort. • Clinical, administrative and quality improvement data.	• Compared to younger patients, older patients had fewer mental health problems, reported less severe alcohol use, fewer outpatient treatment experiences, and were less likely to attend formal outpatient aftercare or contact a sponsor.
Atkinson et al. [23]	• 110 veterans aged 55+ in alcohol treatment. • >90% White, 100% male. • United States.	• Retrospective cohort. • Clinical data (August 1994–July 1998).	• Legal and self/family referrals were more likely to complete treatment than social service referrals. • Patients with a history of alcoholism treatment were more likely to complete treatment than those without a history.
Gordon et al. [15]	• 301 hazardous drinkers. • 15% aged 65+. • Pennsylvania.	• *Post hoc* analysis. • Survey data (October 1995–December 1997).	• Older patients were more likely to be male (87%), have less education (31%), be employed or retired (98%), have fewer days abstinent each month and drink 1–6 standard drinks per day than younger patients. • There was no significant reduction in consumption between interventions or standard care.
Lemke and Moos [17, 21]	• 1296. • Divided equally into those aged 21–39, 40–54, and 55+. • Veteran's Administration (VA) residential alcohol treatment programmes. • In each group: 71% White, 19% married, 31% were dually diagnosed, 26% from 12-step programmes, 40% from cognitive behavioural programmes, and 34% from eclectic programmes. • United States.	• Prospective cohort. • Survey and Treatment records.	• Levels of alcohol dependence were similar for all ages. • Older patients scored lowest on a substance abuse problems scale, cognitive function scale, and treatment motivation scale. • Older patients were least likely to report positive social consequences for drinking and identify quitting costs. • Older patients were most likely to use approach coping to deal with stressful situations, report only a few psychological symptoms, be socially engaged, religious, have positive treatment experiences, high levels of support and low levels of anger and aggression; • Older patients had longest programme stays. • For older patients, psychiatric care did not relate to level of psychological distress at 5-year follow-up. • Although older patients had slightly better indicators at entry, they had somewhat better outcomes at 5-year follow-up.

Study	Sample	Design	Results
Blow et al. [20]	• 90. • In-patients in an elder specific treatment programme. • 85.6% alcohol abuse/dependence diagnosis w/ no other substance abuse disorder, 14.4% alcohol and prescription drug abuse; • 88.8% White, 58.9% male, 42.9% married, 93.8% unemployed. • Midwestern United States.	• Prospective cohort. • Survey/interview.	• 31.1% of participants had ≥1 psychiatric diagnosis. • 57.8% were nicotine dependent, 13.8% were sedative dependent, 6.2% were opiate dependent. • At 6-month follow-up, 55.9% were abstainers, 13.3% were nonbinge drinkers and 26.5% were binge drinkers. • Abstainers, nonbinge drinkers and binge drinkers reduced drinking by 6-month follow-up. • Participants had improvement general health perceptions and were less limited by pain at follow-up. • Emotional distress also declined from baseline to follow-up among abstainers and nonbinge drinkers.
Fleming et al. [16]	• 146. • 33% women. • Wisconsin.	• Prospective cohort. • Physician intervention or standard care.	• Participants consumed an average of 16–17 drinks per week. • Consumption decreased more in the intervention than control group (40 vs 6%, respectively) by 3 months and was maintained in the intervention group through 12 months; • Excessive drinking decreased in the intervention group by 3 months and remained lower at 12 months; • Excessive and binge drinking increased in the control group by 3 months and remained higher at 12 months.
Kraemer et al. [22]	• 284 (56% aged 50+). • VA Alcohol detoxification unit. • 98% White, 98% male, 21% married. • Manchester, NH.	• Retrospective cohort. • Medical records (1 September 1992–31 August 1994).	• Daily consumption, blackouts, and morning 'eye-openers' decreased with age, but consistency in daily consumption increased with age. • Patients aged 70+ had fewer episodes of inpatient detoxification and less formal treatment than younger patients despite a longer duration of heavy alcohol use. • Length of stay in the treatment unit increased with age.

respondents aged ≥60 years (N = 4646), Sacco *et al.* [13] found that 0.34% (N = 22) of current alcohol users had sought alcohol-related services in the past year and that 1.48% (N = 174) contemplated seeking them. Based on multiple alcohol use variables, Sacco *et al.* [13] identified three classes (groups) of drinking-related risk (low, moderate and high). Correlates of being a moderate-risk drinker (compared with the low-risk group) included being a child of an alcoholic, being a previous (but not current) smoker and being a current smoker. Correlates of being a high-risk drinker (compared with the low and moderate-risk groups) were past-year major depression, being a child of an alcoholic and being a current smoker. The investigators further found that 0.10% (N = 6) of low-risk drinkers sought services in the past year, 1.67% (N = 10) of moderate-risk drinkers did so and 7.46% (N = 6) of high-risk drinkers did. This national study demonstrates a low prevalence of alcohol treatment use among high-risk drinkers; of them, 81.88% met criteria for alcohol abuse or dependence and more than a quarter had either a co-morbid depressive (24.90%) or anxiety disorder (8.78%). In the United Kingdom, Christie *et al.* [14] analysed National Health Service (NHS) Trust Community Alcohol Team data (N = 11 829), a data set begun in 1975 that includes information on individuals seeking alcohol-related treatment through a variety of referral sources (e.g. self, family, probation or social services). They found that 585 adults aged ≥60 years received an alcohol treatment assessment from April 1988 to March 2008. While the actual number of assessments for those aged ≥60 years increased over time, with the greatest increase in male assessments, the proportion of assessments for adults aged ≥60 years remained consistent at 6–7%. Most (79%) of the aged ≥60 years drinkers assessed by the NHS drank daily. Taken together, studies suggest a similar proportion of high risk or daily drinkers aged ≥60 years receive services (6–7%) in the United States and United Kingdom.

Few studies report on prevalences of hazardous drinking among older adults in general medical settings. In a *post hoc* analysis of recruitment data (N = 13 438, 20% aged ≥65 years) collected in Western Pennsylvania physician-based clinic waiting rooms from October 1995 to November 1997, Gordon *et al.* [15] found that 7% of adults aged ≥65 years were considered as having engaged in hazardous drinking as defined by the AUDIT (i.e. AUDIT score ≥8) or Quantity/Frequency (QF) criteria (≥16 standard drinks per week for men and ≥12 drinks per week for women). Patients who screened positive for either QF or AUDIT were randomly assigned to either a motivational enhancement intervention (one 45–60 minute and two 10–15 minute sessions using motivational interviewing to assist patients in identifying consequences of drinking and setting goals to reduce alcohol consumption), a brief advice intervention (a single 10–15 minute counselling session advising patient to quit behaviour) or standard care (a variety of services provided by medical offices (e.g. referral, brochures). Each intervention group showed a reduction in alcohol consumption at six and 12 months.

Fleming *et al.* [16] conducted a study to screen hazardous drinking among all patients aged ≥65 years from 1 April 1993 to 1 April 1995 at 24 physician-based clinics. They found that 10.8% of 6073 patients screened positive for hazardous drinking (women >8 drinks/week, men >11 drinks/week, or two positive responses on the CAGE criteria). Patients who screened positive for hazardous drinking were randomized to either a control (received a general health booklet) or intervention group (same booklet and two appointments with their physician to receive intervention following specific study protocol). At three-month follow-up, average weekly alcohol consumption dropped 40% in the intervention group and 6% in the control group. The decrease in the intervention group was maintained at 12 months. Excessive and binge drinking also decreased in the intervention group at three months and remained at a low level at 12 months, while excessive and binge drinking increased in the control group at three months and remained higher at 12 months. The variation in study designs and participants may account for differences in results. Overall, studies suggest that 7–10% of patients aged ≥65 years screen positive for hazardous drinking in a general medical setting, and those who screen positive are able to reduce drinking with assistance.

Studies of clinical or treatment-seeking people suggest that older adults represent an important proportion of patients (16–17%) in substance abuse treatment programmes. As part of a larger Veterans Administration (VA) evaluation project, Lemke and Moos [17] examined the consecutive admissions at 12 VA substance treatment centres across the United States during an undisclosed period and found that, of the 3234 individuals who agreed to participate, 88% (n = 2858) had an ICD-9 alcohol-related diagnosis. By age, 35% were aged 21–39, 49% were aged 40–54 and 16% were aged 55–77. Al-Otaiba et al. [18] examined data from a convenience sample of 181 predominantly White, married, employed, alcohol dependent US women who participated in alcohol treatment studies and found that 17% were aged ≥55 years and 35% were aged 44–55.

Multiple studies focused on the characteristics associated with elders seeking alcohol treatment. Oslin et al. [19] analysed data for 1358 first-time patients aged ≥50 years with an alcohol use disorder diagnosis at two Minnesota inpatient alcohol treatment centres and found that patients aged ≥50 years were predominantly White, male and married. Patients aged ≥50 years were less likely than those aged <50 to be employed or have a college education, but older patients also had fewer mental health problems, reported less severe alcohol use and had fewer outpatient treatment experiences than younger ones. Gordon et al. [15] found patients aged ≥65 years seeking alcohol treatment were predominantly male, less educated and either employed or retired. Those aged ≥65 years seeking treatment were also more likely to have fewer days abstinent from alcohol each month and to drink 1–6 standard drinks per day than patients aged <65. Blow et al. [20] examined 90 predominantly White, male inpatients in a Midwestern elder specific (aged ≥55 years) substance abuse treatment programme with a diagnosis of alcohol abuse/dependence and found that 31.1% of participants had at least one psychiatric diagnosis, 57.8% were nicotine dependent, 13.8% were sedative dependent and 6.2% were opiate dependent. In the United Kingdom, Christie et al. [14] found that, of the 585 adults aged ≥60 years assessed for alcohol treatment, most were White, male, married and retired. Results also showed that women tended to drink for reasons of anxiety, loneliness and depression, whereas men tended to drink for reasons of habit/dependency or anxiety. Taken together, older adults using alcohol treatment are likely to be White, male, less educated and to have co-morbid mental health problems.

Older adults appear to have fewer alcohol problems than younger adults but the decline in cognitive functioning may affect their treatment use. Comparing three equally matched age groups (total n = 1296, age groups = 21–39, 40–54 and 55–77), Lemke and Moos [17] found that veterans aged 55–77 scored lowest on an alcohol abuse problems scale, were the least likely to report positive social consequences for drinking, psychological symptoms, quitting costs (e.g. loneliness, moodiness) or anger and aggression. Older patients were also most likely to use approach coping to deal with stress, be socially engaged, express confidence in abstaining under stress, be religious, report a positive treatment experience and report support. However, patients aged 55–77 had the longest in-treatment stays, lowest cognitive function scores and lowest treatment motivation scores. Lemke and Moos [21] further found fewer patients aged 55–77 received outpatient psychiatric care and were seen for shorter periods than patients aged 40–54, although proportions of dual diagnoses (i.e. alcohol abuse/dependence and mental illness) were similar. The latter suggests that older adults with co-morbid psychiatric problems are underserved.

There is limited information about older women who used substance abuse treatment and the available data show important gender differences in substance abuse treatment profiles and needs. Contrary to the findings from men, older women with alcohol dependence appear to have more alcohol problems than younger women with alcohol dependence. Among the 181 women seeking alcohol dependence treatment, Al-Otaiba et al. [18] found women aged ≥55 years drank more often (77.1%) than those aged 45–55 (72.6%) or aged <45 (61.3%). Women aged ≥55 years reported greater heavy drinking (62.7%) than those aged 45–55 (60.1%) and <45 (49.6%) as well as later age of alcohol use initiation and later age for alcohol abuse or dependence onset. In addition, older women had used fewer types of drugs (specific drug classes not provided), had fewer DSM-IV Axis I mental disorders and fewer heavy drinkers in their social networks when compared to middle aged and younger women. These findings point toward the need to investigate triggers for late onset alcohol use and problems among older women, which may include conditions related to anxiety, loneliness and depression [14]. There is also a clear need to distinguish between late onset versus early onset alcohol abusers to inform prevention and treatment. The early onset group may have more chronic or psychiatric co-morbidities than the late onset group, while the late onset group appears to have predominately alcohol problems. Both will require different treatment services.

Characteristics of older adults presenting for alcohol withdrawal were also described. The risk for experiencing a severe pattern of alcohol withdrawal can increase with age and the older adults may require additional medical treatment than younger adults. Kraemer et al. [22] analysed the medical records of 284 predominantly male, veterans (56% aged ≥50 years) admitted to a New Hampshire VA detoxification unit for alcohol withdrawal and found that daily alcohol consumption, blackouts and use of morning 'eye-openers' decreased with age. However, consistency in daily drinking increased. In addition, adults aged ≥60 years had increased risk for delirium, lethargy and transient dependency in two or more activities of daily living. Those aged 70+ had fewer inpatient alcohol detoxification episodes than younger patients, even though elders had a longer duration of alcohol use. Length of in-treatment stays increased with age, and older patients were restrained and given intravenous fluids more than younger patients. Thus, alcohol dependence symptoms (e.g. withdrawal) occurring in elderly, chronic drinkers and age-related medical conditions can complicate treatment.

Few studies examined alcohol treatment outcomes among older adults and treatment outcomes were inconsistently reported. Some data showed older adults can reduce alcohol consumption with assistance. In a sample of 90 inpatients aged ≥55 years who were diagnosed with DSM-III-R alcohol abuse/dependence, Blow et al. [20] found that, at six-month follow-up, 55.9% were alcohol abstainers, 13.3% were nonbinge drinkers and 26.5% were binge drinkers. Abstainers, nonbinge drinkers and binge drinkers reduced drinking by six-month follow-up, had an improved perception of their health and were less limited by pain. In addition, emotional distress declined from baseline to follow-up for abstainers and nonbinge drinkers. On the other hand, Oslin et al. [19] found older adults aged ≥50 years who received inpatient substance abuse treatment were less likely than younger adults aged <50 to attend formal outpatient aftercare or contact a sponsor. Additional research is needed to elucidate older adults' use of outpatient aftercare care and their long-term treatment outcomes.

Few studies examined the likelihood to complete a treatment programme as an outcome measure. Atkinson et al. [23] explored the correlates of completing alcohol treatment among 110 predominantly White, male US veterans aged ≥55 years who were diagnosed with alcohol dependence. Overall, 40% completed the treatment, and patients referred by the legal system, themselves or family members were more likely to complete treatment than those referred by social services. Atkinson et al. [23] also found that veterans with a history of alcohol abuse treatment were more likely to complete treatment than those without such a history. These findings suggest that legal or familial supervision and treatment readiness may increase older adults' likelihood of completing alcohol treatment. In a study of alcohol treatment among 181 women, Al-Otaiba et al. [18] found younger women aged <45 attended fewer treatment sessions than women aged 45–55 or aged ≥55 years. Although it was unclear why younger women had a lower level of treatment compliance than older women, Al-Otaiba et al. [18] hypothesized that it might be due to therapy more in line with older women's needs or to a lack of motivation among younger women to quit drinking. Their results suggest an association between attending treatment sessions and outcomes. For example, there was a significant interaction effect between age and time in treatment, which suggested that women aged ≥55 years who attended more treatment sessions reduced their percentage of drinking days and of heavy drinking more than younger women who attended fewer sessions. Among veterans, Lemke and Moos [21] found those aged 55–77 had slightly better indicators at entry and better outcomes (e.g. alcohol consumption, problem consequences of drinking and psychological distress) at follow-up than patients aged 19–39 or 40–54.

Taken together, results from a national sample showed that few older high-risk alcohol users used alcohol-related services in the past year. However, screenings of adults aged ≥65 years seeking general health care showed that 7–10% met criteria for hazardous drinking, suggesting that many older adults with alcohol problems may not use alcohol-related services. Clinical samples suggest older adults represent an important proportion of patient populations. Among veterans seeking treatment for an alcohol diagnosis, 16% were aged 55–77. Among women seeking treatment for alcohol dependence, 17% were aged ≥55 years. However, there is a lack of reliable population-based prevalence rates of alcohol treatment use among older adults with an alcohol use disorder. The available data indicate that elder drinkers seeking treatment were predominately White, male, less educated or with mental health problems. Older men in alcohol treatment appear to have fewer alcohol problems than younger men; however, older women in alcohol treatment showed a severe pattern of alcohol use compared to younger women. Older problem drinkers were able to quit or reduce alcohol consumption with intervention to positive outcome, but data on long-term outcomes are lacking. Little is known about treatment use for older ethnic or racial minority adults.

Trend in substance abuse treatment admissions

This section includes drug and alcohol substance abuse treatment admission data by studies that examine the Treatment Episode Data Set (TEDS), summarized in Table 16.4 [24–27]. TEDS is maintained by the Center for Behavioral Health Statistics and Quality, the US Substance Abuse and Mental Health Services Administration (SAMHSA), and includes substance abuse treatment admission data from facilities that receive State funds. Because data reflect treatment admission episodes and not individual data, they may not differentiate multiple admissions for the same person. TEDS data also do not represent admissions to facilities operated by federal agencies (e.g. the VA). It must also be noted that differences in how States provide funds and services can affect data collection.

The treatment admission data indicate an increase in substance abuse treatment use among older adults. Lofwall *et al.* [26] compared TEDS data from 1992 (n = 1.55 million treatment admission episodes) to TEDS data from 2005 (n = 1.85 million treatment admission episodes) and found substance abuse admissions for adults aged 50–54 increased from 3.1 to 6.0% of all identified substance abuse treatment admissions and for those aged ≥55 years from 3.5 to 4.2%. TEDS data from 2001–2005 also showed increased admissions for adults aged ≥50 years, from 8 to 10% (n = 143 900 and n = 184 400, respectively) [25]. Arndt *et al.* [27] compared 1998 to 2008 TEDS data for first-time substance abuse admissions among young adults aged 30–54 (n = 3 547 733 admissions) and older adults aged ≥55 years (n = 258 542 admissions). Results showed that first-time admissions for those aged ≥55 years increased from 2.9 to 4.4%, suggesting a slight increase in substance abuse treatment use by older adults who had not used substance abuse treatment before.

Table 16.4 Studies of alcohol and drug abuse treatment use among older adults

Citation	Sample and location	Design and data	Findings
Arndt et al. [27]	• 3 806 275. • 7% aged 55+. • First time admits. • United States	• Cross-sectional. • Treatment Episode Dataset -Admissions (TEDS). • 1998–2008	• Elder admissions increased 2.86–4.42% from 1998–2008. • Elder admissions increased more among Blacks than whites but less among Latinos than non-Latinos. • Elder self-referrals increased 6.05%, criminal justice referrals decreased 5.85%. • Elders needed alcohol treatment most often, but drug use increased.
Rosen et al. [30]	• 140 (Aged 50+). • Midwestern United States. • 52.1% Black, 64.3% male, 17.9% working.	• Cross-sectional. • Survey data. • Methadone treatment centre.	• 57.1% had a mental health diagnosis, 44.4% had more than one. • Depression was the most common mental health disorder. • 47.1% took a psychotropic medication for their mental health. • 57.7% had poor physical health and 87.1% smoked cigarettes.
Lofwall et al. [26]	• 1.55 million admissions in 1992 and 1.85 million in 2005.	• Cross-sectional. • TEDS-A.	• Aged 50–54 admissions increased from 3.1 to 6.0% 1992–2005, and aged 55+ increased from 3.5 to 4.2% 1992–2005. • There was an increase in poly-substance use admits. • Alcohol abuse admits declined as drug abuse admits increased. • Prescription opioids, marijuana and methamphetamine admits appeared to trend upwards among elders. • 46–47% of drug abuse admits were White and 40% Black in 2005. • Only alcohol abuse admits remained primarily White from 1992–2005. • Elder admissions increased for those with ≥12 years of education and the unemployed.
Neighbors et al. [33]	• 837. • Aged 55+. • Black. • 9.6% met criteria for a mood, anxiety or substance disorder.	• Cross-sectional. • Nat'ional Survey of American Life.	• 20.8% of those who abused alcohol sought services, 5.9% sought mental health services and 20.8% sought general medical care. • 30.3% of those with alcohol dependence sought services, with all 30.3% seeking general medical care. • None abused or were dependent on drugs.

(continued)

Table 16.4 (continued)

Citation	Sample and location	Design and data	Findings
Satre et al. [31]	• 84 (Aged 55+). 92.9% White, 30% female, 59.5% married, 33.7% employed.	• Prospective cohort study. • Survey measures at baseline and 7-year follow-up. • Outpatient addiction treatment.	• 79.8% alcohol dependent, 4.8% drug dependent and 3.6% dependent on alcohol and drugs. • At 7 years: abstinence correlated with 12-step attendance at 5 and 7 years, and length of stay in treatment.
Arndt et al. [24]	• 1051 983 (5.5% aged 55+).	• Cross-sectional. • TEDS. • 2001.	• Male elder admissions 79.84% vs male younger admissions 69.13%. • Black elder admissions 23.24% vs Black younger admissions 28.88%. • Older admissions were more likely to be married, outside the labour force but with income (e.g. retired), and have insurance. • Older individuals were most likely to list alcohol as the only substance abused and to report daily use. • Female elders more likely than males to report high education, live independently, be White, have income and be a first time admit. • Male elders more likely than females to be homeless and list the reason for a lack of income as incarceration.
Lofwall et al. [29]	• 67 (61% aged 50–66). • Johns Hopkins. • Older patients = 66% non-White, 49% female and 44% employed. • Younger patients = 62% non-White, 58% female and 58% employed.	• Cross-sectional. • Survey. • Opioid maintenance.	• Older participants were in treatment longer than younger, had more lifetime years of incarceration, were less likely to receive medical assistance and more likely to have commercial health insurance. • Major depression was the most common diagnosis in both groups. • The older group had fewer positive urine screens for opiates (3.7 vs 6.9%), cocaine (7.8 vs 8.9%), marijuana (3.3 vs 5.0%) and benzodiazepines (5.0 vs 5.5%), but only the difference for opiates was significant (Mann–Whitney U = 324, p = 0.012). • Older participants had poorer health than younger participants and took more prescribed medications (43.9% older patients taking ≥ 3 daily medications vs 3.8% of younger participants).

| Satre et al. [28] | • 925 (7% aged 55+).
 • Kaiser Permanente.
 • Of those 55+, 92% White, 74% male, and 33% employed.
 • Prospective cohort study.
 • Survey.
 • Outpatient chemical dependency | • Older adults were diagnosed with alcohol dependence more than middle aged or younger adults and less likely to be diagnosed with drug dependence.
 • Older adults stayed in treatment longer than younger adults.
 • Elders had fewer close friends than younger or middle aged adults.
 • Elders were less likely than younger adults to report having family or friends who encouraged use and smoke cigarettes.
 • Elders were more likely to be married, report abstinence from alcohol and drugs during the past month and year, and report worse health than younger adults.
 • Elders were less likely than middle aged adults to have ever considered themselves a member of a 12-Step programme.
 • Correlates of abstinence were female gender, greater treatment retention and having no close family or friends who encouraged alcohol or drug use at 5 years.
 • Older women were more likely to be abstinent and stay in treatment longer than older men, and older women were more likely to be abstinent than younger women. |

The TEDS data provide important information about racial/ethnic differences in treatment admissions and recent data suggest increased numbers of substance abuse treatment admissions among older Blacks. Using the 2005 TEDS data, Lofwall *et al.* [26] found that 61% of drug abuse treatment admissions for all ages were White and 24% Black. In the sample aged ≥50 years, a greater proportion of Blacks were admitted for drug abuse than Whites. Therefore, it appears that older Blacks had more drug-related admissions than older Whites. In addition, alcohol abuse was the only admission category that remained the primary problem for Whites in 2005. However, TEDS data from 2001–2005 showed that White admissions increased with age, as Black admissions decreased with age [25]. Comparing 2001 TEDS data for individuals aged ≥55 years (n = 58 073) to data for individuals aged 30–54 (n = 1 043 910), Arndt *et al.* [24] found that older treatment admissions were more predominantly White and that alcohol was the primary substance of abuse. Recently, Arndt *et al.* [27] examined racial/ethnic differences in substance abuse treatment admissions and found a rise in substance abuse treatment (undifferentiated drug and alcohol) admissions among Blacks. Between 1998 and 2008, substance abuse admissions for adults aged ≥55 years increased more among Blacks than Whites but less among Latinos than non-Latinos. Therefore, future research needs to monitor substance abuse treatment use among older Blacks.

Although alcohol was the primary substance of abuse among older adults, the TEDS data suggest an increase in the number of drug abuse related treatment admissions (marijuana, methamphetamine and prescription opioids). Between 1992 and 2005, the number of alcohol treatment admissions (proportions) among adults aged ≥50 years declined as the number of drug abuse admissions increased, particularly for marijuana, methamphetamine and prescription opioids [26]. There was also a marked increase in poly-substance abuse related admissions. Arndt *et al.* [27] also found that, between 1998 and 2008, alcohol was the substance individuals aged ≥55 years sought treatment for most often and that there were some increases in drug abuse treatment admissions. Additionally, cocaine was the substance those aged ≥55 years sought treatment for most after alcohol [27]. TEDS data from 2001–2005 calendar years showed age-related differences in substances of abuse. While alcohol was reported most in admissions for those aged ≥65 years (76% for treatment admission), opioids were reported most in admissions for those aged 50–54 (22%) and 55–59 (19%). Opioids were the substance reported most following alcohol. Adults aged 50–59 had greater admission episodes for cocaine, marijuana and stimulants than elders aged ≥65 years [25].

There are important demographic differences in patterns of substance abuse treatment admissions. First-time (new) treatment admissions were more common in the older group than the younger group, suggesting the presence of late onset substance abuse problems. TEDS data from 2001–2005 calendar years showed that 39–44% of adults aged 50–59 had no prior treatment history, compared with 50–54% of adults aged ≥60 years who had no treatment history [26]. Compared with adults aged 30–54, Arndt *et al.* [24] found those aged ≥55 years were more likely to be male, married, outside the labour force, with health insurance, abusing only alcohol and first-time admissions. In terms of alcohol only admissions, Arndt *et al.* [24] found females aged ≥55 years were more likely than men aged ≥55 years to report a higher level of education, live independently, have income, be a first-time admission and report being a homemaker if outside the labour force. Compared to women aged ≥55 years, men aged ≥55 years were more often homeless, listing incarceration as their reason for a lack of income and listing an earlier age of substance initiation. These data show important differences in socioeconomic status and treatment needs between older women and older men. Given that more women than men were first-time treatment admissions, women may be more likely than men to have late onset substance use problems (mainly alcohol).

The TEDS data also provide the information about how elders entered treatment. Arndt *et al.* [24] found that the proportions of referrals from the criminal justice system and self-referrals were the same for adults aged ≥55 years; in terms of criminal justice referrals, adults aged ≥55 years were more likely to be referred through the courts for a substance related infraction (i.e. driving while intoxicated), while admissions aged <55 were more likely to be required to seek treatment as part of a probation or parole agreement. Lofwall *et al.* [26] found that self and criminal justice referrals were the primary sources for treatment admissions for all ages between 1992 and 2005. Subsequently, Arndt *et al.* [27] found that self-referrals for adults aged ≥55 years increased by 6.05%, while criminal justice referrals decreased 5.85% between 1998 and 2008. Future research could examine whether the rates of self-referrals increase over time and the location of treatment used.

In summary, the proportion of substance abuse admissions by older adults aged ≥50 years in the TEDS data set had increased during 1992 and 2008, with an observed increase from 3 to 4% for adults aged ≥55 years, from 3 to 6% for adults aged 50–54 and from 8 to 10% for adults aged ≥50 years. Alcohol was the primary substance of abuse by adults aged ≥50 years but drug abuse related admissions were on the rise, suggesting that use patterns were changing. Admissions among adults aged ≥50 years were most often White, but drug abuse related treatment admissions increased more among Blacks than Whites. Alcohol-related admissions were the only admissions category that remained primarily for Whites. There were also important gender differences in treatment admission, as more older women than older men were first-time treatment admissions.

Drug abuse treatment use and outcomes

Few studies described older adults already in treatment for substance abuse or dependence and reported outcomes (Table 16.4). Four studies are reported here. Satre *et al.* [28] examined outpatients in treatment for chemical dependency and compared adults aged 55–77 to those aged 40–54 and <40. Lofwall *et al.* [29] determined substance use and mental and physical health of 67 patients aged 50–66 in opioid maintenance treatment. Rosen *et al.* [30] also examined substance use and mental and physical health of 140 men aged ≥50 years in methadone mainte-nance treatment. Outcomes are reported below, including a study that examined abstinence in 84 patients seven years after treatment [31].

Of 925 outpatients in treatment for chemical dependency (7% aged 55–77, 32% aged 40–54) from 1994–1998, Satre *et al.* [28] found that patients aged 55–77 were diagnosed more often with alcohol dependence than with drug dependence compared to patients aged 40–54 or <40. Patients aged 55–77 stayed in treatment longer and were less likely to report family or friends encouraging substance use than those aged < 40. Compared to those aged <40 and those aged 40–54, older adults aged 55–77 had fewer close friends, were less likely to be members of a 12-step programme, less likely to report past-month cigarette smoking, more likely to report past-month or year abstinence and more likely to have worse health. The finding is similar to data from TEDS showing that the older group was more likely to have primary alcohol problems than the younger group and that younger adults were more likely to have alcohol and drug problems.

Lofwall *et al.* [29] compared substance use habits and mental and physical health of 67 opioid maintenance patients aged 50–66 (n = 41, predominantly male, unemployed, non-White) and opioid maintenance patients aged 25–34 (n = 26, predominantly female, non-White, employed). Patients aged 50–66 were in treatment longer, had more lifetime years of incarceration, were less likely to receive medical assistance and more likely to have commercial health insurance than patients aged 25–34. Patients aged 50–66 also had fewer positive urine screens for opiates, cocaine, marijuana or benzodiazepines, were older at initiation for all substances except alcohol, had poorer physical health and took more prescribed medications per day than patients aged 25–34. Patients aged 50–66 also had poorer health-related quality of life in terms of physical functioning, physical health limits, and body pain.

Rosen *et al.* [30] examined substance use, mental health and physical health among 140 predominantly Black, males aged ≥50 years in methadone treatment in the Midwestern Unite States and found 57.1% had mental illness (most often depression), 47.1% took a psychotropic medication, 57.7% had poor physical health and 87.1% smoked cigarettes. Compared to population norms, the 140 methadone patients had poorer self-assessed health. Different from studies on alcohol use, results of Lofwall *et al.* [29] and Rosen *et al.* [30] demonstrate a prevalent rate of poor health or psychiatric co-morbidity among older treatment-seeking opioid-dependent adults.

In terms of treatment outcomes, Satre *et al.* [28] found that correlates of abstinence among outpatients were female gender, treatment retention and no close family or friends who encouraged use. Women aged 55–77 had greater abstinence than men aged 55–77 and women aged <40. Women aged 55–77 also stayed in treatment longer than men aged 55–77. Satre *et al.* [31] examined abstinence for 84 predominantly White, male, married individuals seven years after they received drug and alcohol abuse treatment and found that 30-day abstinence positively correlated with length of stay in treatment. Bivariate analyses also showed that seven-year abstinence correlated with attendance at 12-step meetings at five and seven years. Men were more likely than women to continue to drink and continue to drink heavily (i.e. 5+ drinks per day). Among methadone treatment patients, Rosen *et al.* [30] found that, across 24 months, 76.4% screened positive for illegal drug use at least once. Of those who screened positive, 80.4% did so more than once. In addition, 21% reported binge drinking (i.e. ≥4 alcoholic drinks per day) at least once in the past year. Hence, treatment retention may be associated with better outcomes, and treatment outcomes appear to be better in older women than older men.

In summary, similar to studies of TEDS data, patients aged 55–77 were diagnosed with alcohol dependence more than drug dependence. In line with TEDS data, Arndt et al. [27] found that admits aged ≥55 years were more likely than adults aged 30–54 to have health insurance. This was also found by Lofwall et al. [29] of those in treatment aged 50–66. Similarly, Arndt et al. [24] found that more adults aged ≥55 years reported later substance initiation than adults aged 30–54, as did Lofwall et al. [29] of those in treatment aged 50–66. Compared with younger patients, patients aged ≥50 years stayed in treatment longer and had poor physical health. In addition, abstinence among those aged ≥50 years and ≥55 years were associated with being female and treatment retention.

Substance abuse treatment in general health care settings

Two identified studies also examined the need for elder substance treatment in the general medical settings (Table 16.4). The first used visit data from the Drug Abuse Warning Network (DAWN), a US surveillance system that monitors drug-related emergency department (ED) visits. DAWN data showed that, between 2004 and 2008, there was a 121.1% increase in visits related to use or misuse of pharmaceutical drugs by adults aged ≥50 years (N = 115 803 and N = 256 097, respectively). Of the ED visits by persons aged ≥50 years in 2008, 35.6% were made by adults aged 50–54, 23.2% were by those aged 55–59, 11.9% were by those aged 60–64, 9.6% were by those aged 65–69 and 19.7% were by those aged 70+ [32]. Most visits were made by non-Hispanic Whites (78.1%), with 15.2% made by non-Hispanic Blacks and 5.2% by Hispanics. Female ED admissions were more likely than males to be White and most ED visits related to opioid use were by females. Prescription pain relievers (opioids) accounted for most visits (43.5%), followed by pharmaceutical drugs for anxiety and insomnia treatments (31.8%) and antidepressants (8.6%). Alcohol was involved in 20.4% of drug-related ED visits and visits that included alcohol were most likely to be made by adults aged 50–64 [32].

The second study that examined the need for substance abuse treatment by older adults using general mental or physical health care was by Neighbors et al. [33] who analysed a subsample (n = 837) of Blacks aged ≥55 years respondents to the 2001–2003 National Survey of American Life (NSAL). Neighbors et al. found that 5.9% of Blacks aged ≥55 years with DSM-IV alcohol abuse reported the use of mental health care and 20.8% reported the use of the general medical care for problems with their emotions, nerves, mental health or use of alcohol or drugs in the past 12 months. Of those with DSM-IV alcohol dependence (unweighted n = 6), 30.3% sought general medical care for their emotions, nerves, mental health or use of alcohol or drugs in the past 12 months. The results suggest that older Blacks with alcohol dependence use mental health and substance-related services through general health providers. Although the number of Blacks with an alcohol use disorder is small, this population-based study adds findings for an understudied population.

Discussion and conclusion

Studies showed that elders wanted and were able to quit substance use with assistance. Tobacco studies examined cigarette cessation and lacked prevalence information for elders seeking or using tobacco cessation intervention or treatment. Studies of alcohol use reported that 7–10% of patients aged ≥65 years seeking general health care screened positive for hazardous drinking but studies were dated from the early to mid-1990s. Studies examining patients in treatment for alcohol problems, either an ICD-9 alcohol-related diagnosis or alcohol dependence, found the proportion of those in alcohol treatment aged ≥55 years ranged from 16 to 17%. However, studies focusing on population subgroups, such as veterans, were also dated. TEDS data on admissions to alcohol or drug abuse treatment facilities were more recent and showed increased treatment admissions over time. ED visits related to nonmedical prescription drug use (mainly opioid pain relievers) also increased.

Drug and alcohol abuse treatment studies showed that alcohol was the substance elder adults sought treatment for most often, followed by either opiates (TEDS data 2001–2005) [25] or cocaine (TEDS data 1998 and 2008) [27]; however, alcohol abuse treatment admissions declined over time as drug abuse related treatment admissions increased. Tobacco and alcohol use studies examined treatment among predominantly White individuals. While drug abuse admissions were predominantly White, drug abuse treatment among older Black adults appeared to be increasing. Elders in drug and alcohol abuse treatment differed from their younger counterparts in that they were more likely to be male, outside the labour force, have health insurance, be diagnosed with alcohol dependence, be in poor physical health and be in treatment longer. Elders were also less likely than their younger counterparts to use outpatient substance abuse treatment. Studies of cigarette cessation showed that the vast majority of older smokers aged ≥65 years have not received cessation advice from healthcare providers. Poor health was the most common correlate of receiving advice. Only one study from outside the United States was identified. Findings from Christie *et al.* [14] on adults aged ≥60 years entering alcohol treatment were similar to US studies in finding that the majority of those entering treatment were White, male and married.

The next steps for research include gauging the prevalences of individuals aged ≥50 years with a substance use disorder who use or seek treatment, the extent of those seeking treatment who receive it, and what are the facilitators and barriers to receiving treatment. These prevalence estimates for different age, gender and racial/ethnic groups are needed to gauge the treatment needs and gaps for the growing older populations. Research must also address whether individuals aged ≥50 years with a substance use disorder are aware of their treatment need and know where and how to seek assistance. There may be a lack of knowledge by seniors who may need services for substance use problems. Studies also are needed to examine how co-morbid psychiatric conditions affect treatment use and outcomes for different racial/ethnic groups and to distinguish between early onset versus late onset substance abusers in risk and protective factors in order to inform effective prevention and treatment strategies. Lastly, there is a continuous need to monitor shifting drug use patterns and their impact on treatment use.

References

1. Vincent, G.K. and Velkoff, V.A. (2010) *The Next Four Decades, the Older Population in the United States: 2010 to 2050.* Current Population Reports, P25-1138, US Census Bureau, Washington, DC. 2010.
2. Gfroerer, J., Penne, M., Pemberton, M. and Folsom, R. (2003) Substance abuse treatment need among older adults in 2020: the impact of the aging baby-boom cohort. *Drug Alcohol Depend,* **69**, 127–135.
3. Colliver, J.D., Compton, W.M., Gfroerer, J.C. and Condon, T. (2006) Projecting drug use among aging baby boomers in 2020. *Ann Epidemiol,* **16**, 257–265.
4. Johnson, P.B. and Sung, H.E. (2009) Substance abuse among aging baby boomers: Health and treatment implications. *J Addict Nurs,* **20**, 124–126.
5. Substance Abuse and Mental Health Services Administration (2012) *Results from the 2011 National Survey on Drug Use and Health: Detailed Tables.* Center for Behavioral Health Statistics and Quality, Substance Abuse and Mental Health Services Administration, Rockville MD.
6. Blazer, D.G. and Wu, L.-T. (2011) The epidemiology of alcohol use disorders and subthreshold dependence in a middle-aged and elderly community sample. *Am J Geriatr Psychiatry,* **19**, 685–694.
7. Steinberg, M.B., Akincigil, A., Delnevo, C.D. *et al.* (2006) Gender and age disparities for smoking-cessation treatment. *Am J Prev Med,* **30**, 405–412.
8. Ossip-Klein, D.J., McIntosh, S., Utman, C. *et al.* (2000) Smokers ages 50+: Who gets physician advice to quit? *Prev Med,* **31**, 364–369.
9. Brown, D.W., Croft, J.B., Schenck, A.P. *et al.* (2004) Inpatient smoking-cessation counseling and all-cause mortality among the elderly. *Am J Prev Med,* **26**, 112–118.
10. Watt, C.A., Carosella, A.M., Podgorski, C. and Ossip-Klein, D.J. (2004) Attitudes toward giving smoking cessation advice among nursing staff at a long-term residential care facility. *Psychol Addict Behav,* **18**, 56–63.
11. Hall, S.M., Humfleet, G.L., Gorecki, J.A. *et al.* (2008) Older versus younger treatment-seeking smokers: Differences in smoking behavior, drug and alcohol use, and psychosocial and physical functioning. *Nicotine Tob Res,* **10**, 463–470.
12. Whitson, H.E., Heflin, M.T. and Burchett, B.M. (2006) Patterns and predictors of smoking cessation in an elderly cohort. *JAGS,* **54**, 466–471.
13. Sacco, P., Bucholz, K.K. and Spitznagel, E.L. (2009) Alcohol use among older adults in the National Epidemiologic Survey on Alcohol and Related Conditions: A latent class analysis. *J Stud Alcohol Drugs,* **70**, 829–838.
14. Christie, M.M., Bamber, D., Powell, C. *et al.* (2013) Older adult problem drinkers: Who presents for alcohol treatment. *Aging Ment Health,* **17**(1), 24–32.

15. Gordon, A.J., Conigliaro, J., Maisto, S.A. *et al.* (2003) Comparison of consumption effects of brief interventions for hazardous drinking elderly. *Subst Use Misuse*, **38**, 1017–1035.
16. Fleming, M.F., Manwell, L.B., Barry, K.L. *et al.* (1999) Brief physician advice for alcohol problems in older adults: A randomized community-based trial. *J Fam Pract*, **48**, 378–384.
17. Lemke, S. and Moos, R.H. (2002) Prognosis of older patients in mixed-age alcoholism treatment programs. *J Subst Abuse Treat,* **22**, 33–43.
18. Al-Otaiba, Z., Epstein, E.E., McCrady, B. and Cook, S. (2012) Age-based differences in treatment outcome among alcohol-dependent women. *Psychol Addict Behav*, **26**, 423–431.
19. Oslin, D.W., Slaymaker, V.J., Blow, F.C. *et al.* (2005) Treatment outcomes for alcohol dependence among middle-aged and older adults. *Addict Behav*, **30**, 1431–1436.
20. Blow, F.C., Walton, M.A., Chermack, S.T. *et al.* (2000) Older adult treatment outcome following elder-specific inpatient alcoholism treatment. *J Subst Abuse Treat*, **19**, 67–75.
21. Lemke, S. and Moos, R.H. (2003) Outcomes at 1 and 5 years for older patients with alcohol use disorders. *J Subst Abuse Treat*, **24**, 43–50.
22. Kraemer, K.L., Mayo-Smith, M.F. and Calkins, D.R. (1997) Impact of age on the severity, course, and complications of alcohol withdrawal. *Arch Intern Med,* **157**, 2234–2241.
23. Atkinson, R.M., Misra, S., Ryan, S.C. and Turner, J.A. (2003) Referral paths, patient profiles and treatment adherence of older alcoholic men. *J Subst Abuse Treat,* **25**, 29–35.
24. Arndt, S., Gunter, T.D. and Acion, L. (2005) Older admissions to substance abuse treatment in 2001. *Am J Geriatr Psychiatry*, **13**, 385–392.
25. Substance Abuse and Mental Health Services Administration (2007) *The DASIS Report: Older Adults in Substance Abuse Treatment: 2005*. Office of Applied Studies, Substance Abuse and Mental Health Services Administration, Rockville, MD.
26. Lofwall, M.R., Schuster, A. and Strain, E.C. (2008) Changing profile of abused substances by older persons entering treatment. *J Nerv Ment Dis,* **196**, 898–905.
27. Arndt, S., Clayton, R. and Schultz, S.K. (2011) Trends in substance abuse treatment 1998-2008: Increasing older adult first-time admissions for illicit drugs. *Am J Geriatr Psychiatry*, **19**, 704–711.
28. Satre, D.D., Mertens, J.R., Arean, P.A. and Weisner, C. (2004) Five-year alcohol and drug treatment outcomes of older adults versus middle-aged and younger adults in a managed care program. *Addiction*, **99**, 1286–1297.
29. Lofwall, M.R., Brooner, R.K., Bigelow, G.E. *et al.* (2005) Characteristics of older opioid maintenance patients. *J Subst Abuse Treat,* **28**, 265–272.
30. Rosen, D., Smith, M.L. and Reynolds, C.F. (2008) The prevalence of mental and physical health disorders among older methadone patients. *Am J Geriatr Psychiatry*, **16**, 488–497.
31. Satre, D.D., Blow, F.C., Chi, F.W. and Weisner, C. (2007) Gender differences in seven-year alcohol and drug treatment outcomes among older adults. *Am J Addict*, **16**, 216–221.
32. Substance Abuse and Mental Health Services Administration (2012) *Results from the 2011 National Survey on Drug Use and Health: Mental Health Detailed Tables*. Center for Behavioral Health Statistics and Quality, Substance Abuse and Mental Health Services Administration, Rockville MD.
33. Neighbors, H.W., Woodward, A.T., Bullard, K.M. *et al.* (2008) Mental health service use among older African Americans: The National Survey of American Life. *Am J Geriatr Psychiatry*, **16**, 948–956.

Chapter 17
IMPLICATIONS FOR PRIMARY CARE

Devoshree Chatterjee and Steve Iliffe

Department of Primary Care and Population Health, University College London, UK

Background

The scale and range of substance misuse has changed in the period following the Second World War and is now affecting the health of an ageing population whilst posing a challenge for primary care. In the United States 'baby boomers' (the cohort born between 1945 and 1964) use and misuse alcohol, illicit drugs and psychoactive prescription medicines at a higher rate than previous generations [1]. As a consequence, higher levels of substance misuse are currently being witnessed in the 50–64 age group than in those aged 65 and more [2], but this does not mean that substance misuse declines with advancing age. It was once believed that illicit drug users 'matured' out of their drug use but there is evidence that older heroin users, for example, do not reduce their use as they age [3]. In the United States, it is projected that the number of adults aged 50 or older with substance use disorder will double from 2.8 million (annual average) in 2002–2006 to 5.7 million in 2020 [4].

This could have a substantial impact on health services, through a combination of increasing age-related risks of neurotoxicity and other adverse effects, and the interaction of drugs and alcohol with other age-related co-morbidities [2]. For example, the increasing numbers of older adults amongst the population with renal and liver disease could increase the incidence of adverse effects due to increased drug sensitivity and drug accumulation. In the United States there is already evidence of this cohort effect occurring, with a rapid rise in the numbers of people aged 65–84 being admitted to hospital with drug-related conditions [2].

Implications for primary care

There are a number of implications for primary care services. Firstly, practitioners need to distinguish between different types of substance misuse in the older population [5], because approaches to treatment differ for those whose dominant problem is illicit drug use (with or without alcohol problem drinking) compared with those older people misusing psychoactive prescription medication. Secondly, making

Substance Use and Older People, First Edition.
Edited by Ilana B. Crome, Li-Tzy Wu, Rahul (Tony) Rao and Peter Crome.
© 2015 John Wiley & Sons, Ltd. Published 2015 by John Wiley & Sons, Ltd.

this distinction is difficult because of the lack of clear definitions of psychoactive prescription medicine misuse. In addition, clinical manifestations of substance misuse in older people may be ambiguous, which can create barriers to recognition [6, 7]. Thirdly, the interaction of age-related co-morbidities with substance misuse suggests that long-term condition management is probably the best model for intervention [3] with a spectrum of tailored approaches from prevention messages through minimal advice and structured brief interventions, to formalized treatment [1]. One critical period in which interventions may have an impact is retirement from paid employment [8]. Each of these implications is explored here.

Different populations at risk

Older users of illicit drugs who receive treatment are usually long-term users, beginning their habit before the age of thirty, are more likely to be male and White, and often enter therapy from the criminal justice system [2]. Misuse of psychoactive prescription medicines, on the other hand, is more common amongst women who are socially isolated and who have a history of physical abuse, chronic pain, anxiety or sleep disturbance [1]. Iatrogenic exposure to prescribed medications with potential for misuse may be the single greatest risk factor in this population. It is important to remember the abuse of prescription medications is not confined to those living at home. Older adults in residential and nursing homes, assisted living facilities, as well as hospital inpatients are also at risk of exposure to prescription drugs with abuse potential, particularly in care homes where prescribing may not be as regularly monitored and reviewed.

Benzodiazepine sedative-hypnotics and opioid analgesics are the two major classes of prescription medication subject to abuse in the older population [9, 10]. Appropriate use of opioid medications provides analgesia. However, they produce a sense of euphoria, well being and sedation. As a consequence, they also have the potential for misuse and dependency. Older women who misuse opioids report worse pain severity and more depression symptoms; the psychic effects of opioids may be useful for managing stress and users may not be able to distinguish these psychic effects from analgesia [11].

Although not recommended for long-term use of more than four weeks, a common problem encountered in general practice is repeat prescribing of benzodiazepine hypnotic drugs [12, 13]. This can lead to tolerance, dependency and misuse of this class of drugs. Misuse of long acting benzodiazepines is associated with multiple risks, including falls, drowsiness and ataxia, confusion, impaired psychomotor function, deficits in visuospatial and verbal learning, processing speed, road traffic accidents and risk of dependence [14]. Psychomotor slowing may be especially profound in older people, who may have decreased rates of metabolism or greater susceptibility to central nervous system depression [15].

Dependence may lead to anxiety, depression and cognitive impairment causing further medical and neuropsychiatric morbidity in this vulnerable population [14].

Irritability, aggression, hostility and impulsivity may occur in some older people who take benzodiazepines. This paradoxical disinhibition may be due to disinhibition of behaviour normally contained by social restraints [16].

In one study of 74-year-old women, those who misused psychoactive prescription medicines did not differ greatly from those who do not [17]. They did not have more stresses and did not cope with them differently, but they did experience the stresses more intensely, felt more threatened by them and were more dissatisfied with their own coping. Substance misuse for older women is a complex, dynamic phenomenon shaped by social and personal experiences including violence, mental health disorders and social obligations (like caring for others) [18], and is often unintentional [1].

Screening in primary care

Primary care provides an ideal, albeit challenging, setting in which to screen for misuse of prescribed and illicit drugs in older people. However, substance misuse in older people is often not recognized, or recognized but poorly treated [1]. Many barriers encountered by the clinician (time, knowledge about the patient and their medical history) and created by the patient (denial, communication problems, discomfort realizing or admitting and discussing the problem) need to be overcome to ensure screening for substance misuse is effective. Symptoms of substance misuse, including cognitive impairment and falls, can be easily confused with other conditions of ageing and get missed.

The misuse of prescribed medication may present in many ways. It is important to remember this may not always be deliberate and there may be many contributory factors attributable to the patient and the prescriber leading to this misuse. It may involve patients taking higher doses of prescription drugs or 'borrowing' from a friend or relative. It may also occur when prescribed drugs are taken for a longer duration than desired, resulting in tolerance and dependency, or taken for cases other than the approved indication. Older substance misusers do not show typical addiction features, such as drug seeking behaviour, dose escalation, use to 'get high' or illegal sourcing [6]. This failure to fit stereotypes of drug misuse makes the problem difficult for professionals to recognize and acknowledge [18]. At the same time gender, age and substance misuse intersect to create a stigma that discourages the person from reporting their problem, acknowledging its impact on them and their life, and seeking help [18]. As primary care consultations become more rushed and services become more fragmented, misuse of psychoactive prescription medication may become more difficult to detect.

To offset this risk, primary care practitioners need to find more easily recognizable patterns in clinical presentations of substance misuse in older people [19]. For example, one definition of psychoactive prescription medicine misuse is that it is any maladaptive and persistent use of medication that leads to functional impairment (like worsening gait or cognitive impairment), or to psychological distress including social isolation [6]. Another recognizable pattern is when medication misuse involves deliberately taking prescribed or over-the-counter medicines at higher than recommended doses for extended periods, with hoarding of drugs and combination use with alcohol [5]. These working definitions place substance misuse within familiar clinical frames of age-related functional loss, prescription medicine management and observed behaviour (hoarding, alcohol use).

Scale of benefit

Although older substance misusers are less likely than younger people to declare their problem and seek help [2], they are more likely to benefit from treatment when they do seek it [3, 20]. The more favourable long-term outcomes among older substance misusers are likely to be due to the type of substance dependence, their social networks and gender [21]. Older people tend to have lower levels of dependency, show less hostility and greater abstinence motivation, and stay longer in treatment [22].

The treatment needs of this population are likely to change over time and specific programmes tailored to the treatment of substance abuse in older adults and non-pharmacological therapies, such as cognitive behavioural therapy, improving social support and networks, are important adjuncts to the management of this group. Regular medication reviews are imperative to reduce the risks and consequences related to polypharmacy and drug interactions as contributory factors to misuse of medications.

Co-morbidities and social context

It is important to consider whether patients' pain is adequately controlled in those misusing opioids and benzodiazepine drugs. Persistent pain in older adults can lead to insomnia, depression, anxiety, falls and inappropriate drug use. It may be difficult to distinguish 'pseudo-addiction' in the form of drug seeking behaviour due to poorly controlled pain, from true abuse of prescription medications. It is possible that ensuring pain is adequately controlled will reduce the need for inappropriate use of benzodiazepine drugs and potential for abuse [23].

Retirement from paid employment has a complex relationship with substance misuse, particularly with problem alcohol drinking. High job satisfaction, but also high work stress, predict later alcohol problem drinking [8]. Involuntary exit from the workplace and having wide social networks increase the likelihood of alcohol problem drinking after retirement, at least in men, as do chronic pain and previous history of drug or alcohol misuse. Using the Alcohol-Related Problems Survey (ARPS) screening instrument for alcohol problem drinking in older people, and a FRAMES approach to intervention, may be useful at this transition stage of the life course [24]. The FRAMES approach includes Feedback about risks, emphasis on Responsibility, Advice about changing use, providing a Menu of change strategies, expressing Empathy in communication and promoting Self-efficacy.

Conclusions

It is important for professionals, including doctors, pharmacists and nurses caring for the patient, to be vigilant for the presence of prescription drug abuse in older adults and their associated problems. This is not an easy task, as has been indicated, and there is a need to understand the dynamic phenomenon of substance misuse in later life. Primary care practitioners may need specialist support to manage older patients with substance misuse, especially if complex interventions like FRAMES are used therapeutically.

There is a case for specialist outreach into primary care settings, where primary care practitioners can provide a nonstigmatizing environment in which to work and bring their knowledge of individuals and families to the assessment and management of patients with complex problems. In addition, there is need for more research on factors associated with psychoactive prescription medicine misuse in older people, to elucidate the progress from medical exposure to problematic use [25]. This may best be carried out in community settings with less selected populations.

References

1. Blow, F. and Barry, K. (2012) Alcohol and substance misuse in older adults. *Curr Psychiatry Rep*, **14**, 310–319.
2. Wu, L.-T. and Blazer, D.G. (2011) Illicit and nonmedical drug use among older adults: a review. *J Aging Health*, **23** (3), 481–504.
3. Rosen, D., Hunsaker, A., Albert, S. *et al.* (2011) Characteristics and consequences of heroin use among older adults in the United States: a review of the literature, treatment implications, and recommendations for future research. *Addict Behav*, **36**(4), 279–285.
4. Han, B., Gfroerer, J.C., Colliver, J.D. and Penne, M.A. (2009) Substance use disorder among older adults in the United States in 2020. *Addiction*, **104**(1), 88–96.
5. Gossop, M. and Moos, R. (2008) Substance misuse among older adults: a neglected but treatable problem. *Addiction*, **103**, 347–348.
6. Payne, M., Gething, M., Moore, A. *et al.* (2011) Primary care providers perspectives on psychoactive medication disorders in older adults. *Am J Geriatr Pharmacother*, **9**(3), 164–172.
7. Blazer, D.G. and Wu, L.-T. (2012) Patterns of tobacco use and tobacco-related psychiatric morbidity and substance use among middle-aged and older adults in the United States. *Aging Ment Health*, **16**(3), 296–304. doi: 10.1080/13607863.2011.615739.
8. Kuerbis, A. and Sacco, P. (2012) The impact of retirement on the drinking patterns of older adults: a review. *Addict Behav*, **37**, 587–595.
9. Blazer, D.G. and Wu, L.-T. (2009) Nonprescription use of pain relievers by middle-aged and elderly community-living adults: National Survey on Drug Use and Health. *J Am Geriatr Soc*, **57**(7), 1252–1257.
10. Nkogho Mengue, P.G., Abdous, B., Berbiche, D. *et al.* (2013) Impact benzodiazepine dependence on the use of health services: senior' health study. *Geriatr Psychol Neuropsychiatr Vieil*, **11**(3), 229–236.
11. Park, J. and Lavin, R. (2010) Risk factors associated with opioid medication misuse in community dwelling older adults with chronic pain. *Clin J Pain*, **26**(8), 647–655.

12. Voyer, P., Preville, M., Roussel, M.E. *et al.* (2009) Factors associated with benzodiazepine dependence among community-dwelling seniors. *J Community Health Nurs*, **26**(3), 101–113.

13. Voyer, P., Roussel, M.E., Berbiche, D. and Préville, M. (2010) Effectively detect dependence on benzodiazepines among community-dwelling seniors by asking only two questions. *J Psychiatr Ment Health Nurs*, **17**(4), 328–334.

14. Longo, L. and Johnson, B. (2000) Addiction: Part I. Benzodiazepines – Side effects, abuse risk and alternatives. *Am Fam Physician*, **61**(7), 2121–2128.

15. Ashton, H. (1995) Toxicity and adverse consequences of benzodiazepine use. *Psychiatr Ann*, **25**, 158–165.

16. van der Bijl, P. and Roelofse, J.A. (1991) Disinhibitory reactions to benzodiazepines: a review. *J Oral Maxillofac Surg*, **49**, 519–523.

17. Folkman, S., Bernstein, L. and Lazarus, R. (1987) Stress processes and the misuse of drugs in older adults. *Psychol Aging*, **2**(4), 366–374.

18. Koenig, T. and Crisp, C. (2008) Ethical issues in practice with older women who misuse substances. *Subst Use Misuse*, **43**, 1045–1061.

19. Schonfeld, L., King-Kallimanis, B.L., Duchene, D.M. *et al.* (2010) Screening and brief intervention for substance misuse among older adults: the Florida BRITE project. *Am J Public Health*, **100**(1), 108–114.

20. McGrath, A., Crome, P. and Crome, I. (2005) Substance misuse in the older population. *Postgrad Med J*, **81**, 228–231.

21. Satre, D., Mertens, J., Arean, P. and Weisner, C. (2004) Five-year alcohol and drug treatment outcomes of older adults versus middle-aged and younger adults in a managed care program. *Addiction*, **99**(10):1286–1297.

22. Satre, D., Mertensd, J., Arean, P. and Weisner, C. (2003) Contrasting outcomes of older versus middle-aged and younger chemical dependency in a managed care program. *J Stud Alcohol*, **64**(4): 520–530.

23. Chatterjee, D. and Iliffe, S. (2012) Benzodiazepine use in community-dwelling older people in London – is it related to psychological or physical morbidities? Presentation to the British Geriatrics Society conference, 18 May 2012, Llandudno, UK.

24. Hunter, B. and Lubman, D. (2010) Substance misuse: management in the older population. *Austr Fam Physician*, **39**(10); 738–741.

25. Simoni-Wastila, L. and Keri Yang, H. (2006) Psychoactive drug abuse in older adults. *Am J Geriatr Pharmacother*, **4**(4): 380–394.

Chapter 18

ADDICTION LIAISON SERVICES

Roger Bloor[1,2] and Derrett Watts[1]

[1]North Staffordshire Combined Healthcare NHS Trust, UK
[2]School of Medicine, Keele University, UK

Introduction

Liaison psychiatry is a speciality which has grown from its initial beginnings as a link from psychiatry to general hospitals to aid in the management of issues such as overdose, self-harm and psychosis to a service which encompasses the whole range of mental health issues related to physical illness [1].

The value of liaison psychiatry services within the general hospital setting is well recognized, with an understanding that such services promote the concept of integrated care, which is of key importance in the context of the ageing population [2]. Within the older population, the most common mental disorders seen within a general hospital setting are delirium, dementia and depression. Reviews of older patients seen by psychiatric liaison services have shown that a diagnosis of delirium is associated with a significantly higher mortality than similar patients with a diagnosis of depression [3, 4]. Studies of referral rates to consultation liaison services have shown an increasing rate of referral of older people across a variety of countries and this has a bearing on the training needs and staffing profile of such services [5, 6].

The management of alcohol and drug problems within general hospitals has been suggested as falling within the remit of consultation-liaison psychiatry [7], particularly as the recognition of drug and alcohol problems is often poor within a general hospital setting. One study reported 56% of addiction problems being missed by referring doctors when referring to a liaison service [8]. Studies of referrals to liaison services of patients over 60 years of age have shown that they often have high levels of alcohol intake and significant levels of alcohol related morbidity and mortality; the occurrence of benzodiazepine withdrawal was also seen to be higher in this older population [9, 10].

The use of a specialist addiction liaison nurse working in general medical and surgical wards of a district general hospital has been shown to improve detection and management of patients with alcohol problems, with an 88% rate of completion of alcohol treatment compared with 40% prior to the introduction of the liaison service [11].

Substance Use and Older People, First Edition.
Edited by Ilana B. Crome, Li-Tzy Wu, Rahul (Tony) Rao and Peter Crome.
© 2015 John Wiley & Sons, Ltd. Published 2015 by John Wiley & Sons, Ltd.

Organizing an addiction liaison service to a general hospital

The introduction of specialist alcohol liaison services to general hospitals will not only improve clinical outcomes whilst in hospital but also lead to other benefits, such as the training of staff in alcohol identification and brief interventions. Such services also produce increased awareness and referral into specialist alcohol services [12] and reduce the stigma that patients may experience. The role of liaison teams in facilitating the adoption of new treatment protocols, such as symptom-triggered regimens for the management of alcohol withdrawal, may also shorten hospital admissions and save money [13].

A review of projects in alcohol liaison in the United Kingdom identified eight factors to support the effective delivery of alcohol liaison services [14]:

- Strong strategic partnership support.
- The identification of clinical champions.
- The establishment of a steering group.
- Integration of Alcohol Liaison Nurse (ALN) services within the hospital framework.
- Integration of ALN services within the specialist community treatment system.
- Robust management and clinical support structures – to promote best practice and reduce risk.
- Development of comprehensive policies and procedures – to ensure that the management of problem alcohol use reflects current best practice.
- Comprehensive and accurate data collection and the development of interagency/ interdepartmental data sharing agreements.

To enable such a development of services, a strategic approach involving a range of stakeholders, including primary and secondary health services, public health, commissioners, alcohol services and patient groups, is required [12].

Key features of such services include establishing integrated care pathways, requiring the collaboration of medical and psychiatric teams, General Practitioners and community services. Identifying gaps in skills and offering appropriate training is a key to success in establishing liaison services. The importance of delivering education to general hospital clinical staff with regard to the mental health issues involving older patients has been identified and is seen as one of the roles of Liaison Old Age Psychiatry teams [15].

The planning process includes ensuring that the service is available at the time it is needed, not just within routine working hours The service needs to be adaptable and flexible to enable it to engage with those who have struggled in the past to link in to traditional service models. Particular emphasis should be paid to those who are frequent attendees at accident and emergency care services.

Case vignette 1

A 71-year-old lady living alone was under the care of an Older Persons Psychiatric Team and Community Alcohol Services. She had 15 admissions to hospitals in the previous two years, often linked to falls. She was self-neglecting and considered to be at continuing risk in relation to further falls, fire in the home and walking into roads when intoxicated.

> **Key point**
> Patients with alcohol problems are often admitted for a variety of reasons, including acute intoxication, falls, circulatory problems, liver disease, neglect, malnutrition and a variety of alcohol-related health problems.

An accurate history of her alcohol use was difficult to obtain but she demonstrated signs of dependence.

> **Key point**
> The recognition of drug and alcohol problems is often poor within a general hospital setting.

She had been prescribed citalopram and vitamin B tablets but was not complying well with them. In the light of her many recent admissions to hospital, it was felt she may benefit from admission to a detoxification unit, and with some reluctance she agreed. Two days before this was due to occur, she was admitted to the general hospital with a urinary tract infection and diarrhoea. Continuing liaison (via telephone, electronically and ward visits) occurred between the hospital ward, community alcohol worker, Community Psychiatric Nurse for Older Persons Mental Health and the detoxification unit.

> **Key point**
> Liaison psychiatry services for older adults demonstrate positive outcomes from identification of the alcohol-related problems and referral to community treatment services.

She was deemed medically fit for discharge after four days on the ward. Her alcohol withdrawal symptoms were assessed and no benzodiazepine medication had been required. It was felt that she needed further assessment but agreed that this would be better placed on an older persons ward as she was not demonstrating signs of withdrawal. She was offered access to the group sessions available on the detoxification unit, which she could attend whilst in the older persons ward on the same site.

> **Key point**
> Services for older people with substance misuse problems can be delivered using a model in which older people's services are supported by specialist and community addiction services.

Addiction liaison services for older adults

The provision of nurse-led general psychiatry liaison services within a general hospital setting for older adults has been shown to increase the detection rate of alcohol problems [16]. In terms of improved outcomes from such services a

randomized controlled trial [17] comparing such a service with care as usual concluded that nurse-led mental health liaison services that accept generic problems
may not be effective in reducing levels of morbidity. However, the authors expressed
the view that targeted services for particular diagnostic categories may be effective.
This view is confirmed in a review of outcomes from four liaison psychiatry services for older adults; these showed positive outcomes from identification of the
alcohol-related problems and referral to community treatment services [18].

The need for early specialist intervention for older adults with drug and alcohol
problems within a hospital setting was highlighted in a study of the detection rates
of substance misuse problems in this population by medical staff [19]. The results
indicated that only 3 out of 88 problem users of benzodiazepine, 29 out of 76
smokers and 33 out of 99 problem drinkers were identified by the medical staff.
The authors concluded that drug and alcohol services need to become involved in
the early detection of problems in older adult inpatients.

The provision of a liaison service from an alcohol liaison nurse within a general
hospital inpatient setting for patients over the age of 60 has been described [9]. The
patients seen had been admitted for a variety of reasons, including acute intoxication,
falls, circulatory problems and liver disease. Secondary problems included hypertension, neglect and malnutrition and a variety of alcohol-related health problems.

A comparison of older patients and younger adults referred to a liaison service
within a hospital setting highlighted the fact that older patients were more likely to
be admitted for cardiac or gastrointestinal problems and had a lower rate of admission for infections compared with younger adults. The study, conducted over a
six-year period, showed a low rate of referral to the liaison service with only 1% of
elderly patients being referred for substance abuse opinions. [20]

Reviews of referrals to consultation liaison services of patients over 65 years of
age presenting with delirium have shown that up to 20% are related to benzodiazepine withdrawal [21]. The administration of benzodiazepines and opiates to older
patients within intensive care units has been shown to be a significant factor in
prolonging the period of post-treatment delirium [22].

Essential elements of liaison service provision for older adults

A report on the workforce requirements for Mental Health and Substance Misuse
of older adults concluded that services for this population need to provide [23]:

- Detection
- Diagnosis
- Treatment
- Continuing management
- Monitoring

The report states that these types of services are provided to older adults by 'a
bewildering array of organizations and individuals' and calls for a number of

improvements to services, including systematic outreach services, improved diagnosis and coordination of services by trained personnel with access to speciality consultation.

The systems for delivering appropriate treatment of substance misuse in older adults clearly need to focus on two main areas:

- Detection and Diagnosis
- Treatment and Management

The detection of alcohol use disorders within a general hospital setting has been shown to be improved by the introduction of a consultation liaison service [24]. One of the roles of such a service is to assist the general services by introducing standardized methods of screening and diagnosis.

Liaison services are designed to assist with the treatment and management of patients and can operate on a variety of models. These range from a consultation model, in which the consultant psychiatrist accepts referrals from the treating team, through to integration of liaison staff in the treatment team to enable education input to the team and early detection of problems [25].

The use of validated screening instruments has been shown to improve detection rates of both mental illness and substance misuse in a variety of populations [26], including older adults in the community [27].

Screening for alcohol problems in older adults

The identification of patients of working age suitable for referral to a liaison service has been shown to be problematic [8]; the same pattern is seen in services for older adults [20, 28]. The use of screening instruments such as the CAGE questionnaire improves detection rates in the working age population.

Commonly used screening instruments used in the older adult age group are the CAGE, SMAST-G and AUDIT [29]. A modified form of the CAGE questionnaire omitting the (C), Cut down, question has been trialled for use in older populations and shown to have improved specificity and sensitivity compared with the full CAGE questionnaire [30]. The MAST (Michigan Alcoholism Screening Test) has been used in the detection of alcohol-related problems in older male outpatients with a sensitivity of 91.4% and a specificity of 83.9%; the authors recommended that the MAST should be used in conjunction with a questionnaire to assess the frequency and quantity of alcohol consumption [31]. The shortened version of the MAST, the Short Michigan Alcoholism Screening Test – Geriatric Version (SMAST-G), has been used to detect hazardous or risky alcohol intake in older adults [32]. Using the 10-item SMAST-G or the two-item mini Michigan Alcoholism Screening Test – Geriatric version (MMAST-G) gives a good detection rate compared with the full MAST in elderly patients following acute cerebrovascular accidents [33].

A comparison of the CAGE and the SMAST-G in a community population of older adults concluded that a screening strategy using both instruments would provide a higher detection rate than using the single instruments [34], other studies have suggested that the AUDIT questionnaire is the most effective tool in identifying problems drinkers in older male adults [35].

There is an evidence base for the use of the ARPS (alcohol-related problems survey) in elderly outpatients [36] and in a primary care setting [37]; both studies suggest that the ARPS or shorter form (shARPS) are more sensitive than the AUDIT, SMAST-G or CAGE in identifying older age subjects with alcohol-related problems.

A systematic review of screening for alcohol misuse in primary care patients concluded that the AUDIT is best suited for screening for harmful or hazardous use in the elderly whilst the CAGE is more suited for screening for dependence. The ARPS was seen as having practical implementation problems that if overcome may lead to it being superior to the AUDIT or CAGE [38].

Screening for drug use problems

A number of instruments are available for screening for drug misuse, the Drug Abuse Screening Test (DAST) [39] is available in 10, 20 and 28-item versions, it has moderate to high levels of validity, sensitivity and specificity and has been used in a variety of populations [40]. Administering the 20-item DAST to a sample of drug and alcohol patients, a cut-off score of 5/6 was shown to be the optimal threshold score for detection of DSM-III drug abuse or dependence [41]. Dependence and misuse of prescribed medication is common in this age group, particularly the use of benzodiazepines [42], and screening for inappropriate medication prescribing in older people can be undertaken using screening tools such as STOPP [43]. However, there is a need for the development of age-appropriate screening tools for drug misuse in this age group. The inappropriate prescribing of medications such as benzodiazepines and opiates in this age group increases the risk of hospital admission in frail older patients [44].

Case vignette 2

A 72-year-old widower was admitted to the hospital after suffering a fall at home. He suffered a left hip fracture and was recovering on an orthopaedic ward following surgery.

Key point
Fall-induced fracture is one of the most important cause of hospital admission related to inappropriate prescribing in the elderly.

On the fourth day after surgery the patient developed confusion and became agitated with paranoid delusions and disorientation in time and place.

The family visited later that day and during discussion with the ward staff revealed that the patient regularly took a 'tranquillizer' and had done so since the death of his wife. The General Practitioner was contacted and confirmed that the patient had been taking Diazepam, 5 mg three times per day, for over seven years. Attempts had been made to reduce the dose but this always resulted in a recurrence of his anxiety symptoms.

Key point

Hospital admissions related to potentially inappropriate medication in older patients mainly involves overuse or misuse of benzodiazepines, aspirin and opiates.

A liaison consultation was requested and a diagnosis of benzodiazepine withdrawal was made. A diazepam replacement regime was prescribed, producing a rapid improvement in the patients state within two days.

The patient was given a diagnosis of 'delirium secondary to benzodiazepine dependence' and a discharge plan was formed between between the orthopaedic ward, the Community Addiction Team, a Community Psychiatric Nurse for Older Persons Mental Health, the inpatient addiction treatment unit and the General Practitioner.

Key point

Benzodiazepine withdrawal delirium in older hospitalised patients may be associated with potentially inappropriate prescribing.

The management plan enabled the provision of appropriate support and treatment to reduce the risk of further episodes of withdrawal and a long-term benzodiazepine reduction plan was put in place managed by the General Practitioner with support from the other agencies.

Summary

The early identification and treatment of alcohol and drug problems in older people produces positive outcomes in terms of reduced morbidity and mortality. In addition, there are clear economic benefits from reduced length of hospital stay and decreases in discharge to care settings.

The development of addiction liaison services for working age adults has been shown to improve identification and treatment outcomes. The development of such services for older adults would address the needs of the increasing number of older people with substance misuse problems.

The use of age-appropriate screening tools would assist in the initial detection of problems but investment in research and training in this area is essential if services are to develop in the most efficient manner.

References

1. Ajiboye, P.O. (2007) Consultation-liaison psychiatry: the past and the present. *Afr J Med Med Sci*, **36**(3), 201–205.
2. Verwey, B., van Waarde, J.A., Huyse, F.J. *et al.* (2008) [Consultation-liaison psychiatry and general hospital psychiatry in the Netherlands: on the way to psychosomatic medicine]. *Tijdschr Psychiatr*, **50** Spec no., 139–143.
3. Tsai, M.C., Weng, H.H., Chou, S.Y. *et al.* (2012) One-year mortality of elderly inpatients with delirium, dementia, or depression seen by a consultation-liaison service. *Psychosomatics*, **53**(5), 433–438.
4. Tsai, M.C., Weng, H.H., Chou, S.Y. *et al.* (2012) Three-year mortality of delirium among elderly inpatients in consultation-liaison service. *Gen Hosp Psychiatry*, **34**(1), 66–71.
5. Anderson, D., Nortcliffe, M., Dechenne, S. *et al.* (2011) The rising demand for consultation-liaison psychiatry for older people: comparisons within Liverpool and the literature across time. *Int J Geriatr Psychiatry*, **26**(12), 1231–1235.
6. Schellhorn, S.E., Barnhill, J.W., Raiteri, V. *et al.* (2009) A comparison of psychiatric consultation between geriatric and non-geriatric medical inpatients. *Int J Geriatr Psychiatry*, **24**(10), 1054–1061.
7. Glaser, F.B. (1988) Alcohol and drug problems: a challenge to consultation-liaison psychiatry. *Can J Psychiatry*, **33**(4), 259–63.
8. Smith, G.C., Clarke, D.M. and Handrinos, D. (1995) Recognising drug and alcohol problems in patients referred to consultation-liaison psychiatry. *Med J Aust*, **163**(6), 307, 310–312.
9. Mehta, M.M., Moriarty, K.J., Proctor, D. *et al.* (2006) Alcohol misuse in older people: heavy consumption and protean presentations. *J Epidemiol Community Health*, **60**(12), 1048–1052.
10. Wetterling, T., Backhaus, J. and Junghanns, K. (2002) [Addiction in the elderly – an underestimated diagnosis in clinical practice?]. *Nervenarzt*, **73**(9), 861–866.
11. Hillman, A., McCann, B. and Walker, N.P. (2001) Specialist alcohol liaison services in general hospitals improve engagement in alcohol rehabilitation and treatment outcome. *Health Bull (Edinb)*, **59**(6), 420–423.
12. Moriarty, K., Cassidy, P., Dalton, D. *et al.* (2012) *Alcohol Related Disease: Meeting the Challenge of Improved Quality of Care and Better Resources*. A joint position paper on behalf of the British Society of Gastroenterology, Alcohol Health Alliance and the British Association for the Study of the Liver. British Society of Gastroenterology, London.
13. Lee, T.J.W., Samuel, M., Bewick, L. *et al.* (2012) OC-030 Benefits of introduction of a symptom triggered regimen for management of alcohol withdrawal in a large teaching hospital trust: reduced admission duration and cost savings. *Gut*, **61**(Suppl 2), A13.
14. Pender, J. and Ranzetta, L. (2010) *East Midlands Hospital Alcohol Liasison – Evaluation Report*. Ranzetta Consulting, Stanstead Abbotts, Hertfordshire, UK.
15. Teodorczuk, A., Welfare, M., Corbett, S. and Mukaetova-Ladinska, E. (2010) Developing effective educational approaches for Liaison Old Age Psychiatry teams: a literature review of the learning needs of hospital staff in relation to managing the confused older patient. *Int Psychogeriatr*, **22**(6), 874–885.
16. Anderson, D., Cattell, H. and Bentley, E. (2008) Nurse-led liaison psychiatry service for older adults: service evaluation. *Psychiatr Bull R Coll Psychiatr*, **32**(8), 298–302.
17. Baldwin, R., Pratt, H., Goring, H. *et al.* (2004) Does a nurse-led mental health liaison service for older people reduce psychiatric morbidity in acute general medical wards? A randomised controlled trial. *Age Ageing*, **33**(5), 472–478.

18. Rao, R. (2013) Outcomes from liaison psychiatry referrals for older people with alcohol use disorders in the UK. *Ment Health Subst Use*, **6**(4), 1–7.

19. McInnes, E. and Powell, J. (1994) Drug and alcohol referrals: are elderly substance abuse diagnoses and referrals being missed? *BMJ*, **308**(6926), 444–446.

20. Weintraub, E., Weintraub, D., Dixon, L. *et al.* (2002) Geriatric patients on a substance abuse consultation service. *Am J Geriatr Psychiatry*, **10**(3), 337–342.

21. Moss, J.H. and Lanctot, K.L. (1998) Iatrogenic benzodiazepine withdrawal delirium in hospitalized older patients. *J Am Geriatr Soc*, **46**(8), 1020–1022.

22. Pisani, M.A., Murphy, T.E., Araujo, K.L.B. *et al.* (2009) Benzodiazepine and opioid use and the duration of intensive care unit delirium in an older population. *Crit Care Med*, **37**(1), 177–183.

23. Eden, J., Maslow, K., Le, M. and Blazer, D. (eds) (2012) *The Mental Health and Substance Use Workforce for Older Adults: In Whose Hands?* The National Academies Press, Washinton, DC.

24. Diehl, A., Nakovics, H., Croissant, B. *et al.* (2009) Consultation-liaison psychiatry in general hospitals: improvement in physicians detection rates of alcohol use disorders. *Psychosomatics*, **50**(6), 599–604.

25. Bronheim, H.E., Fulop, G., Kunkel, E.J. *et al.* (1998) The Academy of Psychosomatic Medicine practice guidelines for psychiatric consultation in the general medical setting. *Psychosomatics*, **39**(4), S8–S30.

26. Barnaby, B., Drummond, C., McCloud, A. *et al.* (2003) Substance misuse in psychiatric inpatients: comparison of a screening questionnaire survey with case notes. *BMJ*, **327**(7418), 783–784.

27. Schonfeld, L., King-Kallimanis, B.L., Duchene, D.M. *et al.* (2010) Screening and brief intervention for substance misuse among older adults: the Florida BRITE project. *Am J Public Health*, **100**(1), 108–114.

28. McRee, B. (2012) Open wide! Dental settings are an untapped resource for substance misuse screening and brief intervention. *Addiction*, **107**(7), 1197–1198.

29. Caputo, F., Vignoli, T., Leggio, L. *et al.* (2012) Alcohol use disorders in the elderly: a brief overview from epidemiology to treatment options. *Exp Gerontol*, **47**(6), 411–416.

30. Hinkin, C.H., Castellon, S.A., Dickson-Fuhrman, E. *et al.* (2001) Screening for drug and alcohol abuse among older adults using a modified version of the CAGE. *Am J Addict*, **10**(4), 319–326.

31. Hirata, E.S., Almeida, O.P., Funari, R.R. and Klein, E.L. (2001) Validity of the Michigan Alcoholism Screening Test (MAST) for the detection of alcohol-related problems among male geriatric outpatients. *Am J Geriatr Psychiatry*, **9**(1), 30–34.

32. Naegle, M.A. (2008) Screening for alcohol use and misuse in older adults: using the Short Michigan Alcoholism Screening Test-Geriatric Version. *Am J Nurs*, **108**(11), 50–58; quiz 58–59.

33. Johnson-Greene, D., McCaul, M.E. and Roger, P. (2009) Screening for hazardous drinking using the Michigan Alcohol Screening Test-Geriatric Version (MAST-G) in elderly persons with acute cerebrovascular accidents. *Alcohol Clin Exp Res*, **33**(9), 1555–1561.

34. Moore, A.A., Seeman, T., Morgenstern, H. *et al.* (2002) Are there differences between older persons who screen positive on the CAGE questionnaire and the Short Michigan Alcoholism Screening Test-Geriatric Version? *J Am Geriatr Soc*, **50**(5), 858–862.

35. Ryou, Y.I., Kim, J.S., Jung, J.G. *et al.* (2012) Usefulness of alcohol-screening instruments in detecting problem drinking among elderly male drinkers. *Korean J Fam Med*, **33**(3), 126–133.

36. Fink, A., Tsai, M.C., Hays, R.D. *et al.* (2002) Comparing the alcohol-related problems survey (ARPS) to traditional alcohol screening measures in elderly outpatients. *Arch Gerontol Geriatr*, **34**(1), 55–78.

37. Moore, A.A., Beck, J.C., Babor, T.F. *et al.* (2002) Beyond alcoholism: identifying older, at-risk drinkers in primary care. *J Stud Alcohol*, **63**(3), 316–324.
38. Berks, J. and McCormick, R. (2008) Screening for alcohol misuse in elderly primary care patients: a systematic literature review. *Int Psychogeriatr*, **20**(6), 1090–1103.
39. Skinner, H.A. (1982) The drug abuse screening test. *Addict Behav*, **7**(4), 363–371.
40. Yudko, E., Lozhkina, O. and Fouts, A. (2007) A comprehensive review of the psychometric properties of the Drug Abuse Screening Test. *J Subst Abuse Treat*, **32**(2), 189–198.
41. Gavin, D.R., Ross, H.E. and Skinner, H.A. (1989) Diagnostic validity of the drug abuse screening test in the assessment of DSM-III drug disorders. *Br J Addict*, **84**(3), 301–307.
42. Culberson, J.W. and Ziska, M. (2008) Prescription drug misuse/abuse in the elderly. *Geriatrics*, **63**(9), 22–31.
43. Gallagher, P.F., O'Connor, M.N. and O'Mahony, D. (2011) Prevention of potentially inappropriate prescribing for elderly patients: a randomized controlled trial using STOPP/START criteria. *Clin Pharmacol Ther*, **89**(6), 845–854.
44. Dalleur, O., Spinewine, A., Henrard, S. *et al.* (2012) Inappropriate prescribing and related hospital admissions in frail older persons according to the STOPP and START criteria. *Drugs Aging*, **29**(10), 829–837.

Chapter 19
CURRENT HEALTHCARE MODELS AND CLINICAL PRACTICES

Rahul (Tony) Rao[1], Ilana B. Crome[2,3,4,5], Peter Crome[6] and Finbarr C. Martin[7]

[1] Institute of Psychiatry/South London and Maudsley NHS Foundation Trust, UK
[2] Keele University, UK
[3] Queen Mary University of London, UK
[4] Imperial College University of London, UK
[5] South Staffordshire and Shropshire Healthcare NHS Foundation Trust, UK
[6] Department of Primary Care and Population Health, University College London/Keele University, UK
[7] Guys and St Thomas' NHS Foundation Trust/King's College London, UK

Introduction

The provision of clinical services for older people with substance misuse faces considerable challenges in the form of a growing older population in whom successive cohorts show increasingly higher rates of misuse across a range of substances. For people aged 65 and over in the United States, there has been a 25% increase in the prevalence of binge drinking from 2000 to 2010 [1]. Over the same frame, there have been increases of 43% for alcohol dependence, 143 % for illicit drug misuse and 50% for the nonmedical use of prescription drugs [1].

An ageing population

When the National Health Service was set up in the United Kingdom over 65 years ago, nearly half the population died before the age of 65. Half a century later, it had fallen to around 18% and the chance of surviving from birth to age 85 has more than doubled for men over the last three decades, from 14% in 1980–1982 to 38% in 2009–2011 [2]. Life expectancy at the age of 65 in England and Wales for men in 2009–2011 has risen by 5.1 years since 1980–1982, when it was 13.0 years. Women have seen a smaller increase of 3.8 years since 1980–1982, when it was 17.0 years [2].

The number of people living with one or more long-term medical conditions (LTCs) is increasing; 40% of those 65 and over report two or more self-reported LTCs. However, it is known that mental well-being peaks at ages 65–74 [3]. In spite of this, most people aged 75 and over report three or more LTCs; these account for 55% of GP appointments, 77% of inpatient bed days and around 70% of total

Substance Use and Older People, First Edition.
Edited by Ilana B. Crome, Li-Tzy Wu, Rahul (Tony) Rao and Peter Crome.
© 2015 John Wiley & Sons, Ltd. Published 2015 by John Wiley & Sons, Ltd.

spending on health in England [4]. When the effects of a growing older population with substance misuse are considered, there is cause for concern from both public health and clinical perspectives. Demographic and epidemiological trends are compounded by the additional presence of mental and physical frailty from the effects of ageing, lifestyle, life events and disease combining to render bodily and mental functions impaired, with the resultant diminished functional reserve making the individual vulnerable to decompensation with additional 'minor' illnesses or challenge. This lost resilience may manifest itself as the geriatric syndromes of falls, immobility and confusion, all of which interact adversely with substance misuse.

The realization that the presence of frailty is an important predictive factor for hospitalization, functional decline and death is leading to the creation of clinical pathways in both primary and secondary care. In secondary care, patients requiring admission are more and more being streamed to geriatric medicine wards, where comprehensive assessment (including use of substances) can be undertaken. Such an approach has been shown to reduce mortality and keep patients at home.

There is now a consensus statement defining frailty [5] that also stresses the importance of the reduction of polypharmacy as a potential method of ameliorating this new geriatric giant. How best to identify frail patients and which groups of older people should be screened for its presence remains to be determined [6].

Service development and provision

Clinical practice should ensure that models of care cut across both hospital and community settings, with the latter including independent living (including supported accommodation) and care homes, as well as prison and probation settings, hostels and those for older homeless people. It is also important to bear in mind the needs of Black and ethnic minority groups (e.g. older Irish people), particularly in areas of high socioeconomic deprivation [7].

A particular challenge for service provision is the delivery of integrated care for Substance Misuse and Co-morbid Mental Disorder (SMCD), also known as Dual Diagnosis [8]. This includes a range of substance misuse seen in co-morbid mental disorders, with adverse impacts on both health and social function. Older people with SMCD also show greater service use than those with substance misuse alone. In spite of this observation, there have been few policy drivers to changes in service provision [1, 9].

Identifying clinical need for service development and implementing provision of services is often constrained by the limitation of financial resources but one such model has been developed in the United Kingdom over the past 10 years. This model was developed in response to an increasing clinical burden of alcohol misuse within a mental health of older adult service and necessitated the acquisition of additional knowledge and skills in substance misuse [10]. This service is now able to provide integrated care for older people, with dual diagnosis accompanying alcohol misuse within a mainstream old age psychiatry service, with improved access to service, clinically effective care pathways, robust partnerships with key stakeholders (including working with service users and carers), a workforce skilled to address unmet need and the promotion of health education, prevention and early intervention. It has been one of the few services in the United Kingdom to have provided outcome data on clinical interventions for alcohol misuse [11].

The voluntary sector plays a vital role in complementing mainstream delivery of health services. In the United Kingdom, most of these services are for those aged 50 and above, delivering interventions within a home-based model. Using a summary of older focus client outcomes over 18 months, *Addiction Northern Ireland* found a 60% overall reduction in alcohol misuse accompanied by an improvement in quality of relationships, emotional health and use of time following one-on-one counselling [12]. *Addaction* in Scotland implemented a similar model but also included peer-led counselling and found that 80% of service users had reduced their alcohol intake and showed similar improvements in mental and physical health. The *Foundation 66 Project* in Hammersmith and Fulham in London identified several themes involved in alcohol misuse in older people that included loneliness/social isolation, low mood, loss of status and retirement. Positive outcomes were found using interventions such as offering a drink diary, providing health information, monitoring medication compliance, structuring meal times and using brief advice and motivational interviewing [12].

In each country, the constellation of available, or potentially available, services will differ. Commissioners and providers are likely to establish that there are some consistent characteristics that need to be considered for provision. Services need to be 'older person friendly'. This includes making the referral process easy, ensuring that there are the facilities and information which older people require [13] for addiction issues, including the capability to counter the negativity and negative stereotypes about older people, information which is age specific in content with perhaps simple explanations if required and administered at the pace which is comfortable for older people. In other words, there needs to be a safe, suitable environment that takes account of the person's mobility, sensory, language and literacy needs.

Older people now comprise the majority of hospital inpatients, so knowledge about the relationship of substance use to common presenting problems needs not only to be rooted in the main psychiatric specialties of old age psychiatry, liaison psychiatry and addiction psychiatry but also in accident and emergency medicine, geriatrics, general medicine, general practice and other health professions, for example residential and nursing homes. In the United Kingdom, as in most developed countries, there are few models of service provision specifically for this group of patients. The developing world is even more impoverished.

Integrated care and workforce development

Bartels *et al.* undertook a multisite study to determine whether mental health/substance abuse clinics in primary care were more effective than referral to specialist clinics [14]. 71% of patients engaged in integrated treatment compared with 49% in the enhanced referral model. They concluded that older primary care patients were more likely to accept collaborative mental health treatment within primary care than in substance abuse/mental health clinics, due to improved access. This has implications for service developments in a group that underuse facilities [14].

The US National Academy of Sciences has produced a report that recommends how the workforce can be prepared to meet the needs of older people with mental health and substance use problems [1]. The range of practitioners, from those with minimal education to specialists, was considered. These included: specialists such as general psychiatrists, psychologists, social workers, psychiatric nurses and counsellors; primary care teams, including general physicians, general practitioners, nurses and physician assistants; specialists in the care of older adults, such as geriatricians and geriatric nurses, geriatric psychiatrists, gerontological nurses, geropsychologists and gerontological social workers; care workers who provide support services; peer support providers; and informal care givers, for example family, friends and volunteers. However, their roles were often poorly defined.

It was suggested that as the 'baby boom' generation had had higher mental health service use throughout their lives, it was likely that this would continue, although estimates on which to base accurate predictions were not available.

However, it was concluded that the requirement for specialist providers was far in excess of that which was available, and that this shortage meant that needs would have to be met by a whole range of providers. The report further highlighted the limited opportunities for recruitment to specialization in terms of financial incentives, support and mentorship. Professional training was not mandatory, so that it was inconsistent, and where progress had been made programmes with promise were not disseminated or evaluated, and were therefore at risk of collapse. Strengthening the roles and training of care workers, carers and families was outlined.

The report further stated:

'A persuasive body of evidence, drawn from two decades of research, shows that two common MH/SU disorders among older adults – depression and at-risk drinking – are most effectively addressed when care is organized to include these essential ingredients: (1) systematic outreach and diagnosis; (2) patient and family education and self-management support; (3) provider accountability for outcomes; and (4) close follow-up and monitoring to prevent relapse. Moreover, these elements are best obtained when care is patient centred (integrating patient preferences, needs and strengths), in a location easily accessed by patients (e.g. in primary care, senior centres or patients' homes) and coordinated by trained personnel with access to specialty consultation. There is also evidence suggesting great promise in telehealth and web-based interventions for older adults with MH/SU conditions. Progress in these areas is not likely to be achieved, however, without practice redesign and change in Medicare payment rules. There is a fundamental mismatch between older adults' need for coordinated care and Medicare fee-for service reimbursement that precludes payment of trained care managers and psychiatry consultation. Finally, research on effective delivery of MH/SU care for certain older populations is urgently needed, especially for individuals residing in nursing homes and other residential settings, prisoners, rurally isolated elders and older adults with severe mental illnesses.'

Major hindrances in the implementation of training, treatment and evaluation are the multiple agencies and departments within government, the voluntary sector and private organizations that need to collaborate to agree to deliver education, services and research. Many countries are facing severe reductions in budgets and this further deters motivation to embark on so daunting a task, about which there is only partial awareness.

Conclusions and recommendations

The growing number of older people with substance abuse issues requires a concerted response by commissioners of health and social care services to develop appropriate integrated elder-friendly services. This is particularly so for those with multiple medical and psychiatric co-morbidities who may 'fall between the cracks' of separate services. Services must be accessible, which may mean being home based. This may mean adaptation of present services or the creation of new ones. Flexibility will be required as changes outside the field of addiction are implemented, for example greater community care, better inter-professional working and telemedicine. How best to deliver services must be locally determined but there are some existing models in the health and voluntary sector that may be adapted.

Improvements in the present situation will require:

- Recognition by commissioners that this is an issue that requires remedy and funding.
- Involving service users in the development of local services.
- Training of health and social care staff in substance abuse awareness, recognition, assessment and basic treatment.
- The establishment of clear clinical pathways for referral and long-term support.
- Regular review of substance abuse issues by clinical audit/quality improvement both within designated older persons services and in the wider health service.
- Research to identify best methods of assessment, treatment and service delivery.
- Above all, funding to make this happen.

References

1. Eden, J., Maslow, K., Le, M. and Blazer, D. (eds) (2012) *The Mental Health and Substance Use Workforce for Older Adults: In Whose Hands?* Institute of Medicine of the National Academies, Washington, DC.
2. Office for National Statistics (2013) Interim Life Tables, England and Wales, 2009–2011. http://www.ons.gov.uk/ons/rel/lifetables/interim-life-tables/2009-2011/stb-2009-2011.html (last accessed 13 April 2014).
3. Department of Health (2012) Health Survey for England 2011. https://www.gov.uk/government/publications/health-survey-for-england-2011 (last accessed 13 April 2014).

4. Office for National Statistics (2009) General Household Survey, 2007 Report. http://www.ons.gov.uk/ons/rel/ghs/general-household-survey/2007-report/index.html (last accessed 13 April 2014).

5. Morley, J.E., Vellas, B., Abellan van Kan, G. *et al.* (2013) Frailty consensus: A call to action. *Journal of the American Medical Directors Association*, 14(6), 392–397.

6. Gordon, A.L., Masud, T. and Gladman, J.R. (2014) Now that we have a definition for physical frailty, what shape should frailty medicine take? *Age and Ageing*, 43(1), 8–9.

7. Rao, R. (2006) Alcohol misuse and ethnicity: Hidden populations need specific services—and more research. *British Medical Journal*, 332, 682.

8. Wu, L.-T. and Blazer, D.G. (2013) Substance use disorders and psychiatric comorbidity in mid and later life: a review. *International Journal of Epidemiology* [Epub ahead of print].

9. US Department of Health and Human Services (2002) Promoting older adult health. Publication No. 02-3628, SAMHSA (Substance Abuse and Mental Health Services Administration), Rockville, MD.

10. Rao, R. and Shanks, A. (2011) Development and implementation of a dual diagnosis strategy for older people in south east London. *Advances in Dual Diagnosis*, 4, 28–35.

11. Rao, R. (2013). Outcomes from liaison psychiatry referrals for older people with alcohol use disorders in the UK. *Mental Health and Substance Use*, 6, 362–368.

12. Wadd, S., Lapworth, K., Sullivan, M. *et al.* (2011) Working with older drinkers. Tilda Goldberg Centre for Social Work and Social Care, Luton, UK.

13. Crome, I.B. (2014) Substance misuse and the older person. In: *International Textbook of Substance Abuse Medicine* (eds N. El Guebaly, G. Carra, and M. Galanter). (In press).

14. Bartels, S.J., Coakley, E.H., Zubritsky, C. *et al.* (2004) Improving access to geriatric mental health services: a randomized trial comparing treatment engagement with integrated versus enhanced referral care for depression, anxiety, and at-risk alcohol use. *American Journal of Psychiatry*, 161(8), 1455–1462.

AGE-SPECIFIC TREATMENT INTERVENTIONS AND OUTCOMES

Chapter 20

PHARMACOLOGICAL AND INTEGRATED TREATMENTS IN OLDER ADULTS WITH SUBSTANCE USE DISORDERS

Paolo Mannelli[1], Li-Tzy Wu[1] and Kathleen T. Brady[2]

[1] Department of Psychiatry and Behavioral Sciences, School of Medicine, Duke University Medical Center, USA
[2] South Carolina Clinical and Translational Research Institute, Medical University of South Carolina, USA

Introduction

In the twentieth century, life expectancy has doubled and one-third of the population in western countries will be older than 50 by the middle of the current century [1, 2]. The number of older people (≥50 years) requiring treatment for a substance use disorder will likely triple well before that mark [3]. With additional individuals in this age cohort showing subclinical deteriorating substance abuse conditions [4], unprecedented health care challenges are predicted [5, 6]. Increases in older-age marijuana users and nonmedical users of prescription psychotherapeutic drugs are expected to be large [7, 8]. The service delivery system is unprepared to meet estimated needs [3, 9] and more effective pharmacological treatments addressing the physiological, neurobiological and psychosocial changes associated with ageing are necessary. Pharmacokinetic modifications associated with changes in body composition and renal and hepatic functions consist of increased volume of distribution of lipid-soluble drugs and reduced clearance. These changes lead to prolonged plasma elimination half-life. Pharmacodynamically, age-dependent changes increase sensitivity to drugs. Reduced homeostatic mechanisms prolong the time older adults require to regain steady-state levels following drug administration [10]. Thus, pharmacological treatment should be started at a low dose and titrated slowly. For similar reasons, the limits for safe drinking may need to be reduced compared to younger people, especially among individuals who have co-existing health problems and/or use medications that interact with alcohol [11, 12].

The ageing process affects neurobiological systems involved in reward, mood, cognition and substance use disorders, although clinical consequences have not been well characterized [13]. Anticipatory reward is associated with increased activity of the ventral striatum, the anterior cingulate cortex and the left intraparietal region in young adults, compared to only the left intraparietal region in older adults [14]. Mid-brain dopamine synthesis and prefrontal cortex activity are reduced during ageing [14], dopamine transporter binding decreases [15] in association with dopaminergic and serotonergic receptor loss within the prefrontal cortex and striatum [16, 17]. N-methyl- D-aspartate glutamate receptor density and activity have shown age-related decreases as well in the cortex, striatum and hippocampus [13]. The clinical picture may be further confounded by an older adult's past substance abuse history [13] and present likelihood of use of multiple medications [18].

Despite changes in neurocognitive and physical functioning associated with ageing, older adults are just as likely to engage in treatment as younger individuals; in some cases, they show better compliance and better outcomes [19–21]. Several problems along the therapeutic process have been identified in detection, diagnosis and management of substance use disorders among older adults. Drug use can mimic age-related issues such as confusion and cognitive declines [22, 23]. Inadequate drug and alcohol history taking has been observed in the elderly, with low referral rates and insufficient numbers of specialist drug and alcohol services, and greater use of prescription drugs with potential for misuse to treat chronic or pain-related medical conditions [24–26]. However, sociological factors come into play as barriers to treatment. Loneliness and isolation are common among older individuals and are associated with undetected substance use [27]. Older adults, like other age groups, may be reluctant to seek help with drug use problems due to stigma and shame, and generational effects may render these perceptions more potent than among younger groups [28]. However, in the elderly there is more regular contact with medical services. Thus, primary care and other healthcare services, where the presence and support of the family is likely to be noted, provide a valuable opportunity to screen for substance use problems and plan for intervention [29]. Mental health, substance abuse and general medical care providers can work together to address both the physical and mental health needs of older patients [30], and positive results obtained should be replicated and expanded. There is evidence that age-specific programmes addressing the unique social characteristics of ageing are linked to better treatment outcomes and adherence [31–33], though further 'head-to-head' comparisons with mixed-age treatments are warranted [34].

In summary, there is a shortage of evidence-based indications to guide practitioners in treating substance misuse or abuse in older adults. Elderly people are typically excluded from clinical trials of pharmacotherapy [35]. In this chapter, characteristics and outcomes of available treatments are identified, highlighting the gaps for further research. The management of severe acute intoxication or overdose have not been included, as this does not differ from the general population.

Tobacco

Evidence-based smoking cessation programmes, in particular counselling, medical advice and nicotine replacement therapy, have been found to be safe and effective in older adults [36]. Prescribers, however, may need to be better educated regarding treatment safety and efficacy in order to effectively treat older patients for smoking cessation. A survey of 58 000 physician visits shows no age differences in rates of tobacco counselling, while patients older than 65 years were less likely to receive a prescription for cessation medication [37]. A telephone follow-up survey of 1070 older smokers (ages 65–74) who were prescribed nicotine patches found that 29% reported current seven-day or longer abstinence at six-month follow-up [38]. Similar results were reported six months after free distribution of nicotine replacement therapy [39]. An investigation among urban smokers (n = 34 090) who phoned a toll-free 'quit line' to receive a six-week course of nicotine replacement therapy and had brief follow-up counselling calls, found that more nicotine therapy recipients quit smoking compared with those who did not receive treatment because of mailing errors (33 vs 6%). The highest quit rates after six months were associated with participants older than 65 years (47%).

The evidence on the effects of combination therapy is limited. A 12-week, open randomized clinical trial with two-year follow-up found that cognitive behavioural therapy was more effective than nicotine replacement and bupropion [40]. Pharmacotherapy did not augment and actually reduced the efficacy of cognitive behavioural therapy in 402 smokers aged ≥50 years. In terms of safety, placebo-controlled trials of nicotine patches on older patients with coronary artery disease have found no evidence for an increased risk of cardiac complications [41, 42]. Medications prescribed for smoking cessation have not been extensively studied in controlled trials among older adults and limited safety data are available. In trials of immediate and sustained release bupropion for depression treatment, no overall differences in safety or effectiveness have been observed between older subjects and younger subjects (Prescribing information 2013), but comparable data in smoking cessation are lacking. A reduced maximum dose of 150 mg bupropion daily is often recommended for the elderly [43]. There is no specific dose reduction recommended in older adults for varenicline in smoking cessation treatment except where there is coexisting renal insufficiency [44].

Alcohol

A lower threshold for inpatient treatment of alcohol withdrawal is recommended in older people [45] based on the findings of a protracted and more severe alcohol withdrawal syndrome, and the likelihood of neurological and medical complications in the elderly compared with younger people with equal drinking severity [46, 47]. However, detoxification studies have not consistently identified a relationship between the severity of alcohol withdrawal and age [48, 49]. Benzodiazepines are the treatment of choice for alcohol withdrawal, though doses may need to be reduced in older people [45]. Shorter acting benzodiazepines (e.g. oxazepam, lorazepam) are preferred, especially in the presence of hepatic impairment and concern about accumulation with oversedation [50, 51]. In the absence of high-quality evidence on anti-craving and aversive pharmacological interventions to maintain alcohol abstinence in older people, clinical decisions should rely on the larger adult evidence base and medication adverse events profile [45].

There are concerns about risk of serious adverse effects in older adults prescribed the aversive medication disulfiram due to physical co-morbidities, polypharmacy and the possibility of precipitating a confusional state [27, 52, 53], and cardiovascular concerns in case of alcohol ingestion [54]. However, Zimberg [55] found disulfiram to be safe and effective in a dose of 125 mg per day in medically stable elderly patients. Acamprosate and naltrexone have been considered potential good pharmacological agents for relapse prevention in older adults in terms of safety. Acamprosate is known to have a good safety profile except in renal insufficiency. Dose adjustment may be required in older adults due to age-related reduced kidney function. Naltrexone appears to be safe and well tolerated in older adults. A 12-week double-blind, placebo-controlled study of naltrexone (50 mg per day) in 44 alcohol-dependent subjects over 50 years of age found no difference in frequency of adverse events, including changes in liver enzymes, between placebo and naltrexone-treated groups [56]. There were no significant differences between the placebo and naltrexone-treated groups on abstinence or relapse rates, possibly due to the small sample size and a high drop-out rate (n = 17). Among those individuals exposed to alcohol, those on naltrexone were significantly less likely to relapse than those on placebo.

In a larger naltrexone study, 183 alcohol-dependent individuals were randomly assigned to one of three conditions, including a nonconfrontational behavioural intervention and placebo, and treated for nine months [20]. Participants who were 55 or older demonstrated greater rates of treatment engagement and medication adherence than younger adults. There were no significant differences between groups on abstinence or relapse rates; however, significant interaction effects demonstrated that older patients were more likely to be abstinent and less likely to relapse due to greater therapy and medication adherence. Again, small cell sizes may have impeded the ability to detect main effects.

The high co-morbidity of alcoholism and depression increases the complexity of treatment and is associated with severe disability and morbidity. There has been a general lack of well-controlled large treatment trials of antidepressant medication or psychotherapy in elderly depressed patients with alcohol use disorders [57]. Clinical evidence had suggested that successful treatment of depression among the elderly may lead to reductions in their alcohol use [58]. One controlled trial has examined the effects of naltrexone combined with the antidepressant sertraline for treatment of adults 55 and older with co-occurring major depression and alcohol dependence [59]. Overall, 42% of the 74 participants achieved remission of both depression and alcohol use over the 12-week trial; however, no added benefit was found by combining naltrexone with the antidepressant medication. Initial full responders sustained better overall treatment outcomes at six and twelve months follow-up, compared with partial responders and nonresponders [60]. Relapse to alcohol use was strongly associated with continued depression, confirming the linkage between these disorders in the elderly.

In a recent trial among adults with alcohol dependence, patients treated with the sertraline-naltrexone combination achieved more abstinence from alcohol and delayed relapse to heavy drinking, showing lower likelihood of being depressed at the end of treatment compared with those treated with sertraline or naltrexone alone or with placebo [61]. Further study in older adults may shed light on the utility of a dual pharmacotherapy in the management of co-occurring mood and substance use disorders in this cohort [62]. Other co-morbidities may significantly affect the outcome of problem drinking in older populations. A prospective study in 1291 patients has shown that late middle aged individuals who have more numerous painful medical conditions can reduce alcohol consumption but remain at risk for more frequent episodes of excessive drinking [63]. Clinicians should be alert to drinking problems among their older pain patients, especially men.

Opioids

Opioid agonist substitution therapy is safe and effective among older opioid-dependent patients in helping discontinue drug use with minimal withdrawal discomfort and preventing relapse, although existing studies are insufficient to provide a complete description of patients' needs and anticipate comprehensive health challenges for treatment providers and planners. A retrospective study of 91 older patients enrolled in methadone maintenance treatment found that individuals who remained in treatment showed a statistically significant reduction in drug use as well as reduced psychiatric and legal problems compared to treatment dropouts [64]. Among 165 patients attending an urban methadone treatment programme, older adults were more likely than younger adults to have longer periods of treatment and less likely to report current heroin use and overall drug use, though they had more often a history of alcohol use problems [65]. Firoz and Carlson [66] reviewed the clinical status of 54 older methadone-maintained patients compared with 704 patients under 55 years of age from the same methadone programmes. The older group had improved outcomes on drug use measures at nine months compared with the younger adults. Groups did not significantly differ in medical or psychiatric problems. In another retrospective investigation in a methadone maintenance population, the older group (n = 41) had significantly more medical problems and worse general health than the younger group (n = 96), while both groups showed poor general health compared to population norms [67]. However, low rates of positive urine opioid tests were found in both older and younger patients without age-specific services.

Although it is reported that the ageing of methadone maintained patients can safely coexist with a gradual increase in methadone doses among patients [68], there is no evidence on specific methadone dosing regimens for maintenance treatment in the older cohort. Guidance from the pain management literature recommends reduced opioid doses, a longer time interval between doses and monitoring of creatinine clearance [69]. As maintenance treatment uses daily methadone dosing, slower dose titration and medical monitoring are advisable. Evidence from chronic pain management suggests that methadone may not be the best choice in frail elderly patients, compared with buprenorphine and other analgesics agents [70]. Methadone has a high drug–drug interaction potential, is associated with prolongation of the QT interval and a potential risk of accumulation due to a long elimination half-life [69]. In addition, methadone is difficult to titrate because of its large interindividual variability in pharmacokinetics. In nonopioid dependent elderly individuals, methadone prescription has been associated with a high proportion of emergency department visits for injuries and drug interactions with other central nervous system-active agents [71].

In the absence of specific studies focused on naltrexone and buprenorphine treatment of opioid dependence in older adults, clinical decisions are based on extrapolations from the evidence gathered in the general population. It is important to note that the administration of the opioid antagonist naltrexone in the presence of opioids can trigger significant withdrawal symptoms and delirium-like conditions [72]. The induction to naltrexone treatment is potentially complex in opioid dependence [73]. While the transition from opioid use to antagonist medication can be routinely performed in the outpatient setting, it may require hospitalization in older patients with reduced cognitive and physical abilities, and those with current use of multiple prescription medications. Studies in the treatment of chronic pain suggest that the partial opioid agonist buprenorphine may be an optimal choice for patients with renal dysfunction [69], but studies in opiate-dependent older adults have not been conducted.

Particular attention also is required in the care of older opioid-dependent patients receiving agonist substitution therapy and in need of pharmacotherapy for chronic, noncancer pain. Poor adherence to pain treatment guidelines and inappropriate medication choice have been reported with a single physician management model, making for unsafe and costly interventions not only among opioid-dependent patients but also in the general population [74, 75]. A substance abuse treatment programme of integrated medical-psychiatric stepped care has been proposed, tailoring the level of care to the individual patient's needs [75]. It should be noted that, in contrast to common expectations, older opioid-dependent patients can be reliable historians of their co-morbid pain conditions [76] and may be able to actively take part in the treatment process.

Benzodiazepines

Concerns about inappropriate prescribing of benzodiazepines to older adults have been associated with a high risk of developing dependence, even among those who have no personal history of past addiction problems [77]. Persistent pain, depression and isolation can predispose older adults to benzodiazepine use and dependence [78]. Although the elderly can successfully be withdrawn from chronic benzodiazepine use, they are also more likely to return to using within years of discontinuation [79, 80]. Chronic benzodiazepine use can lead to neuropsychiatric and medical morbidity in older individuals that have high likelihood of multiple underlying medical disorders and polypharmacy [81]. Cognitive effects may range from increased forgetfulness, reduced short-term recall and anterograde amnesia [82], to confusion, learning deficits and dementia [83]. Older patients with long-term benzodiazepine use have more than a twofold increased risk of developing dementia [84]. Symptoms such as agitation, anxiety, confusion, delirium and seizures can occur during withdrawal among patients with benzodiazepine dependence [82]. Thus, either acute/chronic benzodiazepine intoxication or withdrawal may complicate medical and psychiatric assessment, as well as clinical management in older adults.

Unlike research in other drug use disorders, benzodiazepine discontinuation studies of prolonged 'therapeutic dose' have been typically conducted in elderly populations. These usually involve patients in general practice or outpatient settings and have been reviewed in detail [85, 86]. Investigations using minimal interventions and graded discontinuation have proven effectiveness [87]. The addition of psychological interventions such as cognitive behavioural therapy to graded discontinuation have shown increased effectiveness compared with gradual dose reduction alone [88] and may be particularly beneficial where there is low awareness of risk and low motivation to discontinue the medication [89] or problematic insomnia [90, 91]. Chronic 'high dose' benzodiazepine taper and discontinuation, as in the case of alcohol and opioids, requires careful medical management of withdrawal symptoms; the threshold for choosing an inpatient setting should be lower in older adults because of safety concerns. These may include not only avoiding acute symptoms such as delirium and seizures, but also preventing long-term neurocognitive impairment. A population-based study (n = 25 140) has shown that a longer and more careful benzodiazepine taper significantly decreases the risk of dementia symptoms onset among individuals aged 45 and older [92].

Sleep complaints are a common reason for sustained benzodiazepine use and relapse in the elderly [93]. However, elderly long-term benzodiazepine users are more likely to report poor sleep quality than age-matched nonusers with insomnia [94]. Satisfaction with benzodiazepine treatment has been found to be low in a population-based study (n = 15 830) and patterns of frequent use were often associated with worsening of symptoms the prescriber intended to treat, such as insomnia and anxiety [95]. Documented cognitive deficits known to be associated with the use of medications with antihistamine, opioid or anticholinergic properties significantly limits the choice of alternative treatments [96]. In particular, a recent study has shown that older adults who take anticholinergics, a category of drugs that includes many types of over-the-counter sleeping pills and antihistamines, for as little as two months are almost twice as likely to develop lasting memory problems [97]. Safety and efficacy of short-acting 'nonbenzodiazepine' hypnotics has been demonstrated for six to twelve months in patients up to 70 years old [98, 99]. However, there are no studies of their use as a substitute for benzodiazepine treatment of insomnia, and their indication is for a short-term treatment. Among other compounds, prolonged release melatonin has been reviewed in 380 older patients aged ≥55 years and found to be an effective substitute for benzodiazepines in the treatment of insomnia in 30–40% of cases [100]. At this point for the treatment of insomnia in older populations, a proper diagnosis to exclude co-morbid conditions associated with insomnia and the adoption of cognitive behavioural measures and rules of sleep hygiene seem the safest and most effective approach [101], as the use of sleep medications can be associated with rapid onset cognitive impairment and complications from physiological dependence.

Other substances of abuse

There is little evidence to inform the treatment of other substance use disorders, such as stimulant and cannabis use disorders, in older adults. In older adults presenting with symptoms of heart failure, stimulant abuse may have an etiologic role [102]. Pulmonary emphysema [103] and pulmonary talcosis [104] have been described in adults aged ≥50 years intravenously injecting methylphenidate. A significant proportion of emergency department admission episodes of transient ischemic attack and stroke (9%) were associated with positive urine for cocaine in urban patients older than 50 years [105]. An interaction between ageing and chronic cocaine use has been reported on psychomotor speed, attention and memory comparing older abusers (ages 51–70) with younger abusers (ages 21–39) and age-matching controls [106]. Cannabis smoking has been associated with increased respiratory symptoms and acute and chronic bronchitis [107]. A review of the history of tobacco and cannabis use in almost 400 users aged ≥40 years, after performing respiratory tests, determined that smoking both tobacco and cannabis synergistically increases the risks of chronic obstructive pulmonary disease [108]. Psychosocial intervention is the gold standard for stimulants and cannabis use [109]. In the treatment of cocaine dependence, older patients tend to remain in treatment longer and benefit from behavioural measures more than younger patients [110, 111]. In the following section, the evidence supporting various pharmacotherapies showing some preliminary efficacy in the treatments of stimulant and cannabis use disorders, albeit untested in older individuals, is summarized.

Stimulants

A review of the efficacy of psychostimulant drugs for treatment of cocaine dependence, including 16 studies in 1345 patients, found the proportion of patients achieving sustained abstinence from cocaine was higher with dextroamphetamine, bupropion and modafinil, but only at a statistical trend of significance [112]. Using dexamphetamine or methylphenidate as 'substitution' therapy in the treatment of amphetamine dependence has been reported as possibly beneficial in small investigations [113] and descriptive studies [114]. In one pilot randomized clinical trial (n = 41), dexamphetamine was as effective as weekly counselling in reducing amphetamine use [115]. One randomized clinical trial (n = 80) reported that naltrexone (50 mg/day) significantly increased the number of amphetamine-negative urines compared with placebo [116]. In a recent randomized study among 100 polydrug dependent patients, naltrexone implants resulted in higher retention and decreased heroin and amphetamine use [117]. Disulfiram has been shown to enhance the subjective effects of amphetamine [118], while reducing the rewarding effects of cocaine independent of alcohol use [119]. A combination of disulfiram and naltrexone was most likely to result in abstinence from alcohol and cocaine than placebo in 208 polyabusers [120]. Randomized clinical trials have failed to show disulfiram efficacy in treating cocaine abuse among methadone treated patients [121] or have reported only a modest improvement [122]. A recent investigation suggests the use of weight-based disulfiram doses to produce more reliable effects on cocaine use [123]. Vaccines for use in the treatment of stimulant dependence are in development: a cocaine vaccine has been studied in methadone-maintained opioid-dependent patients with the aim of reaching high levels of anti-cocaine antibodies to facilitate cocaine inactivation [124]. While only 38% of patients achieved target levels of antibodies (IgG), those subjects had significantly more cocaine-free urines. The blockade was obtained for a relatively short time and further work on the vaccine is required. Along this line, pre-clinical development of methamphetamine vaccines is continuing [125].

Cannabis

Research related to the pharmacological treatment of cannabis use disorders has mainly focused on alleviation of withdrawal symptoms to aid quit attempts [126, 127]. A controlled trial of the serotonin agonist buspirone (n = 50) showed a trend for participants randomized to buspirone who completed treatment to achieve the first negative cannabis urine test result sooner than those participants treated with placebo [128]. Another randomized clinical trial among 156 cannabis-dependent patients using dronabinol, a synthetic form of the active marijuana component delta-9-tetrahydrocannabinol, showed the medication had good tolerability and improved treatment retention and withdrawal symptoms, although its use was not associated with significantly reduced cannabis use compared with placebo [129]. In a recent randomized trial among 116 cannabis-dependent adolescents, participants receiving the over-the-counter supplement N-acetylcysteine, a glutamate modulator, had more than twice the odds, compared with those receiving placebo, of having negative urine cannabinoid test results during treatment [130].

Future areas of focus for stimulant and cannabis use disorders in older adults include further understanding of the courses and patterns of use during an older adult's lifetime, careful characterization of co-morbid neuropsychiatric and medical disorders, and age-specific pharmacological interventions. Cognitive deficits occur with stimulant and cannabis use disorders. Given the importance of preserving cognitive function in older adults, it is important to determine whether pharmacological interventions specific to older adults are safe and can be helpful in preserving cognitive deficits.

Integrated treatments

Older adults have been excluded from landmark treatment studies in substance use disorders, such as Project *MATCH* [131]. In turn, substance use disorders have been an exclusion criterion in large investigations of mental health management among older people, including *Impact* [132]. In other studies of depression treatment among older patients, such as *Pathways* [133] and *Prospect* [134], alcohol or substance use were not exclusion criteria but were not the subject of secondary outcome analyses. While such omissions are often necessary and reasonable for research reasons, this has prevented the field from gaining further knowledge on evidenced-based practices and pharmacological approaches to substance abuse treatment in ageing adults [34].

Several forms of brief advice and intervention for alcohol and drug abuse have shown to be effective and relatively easy to integrate with the primary care treatment of older patients. In a randomized controlled trial (n = 158), project GOAL (Guiding Older Adult Lifestyles) [135], at-risk drinkers age 65 and older who received two 15-minute sessions of brief physician advice were more likely to have fewer drinks and 'binge drinking' episodes after 12 months. The Health Profiles Project [136] provided a similar successful home-based brief intervention to primary care patients. A telephone disease management programme for depression and/or at-risk drinking offering patients several contacts with a behavioural health expert, was more effective than specialist referral in helping reduce drinking at four months (48 vs 20%) [137]. Lack of significant group differences was likely due to a small sample size (n = 97).

The BRITE (Brief Intervention and Treatment for Elders) project conducted screenings among 3497 older adults aged ≥52 years for alcohol, medications, illicit drug use or misuse and depression to address underuse of mental health services in an age cohort [138]. Counsellors performed the initial intervention, often in the home of the participant, and completed a health promotion workbook within one to five sessions using techniques of motivational interviewing. If brief intervention was determined inadequate, counsellors were given discretion to also implement 16 sessions of cognitive behavioural therapy. Referrals to more intensive treatment for serious substance use disorders were made at any time. Individuals were followed 30 days post-discharge. Among those who screened positive for alcohol use (n = 339), there were significant reductions in the proportion of individuals experiencing alcohol problems and symptoms of alcohol dependence (from 80 to 18.9%). In addition, 32% reported reduced prescription medication misuse (n = 187, 67.9% reported no improvement); 95.8% improved on use of over-the-counter medications (n = 24); and 75% improved on illicit drug use (n = 12) [138]. Unfortunately, no comparison between brief intervention and treatment conditions was reported and no 'treatment as usual' group was included. Given the design and the considerable variation in length and type of the intervention, conclusions cannot be drawn about what component of the intervention was instrumental in producing results, including the frequent contact of patients with programme staff.

The Primary Care Research in Substance Abuse and Mental Health for the Elderly (PRISM-E) study, a large scale, real-world study of the effectiveness of integrating mental health and substance abuse treatment for older people into primary care, identified 2022 depressed or anxious patients aged ≥65 years. Among them, 560 also had an alcohol use disorder. Patients were randomized to receive care from mental health providers in primary care settings or from providers in specialty settings. Bartels and colleagues [30] reported that alcohol users from this study who received the integrated intervention were twice as likely to accept and stay in treatment. Although no evidence suggested a superiority of either model of care in reducing drinking, the magnitude of reduction in alcohol use achieved in primary care was comparable with other intervention studies [139]. The implementation of integrated models of treatment in clinical practice has shown their utility in helping control drinking among older adults with alcohol use and co-morbid psychiatric disorders who are referred to community mental health services following alcohol-related hospitalization [140]. In medically ill older alcoholics, integrated medical and substance abuse outpatient interventions have significantly increased both engagement and prolonged abstinence while medical care alone was effective in inducing initial abstinence, but not long-term attendance of alcoholism treatment [141]. In the PRISM-E study, both the integration and referral groups showed significant improvement in depression and symptom reduction. However, for the subgroup with major depression and more significant symptoms, referral to specialty care was associated with a better outcome [142]. For the interpretation of the last finding, it may be useful to specify that the study design let practitioners provide whatever mental health treatment they thought most appropriate, but it did standardize the treatment provided to at-risk drinkers at integrated sites. The researchers trained practitioners at primary care sites to use a proven intervention consisting of three brief, alcohol-related counselling sessions.

Only one randomized trial has used a nonage-specific brief intervention for hazardous drinking in adults of all ages in a primary care setting [143]. Elderly drinkers, as their nonelderly counterparts, significantly decreased use of alcohol and trends were found for brief intervention to be more efficacious than usual treatment; however, of the 180 elderly individuals identified as hazardous drinkers, only 25% agreed to participate [144].

The integration of multiple interventions, including a personalized report, booklet on alcohol and ageing, drinking diary, advice from the primary care provider and telephone counselling from a health educator, did not contribute to significantly reduce the proportions of at-risk or heavy drinkers after one year among 631 older participants aged ≥55 years in the Healthy Living as You Age (HLAYA) randomized controlled study [145]. However, the complex intervention was associated with early (two week) reduction in amount of drinking, lasting up to 12 months [145].

Some forms of brief intervention have focused on the education of primary care physicians about medication prescribing for the elderly. In a randomized, controlled trial among 1624 physicians, 274 agreed to participate [146]. In the group which received by mail confidential profiles of benzodiazepine prescription use coupled with evidence-based educational bulletins, the proportion of prescriptions were not significantly reduced compared with the control group receiving educational bulletins about anti-hypertension drug prescribing for elderly patients. Improvement in participation has been sought in new trials introducing continuing medical education goals, national database comparisons, pharmacies and web-based pharmaceutical treatment algorithms that provide recommended alternative treatment options [147–149].

Other models of educational interventions have been performed through automated programmes for prescribers and patients. Fink and colleagues [150] compared automated tailored educational material for use specifically for older adults aged ≥65 years in primary care. In total, 665 participants were randomized to interventions where both clinicians and their patients received reports of patients' alcohol intake and patients received a personalized education program, compared with only patients receiving the report and education, or a treatment as usual condition. After one year, drinking was significantly reduced in the patient report group and the combined report group compared with the group receiving treatment as usual.

The importance of collecting and sharing information on a broad base has been highlighted by international projects such as VINTAGE [151]. The declared intent is to fill the knowledge gap and build capacity for the management of alcohol problems in the elderly by collecting examples of good practices for prevention and dissemination of findings to treating personnel and policy makers involved in the field of alcohol, ageing and public health in general.

Conclusion and future directions

In spite of the increasing percentage of the US population in the over 50 age group, there is limited evidence to guide the treatment of substance use disorders in older adults. In the absence of adequate information, pharmacological treatment should follow indications offered by the treatment of the general adult population, with appropriate dose adjustments for age-related pharmacokinetic and pharmacodynamic changes and for psychiatric and physical co-morbidities. In particular, there should be a lower threshold for admission to inpatient treatment for alcohol, benzodiazepine and opioid withdrawal in older people. Clinical pharmacology trials should consistently enrol older adults rather than exclude them, so that specific questions, including optimal opioid substitution regimen for opioid dependence, the use of long-acting/slow-release formulations of opioid antagonist and antagonist medications in opioid and alcohol dependence and the long-term outcome after alcohol or opioid detoxification, can be addressed.

There is a need for safety studies as well as efficacy studies to expand pharmacological options. For example, naltrexone has potential in the treatment of a number of substance abuse conditions, alone or in combination with other agents. Disulfiram is being investigated for its ability to reduce alcohol and stimulant use and impulse control disorders [152, 153]. However, safety of the use of disulfiram in older patients is questionable due to potential side effects [154]. For both of these agents, data concerning their use in older individuals are needed.

In addition to combination pharmacotherapies, future research should include exploration of combined treatments, such as use of medications and psychosocial interventions. While evidence on this subject may be mixed in the general adult population, multiple studies suggesting better compliance with either treatment regimen in older drug abuse patients compared to younger ones are promising. Furthermore, combined treatment research contributes to knowledge about treatment decision making, mechanism of action and potential algorithms for treatment-resistant older substance users.

At this point, structured and individualized screening and brief intervention protocols are among the most cost-effective methods to identify and treat older adults who are using alcohol and/or psychoactive medications/drugs. As interaction with older substance abusers increase, practitioners will be in search of convenient treatment options and a successful integration of these strategies into medical care and community services may help ensure current and future adequate management of co-occurring mental and physical health disorders.

Recent comparisons of population-based data sources document increasing rates of help seeking among older drug users in the last decade [8, 155]. While changes may be easily explained at first with ageing of the 'baby boomers', a generation with significant substance use history, the requests for treatment are growing mostly among recent onset or middle aged drug users, suggesting the existence of different profiles and possibly nonhomogeneous clinical needs [8]. The major challenges ahead are to understand these differences and meet the growing clinical need by implementing quality research and providing effective and affordable treatment as efficiently and effectively as possible.

References

1. United States Census Bureau (2008) *National Population Projections 2009*. Department of Commerce, Washington, DC.
2. Falaschetti, E., Malbut, K. and Primatesta, P. (2002) *Health Survey for England 2000: The General Health of Older People and Their Use of Health Services*. The Stationery Office, London.
3. Han, B., Gfroerer, J.C., Colliver, J.D. and Penne, M.A. (2009) Substance use disorder among older adults in the United States in 2020. *Addiction*, **104**(1), 88–96.
4. Blazer, D.G. and Wu, L.-T. (2011) The epidemiology of alcohol use disorders and subthreshold dependence in a middle-aged and elderly community sample. *American Journal of Geriatric Psychiatry*, **19**(8), 685–694.
5. Patterson, T.L. and Jeste, D.V. (1999) The potential impact of the baby-boom generation on substance abuse among elderly persons. *Psychiatric Services*, **50**(9), 1184–1188.
6. Rothrauff, T.C., Abraham, A.J., Bride, B.E. and Roman, P.M. (2011) Substance abuse treatment for older adults in private centers. *Substance abuse: official publication of the Association for Medical Education and Research in Substance Abuse*, **32**(1), 7–15.
7. Lin, J., Karno, M., Grella, C. *et al.* (2011) Alcohol, tobacco, and nonmedical drug use disorders in U.S. Adults aged 65 years and older: data from the 2001–2002 National Epidemiologic Survey of Alcohol and Related Conditions. *American Journal of Geriatric Psychiatry*, **19**(3), 292–299.
8. Wu, L.-T. and Blazer, D.G. (2011) Illicit and nonmedical drug use among older adults: a review. *Journal of Aging and Health*, **23**(3), 481–504.
9. Gfroerer, J., Penne, M., Pemberton, M. and Folsom, R. (2003) Substance abuse treatment need among older adults in 2020: the impact of the aging baby-boom cohort. *Drug and Alcohol Dependence*, **69**(2), 127–135.
10. Mangoni, A.A. and Jackson, S.H. (2004) Age-related changes in pharmacokinetics and pharmacodynamics: basic principles and practical applications. *British Journal of Clinical Pharmacology*, **57**(1), 6–14.
11. Crome, I., Li, T.K., Rao, R. and Wu, L.-T. (2012) Alcohol limits in older people. *Addiction*, **107**(9), 1541–1543.

12. Moos, R.H., Brennan, P.L., Schutte, K.K. and Moos, B.S. (2004) High-risk alcohol consumption and late-life alcohol use problems. *American Journal of Public Health*, 94(11), 1985–1991.

13. Dowling, G., Weiss, S. and Condon, T. (2008) Drugs of abuse and the aging brain. *Neuropsychopharmacology*, 33(2), 209–218.

14. Dreher, J., Meyer-Lindenberg, A., Kohn, P. and Berman, K. (eds) (2008) *Age-Related Changes in Midbrain Dopaminergic Regulation of the Human Reward System*. National Academy of Sciences USA, Washington, DC.

15. Volkow, N., Fowler, J., Wang, G. *et al.* (1994) Decreased dopamine transporters with age in health human subjects. *Annals of Neurology*, 36(2), 237–239.

16. Marschner, A., Mell, T., Wartenburger, I. *et al.* (2005) Reward-based decision-making and aging. *Brain Research Bulletin*, 67(5), 382–390.

17. Wang, G., Volkow, N., Logan, J. *et al.* (1995) Evaluation of age-related changes in serotonin 5-HT2 and dopamine D2 receptor availability in healthy human subjects. *Life Sciences*, 56(14), 249–253.

18. Buck, M., Atreja, A., Brunker, C. *et al.* (2009) Potentially inappropriate medication prescribing in outpatient practices: prevalence and patient characteristics based on electronic health records. *American Journal of Geriatric Pharmacotherapeutics*, 7(2), 84–92.

19. Moy, I., Crome, P. and Crome, I. (2011) Systematic and narrative review of treatment for older people with substance problems. *European Geriatric Medicine*, 2, 212–236.

20. Oslin, D.W., Pettinati, H. and Volpicelli, J.R. (2002) Alcoholism treatment adherence: older age predicts better adherence and drinking outcomes. *The American Journal of Geriatric Psychiatry: official journal of the American Association for Geriatric Psychiatry*, 10(6), 740–747.

21. Satre, D.D., Mertens, J.R., Arean, P.A. and Weisner, C. (2004) Five-year alcohol and drug treatment outcomes of older adults versus middle-aged and younger adults in a managed care program. *Addiction*, 99(10), 1286–1297.

22. Beresford, T. (1995) Alcoholic elderly: Prevalence, screening, diagnosis, and prognosis. In: *Alcohol and Aging* (eds T. Beresford and E. Gomberg). Oxford University Press, New York, pp. 3–18.

23. Substance Abuse and Mental Health Services Administration (1998) *Substance Abuse Among Older Adults*. Center for Substance Abuse Treatment, Substance Abuse and Mental Health Services Administration, Rockville, MD.

24. Gottlieb, S.H. (2004) Measure, don't pour. Alcohol and drug interactions. *Diabetes Forecast*, 57(8), 33–35.

25. McInnes, E. and Powell, J. (1994) Drug and alcohol referrals: are elderly substance abuse diagnoses and referrals being missed? *British Medical Journal*, 308(6926), 444–446.

26. Simoni-Wastila, L. and Yang, H.K. (2006) Psychoactive drug abuse in older adults. *The American Journal of Geriatric Pharmacotherapy*, 4(4), 380–394.

27. Schonfeld, L., Dupree, L. and Rohrer, G. (1995) Age-specific differences between younger and older alcohol abusers. *Journal of Clinical Geropsychology*, 1, 219–227.

28. Jimenez, D.E., Bartels, S.J., Cardenas, V. and Alegria, M. (2013) Stigmatizing attitudes toward mental illness among racial/ethnic older adults in primary care. *International Journal of Geriatric Psychiatry*, 28(10):1061–1068.

29. Wolff, J.L. and Roter, D.L. (2011) Family presence in routine medical visits: a meta-analytical review. *Social Science Medicine*, 72(6), 823–831.

30. Bartels, S.J., Coakley, E.H., Zubritsky, C. *et al.* (2004) Improving access to geriatric mental health services: a randomized trial comparing treatment engagement with integrated versus enhanced referral care for depression, anxiety, and at-risk alcohol use. *The American Journal of Psychiatry*, 161(8), 1455–1462.

31. Blow, F., Walton, M., Chermack, S. *et al.* (2000) Older adult treatment outcome following elder-specific inpatient alcoholism treatment. *Journal of Substance Abuse Treatment*, **19**(1), 67–75.

32. Kashner, T.M., Rodell, D.E., Ogden, S.R. *et al.* (1992) Outcomes and costs of two VA inpatient treatment programs for older alcoholic patients. *Hospital & Community Psychiatry*, **43**(10), 985–989.

33. Kofoed, L.L., Tolson, R.L., Atkinson, R.M. *et al.* (1987) Treatment compliance of older alcoholics: an elder-specific approach is superior to "mainstreaming". *Journal of Studies on Alcohol*, **48**(1), 47–51.

34. Kuerbis, A. and Sacco, P. (2013) A review of existing treatments for substance abuse among the elderly and recommendations for future directions. *Substance Abuse: Research and Treatment*, **7**, 13–37.

35. Schmucker, D. and Vesel, E. (2002) Are the elderly underrepresented in clinical drug trials. *Journal of Clinical Pharmacology*, **162**(15), 1682–1698.

36. Abdullah, A.S. and Simon, J.L. (2006) Health promotion in older adults: evidence-based smoking cessation programs for use in primary care settings. *Geriatrics*, **61**(3), 30–34.

37. Steinberg, M.B., Akincigil, A., Delnevo, C.D. *et al.* (2006) Gender and age disparities for smoking-cessation treatment. *American Journal of Preventive Medicine*, **30**(5), 405–412.

38. Orleans, C.T., Resch, N., Noll, E. *et al.* (1994) Use of transdermal nicotine in a state-level prescription plan for the elderly. A first look at 'real-world' patch users. *JAMA: the journal of the American Medical Association*, **271**(8), 601–607.

39. Miller, N., Frieden, T.R., Liu, S.Y. *et al.* (2005) Effectiveness of a large-scale distribution programme of free nicotine patches: a prospective evaluation. *Lancet*, **365**(9474), 1849–1854.

40. Hall, S.M., Humfleet, G.L., Munoz, R.F. *et al.* (2009) Extended treatment of older cigarette smokers. *Addiction*, **104**(6), 1043–1052.

41. Joseph, A.M., Norman, S.M., Ferry, L.H. *et al.* (1996) The safety of transdermal nicotine as an aid to smoking cessation in patients with cardiac disease. *The New England Journal of Medicine*, **335**(24), 1792–1798.

42. Tzivoni, D., Keren, A., Meyler, S. *et al.* (1998) Cardiovascular safety of transdermal nicotine patches in patients with coronary artery disease who try to quit smoking. *Cardiovascular Drugs and Therapy / sponsored by the International Society of Cardiovascular Pharmacotherapy*, **12**(3), 239–244.

43. Sweet, R.A., Pollock, B.G., Kirshner, M. *et al.* (1995) Pharmacokinetics of single- and multiple-dose bupropion in elderly patients with depression. *Journal of Clinical Pharmacology*, **35**(9), 876–884.

44. Faessel, H.M., Obach, R.S., Rollema, H. *et al.* (2010) A review of the clinical pharmacokinetics and pharmacodynamics of varenicline for smoking cessation. *Clinical Pharmacokinetics*, **49**(12), 799–816.

45. NICE (2011) *Alcohol Dependence and Harmful Alcohol Use*. NICE (National Institute for Health and Clinical Excellence), London.

46. Brower, K.J., Mudd, S., Blow, F.C. *et al.* (1994) Severity and treatment of alcohol withdrawal in elderly versus younger patients. *Alcoholism, Clinical and Experimental Research*, **18**(1), 196–201.

47. Caputo, F., Vignoli, T., Leggio, L. *et al.* (2012) Alcohol use disorders in the elderly: a brief overview from epidemiology to treatment options. *Experimental Gerontology*, **47**(6), 411–416.

48. Wetterling, T., Driessen, M., Kanitz, R.D. and Junghanns, K. (2001) The severity of alcohol withdrawal is not age dependent. *Alcohol and Alcoholism*, **36**(1), 75–78.

49. Wojnar, M., Wasilewski, D., Zmigrodzka, I. and Grobel, I. (2001) Age-related differences in the course of alcohol withdrawal in hospitalized patients. *Alcohol and Alcoholism*, **36**(6), 577–583.

50. Mayo-Smith, M.F., Beecher, L.H., Fischer, T.L. *et al.* (2004) Management of alcohol withdrawal delirium. An evidence-based practice guideline. *Archives of Internal Medicine*, **164**(13), 1405–1412.

51. Ntais, C., Pakos, E., Kyzas, P. and Ioannidis, J.P. (2005) Benzodiazepines for alcohol withdrawal. *Cochrane Database of Systematic Reviews* 3 (Art. No.: CD005063). doi: 10.1002/14651858.CD005063.pub3.

52. Dufour, M. and Fuller, R.K. (1995) Alcohol in the elderly. *Annual Reviews in Medicine*, **46**, 123–132.

53. Dunne, F.J. (1994) Misuse of alcohol or drugs by elderly people. *British Medical Journal*, **308**(6929), 608–609.

54. Barrick, C. and Connors, G.J. (2002) Relapse prevention and maintaining abstinence in older adults with alcohol-use disorders. *Drugs & Aging*, **19**(8), 583–594.

55. Zimberg, S. (2005) Alcoholism and substance abuse in older adults. In: *Clinical Textbook of Addictive Disorders* (eds R. Frances, S. Miller and A. Mack), 3rd edn. Guilford, New York, pp. 396–410.

56. Oslin, D., Liberto, J.G., O'Brien, J. and Krois, S. (1997) Tolerability of naltrexone in treating older, alcohol-dependent patients. *The American Journal on Addictions / American Academy of Psychiatrists in Alcoholism and Addictions*, **6**(3), 266–270.

57. Devanand, D.P. (2002) Comorbid psychiatric disorders in late life depression. *Biological Psychiatry*, **52**(3), 236–242.

58. Oslin, D.W., Katz, I.R., Edell, W.S. and Ten Have, T.R. (2000) Effects of alcohol consumption on the treatment of depression among elderly patients. *The American Journal of Geriatric Psychiatry: official journal of the American Association for Geriatric Psychiatry*, **8**(3), 215–220.

59. Oslin, D.W. (2005) Treatment of late-life depression complicated by alcohol dependence. *The American Journal of Geriatric Psychiatry: official journal of the American Association for Geriatric Psychiatry*, **13**(6), 491–500.

60. Gopalakrishnan, R., Ross, J., O'Brien, C. and Oslin, D. (2009) Course of late-life depression with alcoholism following combination therapy. *Journal of Studies on Alcohol and Drugs*, **70**(2), 237–241.

61. Pettinati, H.M., Oslin, D.W., Kampman, K.M. *et al.* (2010) A double-blind, placebo-controlled trial combining sertraline and naltrexone for treating co-occurring depression and alcohol dependence. *The American Journal of Psychiatry*, **167**(6), 668–675.

62. Pettinati, H.M., O'Brien, C.P. and Dundon, W.D. (2013) Current status of co-occurring mood and substance use disorders: a new therapeutic target. *The American Journal of Psychiatry*, **170**(1), 23–30.

63. Brennan, P.L., Schutte, K.K., SooHoo, S. and Moos, R.H. (2011) Painful medical conditions and alcohol use: a prospective study among older adults. *Pain Medicine*, **12**(7), 1049–1059.

64. Fareed, A., Casarella, J., Amar, R. *et al.* (2009) Benefits of retention in methadone maintenance and chronic medical conditions as risk factors for premature death among older heroin addicts. *Journal of Psychiatric Practice*, **15**(3), 227–234.

65. Rajaratnam, R., Sivesind, D., Todman, M. *et al.* (2009) The aging methadone maintenance patient: treatment adjustment, long-term success, and quality of life. *Journal of Opioid Management*, **5**(1), 27–37.

66. Firoz, S. and Carlson, G. (2004) Characteristics and treatment outcome of older methadone-maintenance patients. *The American Journal of Geriatric Psychiatry: official journal of the American Association for Geriatric Psychiatry*, **12**(5), 539–541.

67. Lofwall, M.R., Brooner, R.K., Bigelow, G.E. *et al.* (2005) Characteristics of older opioid maintenance patients. *Journal of Substance Abuse Treatmen,* **28**(3), 265–272.
68. Dursteler-MacFarland, K.M., Vogel, M., Wiesbeck, G.A. and Petitjean, S.A. (2011) There is no age limit for methadone: a retrospective cohort study. *Substance Abuse Treatment, Prevention, and Policy,* **6**, 9.
69. Pergolizzi, J., Boger, R.H., Budd, K. *et al.* (2008) Opioids and the management of chronic severe pain in the elderly: consensus statement of an International Expert Panel with focus on the six clinically most often used World Health Organization Step III opioids (buprenorphine, fentanyl, hydromorphone, methadone, morphine, oxycodone). *Pain Practice: the official journal of World Institute of Pain,* **8**(4), 287–313.
70. van Ojik, A., Jansen, P., Brouwers, J. and van Roon, E. (2012) Treatment of chronic pain in older people: evidence-based choice of strong-acting opioids. *Drugs & Aging,* **29**(8), 615–625.
71. Blackwell, S., Montgomery, M., Waldo, D. *et al.* (2003) National study of medications associated with injury in elderly Medicare/Medicaid dual enrollees during 2003. *Journal of the American Pharmaceutical Association,* **49**(6), 751–759.
72. Mannelli, P., Peindl, K. and Wu, L.-T. (2011) Pharmacological enhancement of naltrexone treatment of opioid dependence: a review. *Substance Abuse and Rehabilitation,* **2011**(2), 113–123.
73. Sigmon, S.C., Bisaga, A., Nunes, E.V. *et al.* (2012) Opioid detoxification and naltrexone induction strategies: recommendations for clinical practice. *The American Journal of Drug and Alcohol Abuse,* **38**(3), 187–199.
74. Cicero, T.J., Wong, G., Tian, Y. *et al.* (2009) Co-morbidity and utilization of medical services by pain patients receiving opioid medications: data from an insurance claims database. *Pain,* **144**(1–2), 20–27.
75. Clark, M.R., Stoller, K.B. and Brooner, R.K. (2008) Assessment and management of chronic pain in individuals seeking treatment for opioid dependence disorder. *Canadian Journal of Psychiatry/Revue Canadienne de Psychiatrie,* **53**(8), 496–508.
76. Barry, D.T., Beitel, M., Garnet, B. *et al.* (2009) Relations among psychopathology, substance use, and physical pain experiences in methadone-maintained patients. *The Journal of Clinical Psychiatry,* **70**(9), 1213–1218.
77. Pinsker, H. and Suljaga-Petchel, K. (1984) Use of benzodiazepines in primary-care geriatric patients. *Journal of the American Geriatrics Society,* **32**(8), 595–597.
78. Madhusoodanan, S. and Bogunovic, O.J. (2004) Safety of benzodiazepines in the geriatric population. *Expert Opinion on Drug Safety,* **3**(5), 485–493.
79. Rickels, K., Case, W.G., Schweizer, E. *et al.* (1991) Long-term benzodiazepine users 3 years after participation in a discontinuation program. *The American Journal of Psychiatry,* **148**(6), 757–761.
80. Schweizer, E., Case, W.G. and Rickels, K. (1989) Benzodiazepine dependence and withdrawal in elderly patients. *The American Journal of Psychiatry,* **146**(4), 529–531.
81. Ballentine, N.H. (2008) Polypharmacy in the elderly: maximizing benefit, minimizing harm. *Critical Care Nursing Quarterly,* **31**(1), 40–45.
82. Bogunovic, O.J. and Greenfield, S.F. (2004) Practical geriatrics: Use of benzodiazepines among elderly patients. *Psychiatric Services,* **55**(3), 233–235.
83. Caplan, J.P., Epstein, L.A., Quinn, D.K. *et al.* (2007) Neuropsychiatric effects of prescription drug abuse. *Neuropsychology Review,* **17**(3), 363–380.
84. Chen, P.L., Lee, W.J., Sun, W.Z. *et al.* (2012) Risk of dementia in patients with insomnia and long-term use of hypnotics: a population-based retrospective cohort study. *PloS One,* **7**(11), e49113.

85. Oude Voshaar, R., Couvée, J., Van Balkom, A. *et al.* (2006a) Strategies for discontinuing long-term benzodiazepine use: meta-analysis. *British Journal of Psychiatry*, **189**, 213–220.
86. Parr, J.M., Kavanagh, D.J., Cahill, L. *et al.* (2009) Effectiveness of current treatment approaches for benzodiazepine discontinuation: a meta-analysis. *Addiction*, **104**(1), 13–24.
87. Belanger, L., Morin, C.M., Bastien, C. and Ladouceur, R. (2005) Self-efficacy and compliance with benzodiazepine taper in older adults with chronic insomnia. *Health Psychology: official journal of the Division of Health Psychology, American Psychological Association*, **24**(3), 281–287.
88. Oude Voshaar, R.C., Krabbe, P.F., Gorgels, W.J. *et al.* (2006b) Tapering off benzodiazepines in long-term users: an economic evaluation. *PharmacoEconomics*, **24**(7), 683–694.
89. Cook, J.M., Biyanova, T., Thompson, R. and Coyne, J.C. (2007) Older primary care patients' willingness to consider discontinuation of chronic benzodiazepines. *General Hospital Psychiatry*, **29**(5), 396–401.
90. Baillargeon, L., Landreville, P., Verreault, R. *et al.* (2003) Discontinuation of benzodiazepines among older insomniac adults treated with cognitive-behavioural therapy combined with gradual tapering: a randomized trial. *CMAJ: Canadian Medical Association Journal/journal de l'Association Medicale Canadienne*, **169**(10), 1015–1020.
91. Morin, C.M., Bastien, C., Guay, B. *et al.* (2004) Randomized clinical trial of supervised tapering and cognitive behavior therapy to facilitate benzodiazepine discontinuation in older adults with chronic insomnia. *The American Journal of Psychiatry*, **161**(2), 332–342.
92. Wu, C.S., Ting, T.T., Wang, S.C. *et al.* (2011) Effect of benzodiazepine discontinuation on dementia risk. *American Journal of Geriatric Psychiatry*, **19**(2), 151–159.
93. Stowell, K.R., Chang, C.C., Bilt, J. *et al.* (2008) Sustained benzodiazepine use in a community sample of older adults. *Journal of the American Geriatrics Society*, **56**(12), 2285–2291.
94. Beland, S.G., Preville, M., Dubois, M.F. *et al.* (2011) The association between length of benzodiazepine use and sleep quality in older population. *International Journal of Geriatric Psychiatry*, **26**(9), 908–915.
95. Nordfjaern, T. (2013) Prospective associations between benzodiazepine use and later life satisfaction, somatic pain and psychological health among the elderly. *Human Psychopharmacology*, **28**(3), 248–257.
96. Tannenbaum, C., Paquette, A., Hilmer, S. *et al.* (2012) A systematic review of amnestic and non-amnestic mild cognitive impairment induced by anticholinergic, antihistamine, GABAergic and opioid drugs. *Drugs & Aging*, **29**(8), 639–658.
97. Cai, X., Campbell, N. and Khan, B. (2013) Long-term anticholinergic use and the aging brain. *Alzheimer's & Dementia*, **9**(4), 377–385.
98. Ancoli-Israel, S., Richardson, G.S., Mangano, R.M. *et al.* (2005) Long-term use of sedative hypnotics in older patients with insomnia. *Sleep Medicine*, **6**(2), 107–113.
99. McCrae, C.S., Ross, A., Stripling, A. and Dautovich, N.D. (2007) Eszopiclone for late-life insomnia. *Clinical Interventions in Aging*, **2**(3), 313–326.
100. Kunz, D., Bineau, S., Maman, K. *et al.* (2012) Benzodiazepine discontinuation with prolonged-release melatonin: hints from a German longitudinal prescription database. *Expert Opinion on Pharmacotherapy*, **13**(1), 9–16.
101. Neikrug, A.B. and Ancoli-Israel, S. (2010) Sleep disorders in the older adult – a mini-review. *Gerontology*, **56**(2), 181–189.
102. Freedland, K.E. and Carney, R.M. (2000) Psychosocial considerations in elderly patients with heart failure. *Clinics in Geriatric Medicine*, **16**(3), 649–661.

103. Stern, E.J., Frank, M.S., Schmutz, J.F. *et al.* (1994) Panlobular pulmonary emphysema caused by i.v. injection of methylphenidate (Ritalin): findings on chest radiographs and CT scans. *American Journal of Roentgenology,* 162(3), 555–560.

104. Ward, S., Heyneman, L.E., Reittner, P. *et al.* (2000) Talcosis associated with IV abuse of oral medications: CT findings. *American Journal of Roentgenology.* 174(3), 789–793.

105. Silver, B., Miller, D., Jankowski, M. *et al.* (2013) Urine toxicology screening in an urban stroke and TIA population. *Neurology,* 80(18), 1702–1709.

106. Kalapatapu, R.K., Vadhan, N.P., Rubin, E. *et al.* (2011) A pilot study of neurocognitive function in older and younger cocaine abusers and controls. *The American Journal on Addictions / American Academy of Psychiatrists in Alcoholism and Addictions,* 20(3), 228–239.

107. Underner, M., Urban, T., Perriot, J. *et al.* (2013) [Cannabis use and impairment of respiratory function]. *Revue des maladies respiratoires,* 30(4), 272–285.

108. Tan, W.C., Lo, C., Jong, A. *et al.* (2009) Marijuana and chronic obstructive lung disease: a population-based study. *CMAJ: Canadian Medical Association Journal /journal de l'Association Medicale Canadienne,* 180(8), 814–820.

109. Dutra, L., Stathopoulou, G., Basden, S.L. *et al.* (2008) A meta-analytic review of psychosocial interventions for substance use disorders. *The American Journal of Psychiatry,* 165(2), 179–187.

110. Weiss, L. and Petry, N.M. (2013) Older methadone patients achieve greater durations of cocaine abstinence with contingency management than younger patients. *American Journal of Addiction,* 22(2), 119–126.

111. Weiss, L.M. and Petry, N.M. (2011) Interaction effects of age and contingency management treatments in cocaine-dependent outpatients. *Experimental and Clinical Psychopharmacology,* 19(2), 173–181.

112. Castells, X., Casas, M., Perez-Mana, C. *et al.* (2010) Efficacy of psychostimulant drugs for cocaine dependence. *Cochrane Database of Systematic Reviews* 2 (Art. No.: CD007380). doi: 10.1002/14651858.CD007380.pub3.

113. Elkashef, A., Vocci, F., Hanson, G. *et al.* (2008) Pharmacotherapy of methamphetamine addiction: an update. *Substance Abuse: official publication of the Association for Medical Education and Research in Substance Abuse,* 29(3), 31–49.

114. Lingford-Hughes, A.R., Welch, S. and Nutt, D.J. (2004) Evidence-based guidelines for the pharmacological management of substance misuse, addiction and comorbidity: recommendations from the British Association for Psychopharmacology. *Journal of Psychopharmacology,* 18(3), 293–335.

115. Shearer, J., Wodak, A., Mattick, R.P. *et al.* (2001) Pilot randomized controlled study of dexamphetamine substitution for amphetamine dependence. *Addiction,* 96(9), 1289–1296.

116. Jayaram-Lindstrom, N., Hammarberg, A., Beck, O. and Franck, J. (2008) Naltrexone for the treatment of amphetamine dependence: a randomized, placebo-controlled trial. *The American Journal of Psychiatry,* 165(11), 1442–1448.

117. Tiihonen, J., Krupitsky, E., Verbitskaya, E. *et al.* (2012) Naltrexone implant for the treatment of polydrug dependence: a randomized controlled trial. *The American Journal of Psychiatry,* 169(5), 531–536.

118. Sofuoglu, M., Poling, J., Waters, A. *et al.* (2008) Disulfiram enhances subjective effects of dextroamphetamine in humans. *Pharmacology, Biochemistry, and Behavior,* 90(3), 394–398.

119. Baker, J.R., Jatlow, P. and McCance-Katz, E.F. (2007) Disulfiram effects on responses to intravenous cocaine administration. *Drug and Alcohol Dependence,* 87(2–3), 202–209.

120. Pettinati, H.M., Kampman, K.M., Lynch, K.G. *et al.* (2008) A double blind, placebo-controlled trial that combines disulfiram and naltrexone for treating co-occurring cocaine and alcohol dependence. *Addictive Behaviors*, **33**(5), 651–667.

121. Oliveto, A., Poling, J., Mancino, M.J. *et al.* (2011) Randomized, double blind, placebo-controlled trial of disulfiram for the treatment of cocaine dependence in methadone-stabilized patients. *Drug and Alcohol Dependence*, **113**(2–3), 184–191.

122. Carroll, K.M., Nich, C., Shi, J.M. *et al.* (2012) Efficacy of disulfiram and Twelve Step Facilitation in cocaine-dependent individuals maintained on methadone: a randomized placebo-controlled trial. *Drug and Alcohol Dependence*, **126**(1–2), 224–231.

123. Haile, C.N., De La Garza, R., 2nd, Mahoney, J.J., 3rd, *et al.* (2012) The impact of disulfiram treatment on the reinforcing effects of cocaine: a randomized clinical trial. *PloS One*, **7**(11), e47702.

124. Martell, B.A., Orson, F.M., Poling, J. *et al.* (2009) Cocaine vaccine for the treatment of cocaine dependence in methadone-maintained patients: a randomized, double-blind, placebo-controlled efficacy trial. *Archives of General Psychiatry*, **66**(10), 1116–1123.

125. Kosten, T., Domingo, C., Orson, F. and Kinsey, B. (2013) Vaccines against stimulants: Cocaine and Methamphetamine. *British Journal of Clinical Pharmacology*, **77**(2), 368–374.

126. Budney, A.J., Hughes, J.R., Moore, B.A. and Vandrey, R. (2004) Review of the validity and significance of cannabis withdrawal syndrome. *The American Journal of Psychiatry*, **161**(11), 1967–1977.

127. Hart, C.L. (2005) Increasing treatment options for cannabis dependence: a review of potential pharmacotherapies. *Drug and Alcohol Dependence*, **80**(2), 147–159.

128. McRae-Clark, A.L., Carter, R.E., Killeen, T.K. *et al.* (2009) A placebo-controlled trial of buspirone for the treatment of marijuana dependence. *Drug and Alcohol Dependence*, **105**(1–2), 132–138.

129. Levin, F.R., Mariani, J.J., Brooks, D.J. *et al.* (2011) Dronabinol for the treatment of cannabis dependence: a randomized, double-blind, placebo-controlled trial. *Drug and Alcohol Dependence*, **116**(1–3), 142–150.

130. Gray, K.M., Carpenter, M.J., Baker, N.L. *et al.* (2012) A double-blind randomized controlled trial of N-acetylcysteine in cannabis-dependent adolescents. *The American Journal of Psychiatry*, **169**(8), 805–812.

131. Project MATCH Research Group (1997) Project MATCH secondary a priori hypotheses. *Addiction*, **92**(12), 1671–1698.

132. Unutzer, J., Katon, W., Callahan, C.M. *et al.* (2002) Collaborative care management of late-life depression in the primary care setting: a randomized controlled trial. *JAMA: the journal of the American Medical Association*, **288**(22), 2836–2845.

133. Katon, W.J., Von Korff, M., Lin, E.H. *et al.* (2004) The Pathways Study: a randomized trial of collaborative care in patients with diabetes and depression. *Archives of General Psychiatry*, **61**(10), 1042–1049.

134. Bruce, M.L., Ten Have, T.R. and Reynolds, C.F., 3rd, *et al.* (2004) Reducing suicidal ideation and depressive symptoms in depressed older primary care patients: a randomized controlled trial. *JAMA: the journal of the American Medical Association*, **291**(9), 1081–1091.

135. Fleming, M.F., Manwell, L.B., Barry, K.L. *et al.* (1999) Brief physician advice for alcohol problems in older adults: a randomized community-based trial. *The Journal of Family Practice*, **48**(5), 378–384.

136. Blow, F.C. and Barry, K.L. (2000) Older patients with at-risk and problem drinking patterns: new developments in brief interventions. *Journal of Geriatric Psychiatry and Neurology*, **13**(3), 115–123.

137. Oslin, D.W., Sayers, S., Ross, J. *et al.* (2003) Disease management for depression and at-risk drinking via telephone in an older population of veterans. *Psychosomatic Medicine*, 65(6), 931–937.

138. Schonfeld, L., King-Kallimanis, B.L., Duchene, D.M. *et al.* (2010) Screening and brief intervention for substance misuse among older adults: the Florida BRITE project. *American Journal of Public Health*, 100(1), 108–114.

139. Oslin, D.W., Grantham, S., Coakley, E. *et al.* (2006) PRISM-E: comparison of integrated care and enhanced specialty referral in managing at-risk alcohol use. *Psychiatric Services,* 57(7), 954–958.

140. Rao, R. (2013) Outcomes from liaison psychiatry referrals for older people with alcohol use disorders in the UK. *Mental Health and Substance Use*, 6(4), 1–7.

141. Willenbring, M.L. and Olson, D.H. (1999) A randomized trial of integrated outpatient treatment for medically ill alcoholic men. *Archives of Internal Medicine*, 159(16), 1946–1952.

142. Krahn, D.D., Bartels, S.J., Coakley, E. *et al.* (2006) PRISM-E: comparison of integrated care and enhanced specialty referral models in depression outcomes. *Psychiatric Services,* 57(7), 946–953.

143. Maisto, S.A., Conigliaro, J., McNeil, M. *et al.* (2001) Effects of two types of brief intervention and readiness to change on alcohol use in hazardous drinkers. *Journal of Studies on Alcohol*, 62(5), 605–614.

144. Gordon, A.J., Conigliaro, J., Maisto, S.A. *et al.* (2003) Comparison of consumption effects of brief interventions for hazardous drinking elderly. *Substance Use & Misuse*, 38(8), 1017–1035.

145. Moore, A.A., Blow, F.C., Hoffing, M. *et al.* (2011) Primary care-based intervention to reduce at-risk drinking in older adults: a randomized controlled trial. *Addiction,* 106(1), 111–120.

146. Pimlott, N.J., Hux, J.E., Wilson, L.M. *et al.* (2003) Educating physicians to reduce benzodiazepine use by elderly patients: a randomized controlled trial. *CMAJ: Canadian Medical Association Journal/journal de l'Association Medicale Canadienne*, 168(7), 835–839.

147. Clyne, B., Bradley, M.C., Smith, S.M. *et al.* (2013) Effectiveness of medicines review with web-based pharmaceutical treatment algorithms in reducing potentially inappropriate prescribing in older people in primary care: a cluster randomized trial (OPTI-SCRIPT study protocol). *Trials*, 14, 72.

148. Martin, P., Tamblyn, R., Ahmed, S. and Tannenbaum, C. (2013) An educational intervention to reduce the use of potentially inappropriate medications among older adults (EMPOWER study): protocol for a cluster randomized trial. *Trials*, 14, 80.

149. Straand, J., Fetveit, A., Rognstad, S. *et al.* (2006) A cluster-randomized educational intervention to reduce inappropriate prescription patterns for elderly patients in general practice – The Prescription Peer Academic Detailing (Rx-PAD) study [NCT00281450]. *BMC Health Services Research*, 6, 72.

150. Fink, A., Elliott, M.N., Tsai, M. and Beck, J.C. (2005) An evaluation of an intervention to assist primary care physicians in screening and educating older patients who use alcohol. *Journal of the American Geriatrics Society*, 53(11), 1937–1943.

151. Galluzzo, L., Scafato, E., Martire, S. *et al.* (2012) Alcohol and older people. The European project VINTAGE: good health into older age. Design, methods and major results. *Annali dell'Istituto Superiore di Sanita'*, 48(3), 221–231.

152. Mutschler, J. and Kiefer, F. (2013) [Mechanism of action of disulfiram and treatment optimization in prevention of recurrent alcoholism]. *Praxis*, 102(3), 139–146.

153. Suh, J.J., Pettinati, H.M., Kampman, K.M. and O'Brien, C.P. (2006) The status of disulfiram: a half of a century later. *Journal of Clinical Psychopharmacology*, 26(3), 290–302.

154. Huffman, J.C. and Stern, T.A. (2003) Disulfiram use in an elderly man with alcoholism and heart disease: a discussion. *Primary Care Companion to the Journal of Clinical Psychiatry*, 5(1), 41–44.
155. Sacco, P., Kuerbis, A., Goge, N. and Bucholz, K. (2013) Help seeking for drug and alcohol problems among adults age 50 and older: A comparison of the NLAES and NESARC surveys. *Drug and Alcohol Dependence*, **131**(1–2), 157–161.

Chapter 21

THE ASSESSMENT AND PREVENTION OF POTENTIALLY INAPPROPRIATE PRESCRIBING

Denis O'Mahony

Department of Medicine (Geriatrics), University College Cork, Ireland

Introduction

Inappropriate prescribing (IP) is generally defined as [1]:

 (i) prescribing of drugs that are potentially dangerous in terms of heightened risk of adverse drug reactions (ADRs) and adverse drug events (ADEs);
 (ii) prescribing of drugs that are ineffective for the patient's condition;
 (iii) prescribing of drugs that are excessively costly;
 (iv) prescribing of drugs for too long or too short a time period;
 (v) prescribing without a clear indication; or
 (vi) failure to prescribe appropriate medication despite a clear indication for that medication and the absence of a contraindication.

Prescription of potentially inappropriate medications (PIMs) is a prevalent public health problem that affects older people globally. A PIM is a drug whose prescription carries a risk of an adverse event that outweighs its clinical benefit, particularly when there is evidence in favour of a safer or more effective alternative therapy for the same condition. PIMs are identified in 13–21% of people aged over 65 in primary care, 25–50% of acutely ill older people in hospital and in 37–60% of frailer older people in the nursing home care setting [2]. Inappropriate prescribing is an added burden on the expanding population of frailer older people worldwide and is also a major drain on healthcare resources. For these reasons, researchers in recent years have examined various ways of defining, detecting and preventing PIMs in older people.

Substance Use and Older People, First Edition.
Edited by Ilana B. Crome, Li-Tzy Wu, Rahul (Tony) Rao and Peter Crome.
© 2015 John Wiley & Sons, Ltd. Published 2015 by John Wiley & Sons, Ltd.

Inappropriate psychotropic use in elderly patients

Psychiatric medications are often prescribed inappropriately in older people. A recent study by Hamilton *et al.* [3] examining the prevalence rate of IP in 600 older people at the point of admission to hospital for treatment of acute unselected illness, noted prescription of potentially inappropriate benzodiazepines in 56 patients with recurrent falls (9.3%), long half-life benzodiazepines in 48 patients (8%), opioids in 18 patients (3%) and neuroleptic antipsychotics in 16 patients (2.7%). Given the abuse potential of benzodiazepines and opioids in particular, these data indicate that inappropriate prescribing practices probably contribute not only to abuse of these medication classes but also physical morbidity as well, particularly in the form of falls and injuries. Older people taking daily psychotropic medication experience a consistent and significant increased risk of falls and injury [4]. Thus, in the case of older fallers, physicians should make specific inquiry about overt and surreptitious use of any psychotropic medication, whether or not it is specifically prescribed for the patient, as there may be undetected abuse of psychotropics underlying recurrent falls. There is evidence that withdrawal of inappropriate psychotropic medications reduces the risk of falls [5, 6].

Recent studies indicate that IP is commonly found among older people with dementia. Montastruc *et al.* [7] have shown that almost 47% of older French patients with Alzheimer's disease receive one or more PIMs. The most commonly prescribed PIMs were cerebral vasodilators, drugs with anticholinergic effects and long half-life benzodiazepines. Gustafsson *et al.* [8] recently found that almost one-third of older people with dementia living in special care dementia units in Sweden were prescribed antipsychotic drugs. In only 39% of cases were the antipsychotics prescribed according to national guidelines. Manthey *et al.* [9] have shown that inappropriate use of prescription benzodiazepines is independently associated with old age and chronic illness. A recent German study by Berger *et al.* [10] has shown that inappropriate medication (Beers criteria) was detected in 40% of older people with generalized anxiety disorder; mostly these were psychotropics, particularly benzodiazepines.

Alcohol abuse is underrecognized in older people and generally causes more physical harm than in younger people [11]. Alcohol abuse combined with IP is a particularly toxic mixture for older people. Both conditions compound physical ailments, may worsen nutritional status and exacerbate the ill-effects of the other disorder. Alcohol abuse is also associated with medication use errors by the patient, adding to the burden of drug-related problems of older people. In the United States, Phillips *et al.* [12] have found a marked increase in mortality from fatal medication errors combined with alcohol and/or illicit drug abuse in the period 1983–2004. Liver disease resulting from alcohol abuse increases the risk of adverse drug reactions of medications that are metabolized by the liver. Abrupt withdrawal of alcohol or benzodiazepines after long-term abuse by older people is just as likely to result in withdrawal syndromes as in younger people. However, in older people, alcohol withdrawal syndromes tend to be more severe [13, 14] and are more likely to be misdiagnosed as acute confusional states caused by other disorders, in particular in those older people with multiple chronic disorders. Undiagnosed alcohol withdrawal presents a risk of Wernicke/Korsakoff syndrome in older alcohol abusers in whom diagnosis may be delayed unless the diagnosis is considered in the context of detectable alcohol abuse. Alcohol abuse should always be considered in cases of acute confusion in older people where the cause is not clear-cut.

Although there is a greater problem with underuse of opioids for moderate to severe pain in older people [15], there is increasing recognition of inappropriate use and abuse of opioids in many older patients in recent years [16]. Recent analysis of opioid abuse in the Unites States indicates that the majority of people who abuse opioids take prescription opioids rather than illicit opioids, although the problem is proportionately much greater in younger people than in older people [17].

Implicit IP criteria

The salient point about IP criteria is to what extent it is possible to:

- detect common instances of IP;
- improve medication appropriateness;
- prevent ADRs and ADEs.

Broadly speaking, there are two types of IP criteria, that is implicit criteria and explicit criteria. Implicit criteria are based on clinical judgement and usually refer to quality indicators of prescribing that a doctor or a pharmacist can apply to any prescription. Because implicit IP criteria are not specific to any particular disease or drug, they require knowledge of pharmacotherapy in the person applying them. The best known set of implicit IP criteria is the Medication Appropriateness Index (MAI), developed by Hanlon and colleagues and first published in 1992 [18]. The MAI considers:

- drug indication;
- drug effectiveness for the indicated condition;
- correctness of drug dose;
- correctness of directions of drug administration;
- practicality of drug taking directions;
- drug–drug interactions;
- drug–disease interactions;
- duplication with other drugs;
- duration of drug therapy;
- drug cost (compared to alternative drugs of equal utility).

The MAI can be operationalized with a weighted score range of 0 to 18 for each drug. At the present time, it is the only implicit IP assessment tool in the literature designed specifically to assess and measure medication appropriateness from the viewpoint of implicit IP criteria. The MAI is often used alongside the Assessment of

Underutilization of Medication (AUM) tool, which provides a means of measuring inappropriate underuse of medication in individual cases [19]. To apply the AUM, one must have a detailed list of the patient's medical conditions and current medications, as well as knowledge of drug indications. In essence, the AUM poses the fundamental question: Is an indicated drug omitted without a valid reason in this case? ACOVE (Assessing Care Of Vulnerable Elders) provides another set of medication underuse criteria described in the literature [20, 21]. However, ACOVE underuse criteria have not found their way into routine clinical usage.

Explicit IP criteria

Explicit IP criteria are essentially criteria-based and spell out very specifically certain drugs/drug classes to be avoided in particular situations in order to avoid drug–disease and drug–drug adverse interactions. An example is the prescription of diazepam in an older person with a history of recurrent nonsyncopal falls due to osteoarthritis of the hips and knees; in this case, diazepam is likely to increase the risk of falls further and is, therefore, likely to be inappropriate. There are several sets of explicit IP criteria in the literature. These have recently been reviewed in detail by O'Connor *et al.* [22]. Beers criteria are the most cited explicit IP criteria in the literature to date. They were first published in 1991 [23] and have undergone three further iterations since then, most recently in 2012 [24–26].

A recent review by Levy *et al.* [27] examined the various sets of explicit IP criteria published since 2003, when the third iteration of Beers criteria appeared in the literature. This review examined Beers criteria, the French Consensus Panel list [28], STOPP (Screening Tool of Older Persons' Prescription) and START (Screening Tool to Alert doctors to Right Treatment) [29], the Australian Prescribing Indicators tool [30] and the Norwegian General Practice (NORGEP) Criteria [31]. The reviewers concluded that 'although no criteria may ever be globally applicable, STOPP and START make significant advances'. Another recent review by Corsonello *et al.* [32] commented that STOPP/START criteria had greater ability to predict ADRs and to prevent potentially inappropriate prescribing compared to Beers criteria.

This endorsement of STOPP/START criteria over Beers criteria is largely based on a study by Hamilton *et al.* [33], which showed that PIMs were significantly associated with incident ADEs in a prospective study of 600 elderly patients at the point of hospital admission with acute illness, whilst Beers criteria (2003 iteration) showed no significant association with identified ADEs. In the same study, patients who were prescribed one or more STOPP criteria PIMs were 2.54 times more likely to experience an ADE compared to patients who were not taking STOPP criteria PIMs. This was an important finding, since the lack of significant association between incident ADEs in older patients and Beers criteria PIMs in the hospital setting concurred with two larger scale previous studies that also found no significant association between 2003 Beers criteria PIMs and ADRs [34, 35]. At the time of writing this chapter, it is uncertain whether the recently updated fourth iteration of Beers criteria [26] has surmounted this lack of association with ADRs seen in the 2003 version of the criteria. This is a very important consideration for any set of IP criteria designed for older people, since the prime purpose of all IP criteria is to identify PIMs *in order to prevent ADRs and ADEs*. Any set of explicit IP criteria that does not display this fundamental characteristic is unlikely to be of value in the routine clinical setting.

The full set of STOPP/START criteria was first published in 2008, following Delphi consensus validation by a group of 18 Irish experts [36]; STOPP and START criteria are listed in Boxes 21.1 and 21.2. STOPP (Screening Tool of Older Persons' Prescriptions) criteria have been applied in a variety of clinical settings and compared directly to Beers criteria (2003 version). These studies show high rates of PIMs, increasing in prevalence from primary care to the acute hospital to the nursing home setting (Table 21.1) [2]. Similarly, potential prescribing omissions (PPOs) according to START (Screening Tool to Alert doctors to Right Treatment) criteria are also highly prevalent in these clinical settings (Table 21.2) [2].

Applying STOPP/START criteria as an intervention

Following the initial PIM and PPO prevalence studies showing high rates of potential IP in various clinical settings, STOPP/START criteria were further evaluated as potentially useful clinical interventions in the hospital setting, applied to acutely ill older patients. Gallagher *et al.* performed a single-centre randomized controlled trial (RCT) in 400 hospitalized acutely ill elderly patients, half of whom had their medications screened using STOPP/START criteria at a single time point within 24 hours of their admission; the other patients received 'standard' pharmaceutical care [37]. The primary outcome measure was medication appropriateness, as measured by MAI and AUM. The study showed highly significant improvements in group mean MAI and AUM scores within the index hospital admission, which were sustained to the end of the follow-up period of six months post-discharge (Figures 21.1a and 21.1b).

After this RCT had demonstrated the powerful effect of STOPP/START on medication appropriateness, a further single-centre RCT has examined the effect of STOPP/START criteria on incident ADRs in older people hospitalized with acute unselected illness. O'Connor *et al.* [38] have recently completed a single-centre RCT in which 732 acutely ill elderly patients admitted to hospital were randomized to either (a) screening of their medication using STOPP/START criteria with identified PIMs and PPOs signalled to their attending doctors or (b) 'standard' pharmaceutical care. Patients were excluded from the trial if they were admitted directly to the psychiatric department or the intensive therapy unit, had attended a geriatrician or a clinical pharmacologist in the previous 12 months, were considered terminally ill or had an expected hospital stay of less than 48 hours. The details of co-morbid illnesses, co-morbidity burden using the Charlson Comorbidity Index, functional status using the Barthel Index, concurrent medications and doses, serum biochemistry profile (including estimated GFR) and cognitive status were recorded in each patient. Within 48 hours of admission, STOPP/START criteria were applied to

Box 21.1 STOPP (Screening Tool of Older Persons' Prescriptions) criteria

The following drug prescriptions are potentially inappropriate in persons aged ≥65 years of age [36].

A. *Cardiovascular system*
  1. Digoxin at a long-term dose >125 µg/day with impaired renal function.*
  2. Loop diuretic for dependent ankle oedema only, that is no clinical signs of heart failure.
  3. Loop diuretic as first-line monotherapy for hypertension.
  4. Thiazide diuretic with a history of gout.
  5. Noncardioselective beta blocker with Chronic Obstructive Pulmonary Disease (COPD).
  6. Beta-blocker in combination with verapamil.
  7. Use of diltiazem or verapamil with NYHA Class III or IV heart failure.
  8. Calcium channel blockers with chronic constipation.
  9. Use of aspirin and warfarin in combination without histamine H2 receptor antagonist (except cimetidine because of interaction with warfarin) or proton pump inhibitor (PPI).
  10. Dipyridamole as monotherapy for cardiovascular secondary prevention.
  11. Aspirin with a past history of peptic ulcer disease without histamine H2 receptor antagonist or proton pump inhibitor.
  12. Aspirin at dose >150 mg day.
  13. Aspirin with no history of coronary, cerebral or peripheral vascular symptoms or occlusive event.
  14. Aspirin to treat dizziness not clearly attributable to cerebrovascular disease.
  15. Warfarin for first, uncomplicated deep venous thrombosis for >6 months.
  16. Warfarin for first uncomplicated pulmonary embolus for >12 months.
  17. Aspirin, clopidogrel, dipyridamole or warfarin with concurrent bleeding disorder.

B. *Central nervous system and psychotropic drugs*
  1. Tricyclic antidepressants (TCA's) with dementia.
  2. TCA's with glaucoma.
  3. TCA's with cardiac conductive abnormalities.
  4. TCA's with constipation.
  5. TCA's with an opiate or calcium channel blocker.
  6. TCA's with prostatism or prior history of urinary retention.
  7. Long-term (i.e. >1 month), long-acting benzodiazepines, for example chlordiazepoxide, flurazepam, nitrazepam, chlorazepate and benzodiazepines with long-acting metabolites (e.g. diazepam).
  8. Long-term (i.e. >1 month) neuroleptics as long-term hypnotics.

9. Long-term neuroleptics in those with Parkinsonism.
10. Phenothiazines in patients with epilepsy.
11. Anticholinergics to treat extra-pyramidal side effects of neuroleptic medications.
12. Selective serotonin re-uptake inhibitors (SSRI's) with a history of clinically significant hyponatraemia.
13. Prolonged use (>1week) of first generation antihistamines, that is diphenydramine, cyclizine, chlorpheniramine, promethazine.

C. *Gastrointestinal system*
1. Diphenoxylate, loperamide or codeine phosphate for treatment of diarrhoea of unknown cause.
2. Diphenoxylate, loperamide or codeine phosphate for treatment of severe infective gastroenteritis, that is bloody diarrhoea, high fever or severe systemic toxicity.
3. Prochlorperazine (Stemetil) or metoclopramide with Parkinsonism.
4. PPI for peptic ulcer disease at full therapeutic dosage for > 8weeks.
5. Anticholinergic antispasmodic drugs with chronic constipation.

D. *Respiratory system*
1. Theophylline as monotherapy for COPD.
2. Systemic corticosteroids instead of inhaled corticosteroids for maintenance therapy in moderate–severe COPD.
3. Nebulised ipratropium with glaucoma.

E. *Musculoskeletal system*
1. Nonsteroidal anti-inflammatory drug (NSAID) with history of peptic ulcer disease or GI bleeding, unless with concurrent H2 receptor antagonist, PPI or misoprostol.
2. NSAID with moderate–severe hypertension.
3. NSAID with heart failure.
4. Long-term use of NSAID (>3months) for symptom relief of mild osteoarthtitis.
5. Warfarin and NSAID together.
6. NSAID with chronic renal failure.*
7. Long-term corticosteroids (>3months) as monotherapy for rheumatoid arthritis or osteoarthritis.
8. Long-term NSAID or colchicine for chronic treatment of gout where no contraindication to allopurinol.

F. *Urogenital system*
1. Bladder antimuscarinic drugs with dementia.
2. Antimuscarinic drugs with chronic glaucoma.
3. Antimuscarinic drugs with chronic constipation.

4. Antimuscarinic drugs with chronic prostatism.
5. Alpha blockers in males with frequent incontinence.
6. Alpha blockers with long-term urinary catheter.

G. *Endocrine system*
1. Glibenclamide or chlorpropamide with type 2 diabetes mellitus (DM).
2. Beta blockers in those with DM and frequent hypoglycaemic episodes.
3. Oestrogens with a history of breast cancer or venous thromboembolism.
4. Oestrogens without progestogen in patients with intact uterus.

H. *Drugs that adversely affect those prone to falls*
1. Benzodiazepines.
2. Neuroleptic drugs.
3. First generation antihistamines.
4. Vasodilator drugs with persistent postural hypotension.
5. Long-term opiates.

I. *Analgesic drugs*
1. Use of long-term powerful opiates, for example morphine or fentanyl, as first line therapy for mild–moderate pain.
2. Regular opiates for >2 weeks in those with chronic constipation without concurrent laxative.
3. Long-term opiates in those with dementia unless indicted for palliative care or management of moderate/severe chronic pain syndrome.

J. *Duplicate drug classes*
1. Any duplicate drug class prescription, for example concurrent opiates, NSAID's, SSRI's, loop diuretics, ACE inhibitors.

*eGFR <50 ml/min/1.73 m^2.

Box 21.2 START (Screening Tool to Alert to Right Treatment) criteria

These medications should be considered for people ≥65 years of age with the following conditions, where no contraindication to prescription exists [36].

A. *Cardiovascular system*
1. Warfarin in the presence of chronic atrial fibrillation.
2. Aspirin in the presence of chronic atrial fibrillation, where warfarin is contraindicated but not aspirin.
3. Aspirin or clopidogrel with a history of atherosclerotic coronary, cerebral or peripheral vascular disease in patients with sinus rhythm.
4. Antihypertensive therapy where systolic blood pressure is consistently >160 mmHg.

5. Statin therapy with a history of coronary, cerebral or peripheral vascular disease, where functional status remains independent for activities of daily living and life expectancy is >5 years.
6. Angiotensin Converting Enzyme (ACE) inhibitor with chronic heart failure.
7. ACE inhibitor following acute myocardial infarction.
8. Beta blocker with chronic stable angina.

B. *Respiratory system*
1. Regular inhaled beta 2 agonist or anticholinergic for mild to moderate asthma or COPD.
2. Regular inhaled corticosteroid for moderate-severe asthma or COPD, where predicted FEV1 < 50%.
3. Home continuous oxygen with documented chronic type 1 respiratory failure or type 2 respiratory failure.

C. *Central nervous system*
1. L-DOPA in idiopathic Parkinson's disease with functional impairment and disability.
2. Antidepressant with moderate–severe depressive symptoms.

D. *Gastrointestinal system*
1. Proton pump inhibitor with severe Gastro-Oesophageal Reflux Disease or peptic stricture requiring dilatation.
2. Fibre supplement for chronic, symptomatic diverticular disease with constipation.

E. *Musculoskeletal system*
1. Disease-modifying anti-rheumatic drug (DMARD) with active rheumatoid disease lasting >12 weeks.
2. Bisphosphonates in patients taking maintenance corticosteroid therapy.
3. Calcium/Vitamin D supplement in patients with osteoporosis (fragility fracture, dorsal kyphosis).

F. *Endocrine system*
1. Metformin with type 2 diabetes +/– metabolic syndrome (in the absence of renal impairment*).
2. ACE inhibitor or ARB in diabetes with nephropathy, that is proteinuria or micoralbuminuria +/– renal impairment.*
3. Antiplatelet therapy in diabetes mellitus with co-existing cardiovascular risk factors.
4. Statin therapy in diabetes mellitus if co-existing major cardiovascular risk factors present.

*eGFR <50 ml/min/1.73 m^2.

Table 21.1 Prevalence rates of potentially inappropriate medications (PIMs) in older patient groups in various clinical settings according to STOPP criteria and Beers [2]

Setting	PIM rate (STOPP criteria) (%)	PIM rate (Beers criteria*) (%)
Primary care	21	12–20
Hospital	35	14–66
Nursing home	60	37

*Third iteration

Table 21.2 Prevalence rates of potential prescribing omissions (PPOs) in older patient groups in various clinical settings [2]

Setting	PPO rate (START criteria) (%)
Primary care	23
Hospital	44–59
Nursing home	42–60

(a)

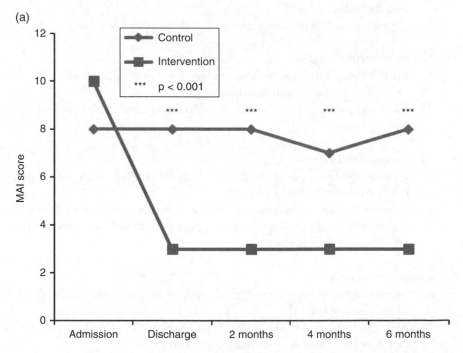

Figure 21.1a Effect of application of STOPP criteria within 48 hours of acute hospital admission (intervention) on medication appropriateness (MAI score) in older patients compared to normal pharmaceutical care (control). The highly significant improvement in group mean MAI score in the intervention group was rapid and was maintained to the end of a six-month follow-up interval (medication appropriateness improves as MAI score decreases) [37].

(b)

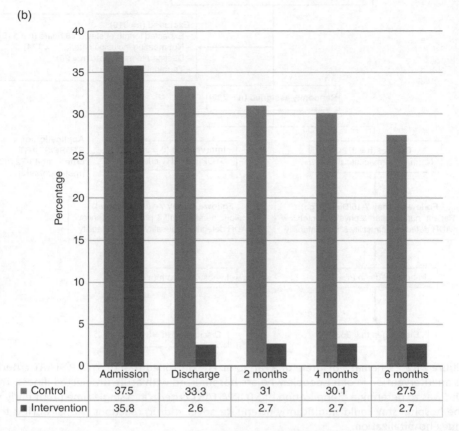

	Admission	Discharge	2 months	4 months	6 months
■ Control	37.5	33.3	31	30.1	27.5
■ Intervention	35.8	2.6	2.7	2.7	2.7

Figure 21.1b Effect of application of START criteria shortly after hospital admission in acutely ill older people. Over one-third of patients had at least one potential prescribing omission according to Assessment of Underutilization of Medication (AUM) criteria. After application of START criteria, the inappropriate underutilization of medication rate in the intervention group fell to under 3%; this beneficial effect was maintained to the end of six-months' follow-up [37].

the intervention patients' (n = 360) medications. Details of identified PIMs and PPOs were presented to a member of the attending medical team, reinforced by direct discussion with the primary researcher. The primary outcome measure was incident nontrivial ADRs during the index hospital stay. Ascertainment of ADRs took place between day 7 and day 10 or at discharge, whichever came first. The RCT profile is summarized in Figure 21.2. The results of the RCT are illustrated in Table 21.3. These show an ADR incidence of 23.9% in the control group compared to 12.5% in the intervention group, that is an absolute risk reduction in ADRs of 11.4%. The number of patients needed to treat with STOPP/START criteria to prevent one non-trivial ADR during hospitalization with acute illness was 9. No other set of IP criteria used an intervention has shown a comparable level of ADR risk reduction. For this reason, STOPP/START criteria may be considered more clinically relevant than Beers criteria and the other sets of IP criteria referred to above.

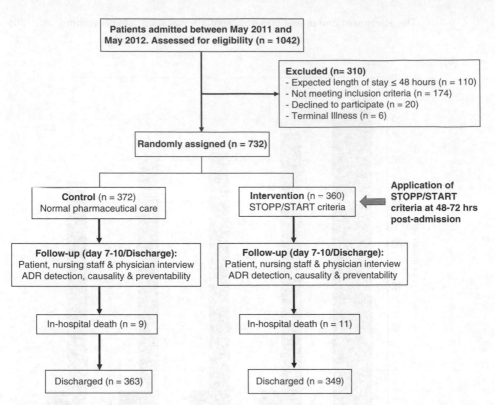

Figure 21.2 Schematic diagram of a randomized controlled trial of STOPP/START criteria as an intervention in older people who are hospitalized with acute unselected illness. The aim was to determine if application of STOPP/START criteria at a single time point early in the hospital stay could significantly attenuate adverse drug reactions (ADRs) during the index hospitalization.

Table 21.3 Results of a randomized controlled trial (Figure 21.2) comparing the adverse drug reaction (ADR) rates in older people with acute illness receiving either standard pharmaceutical care (control) or adjustment of their medication according to STOPP/START criteria advice offered to their attending doctors at a single time point early in the index hospitalization (intervention) [38]

Study Arm	Number (%) of patients with at least one instance of IP according to STOPP/START criteria at randomization	Number (%) of ADRs attributable to medications listed in STOPP/START criteria	Number (%) of ADRs *not* attributable to medications listed in STOPP/START	Total number of ADRs
Control (n = 372)	158 (42.5%)	51 (57%)	38 (43%)	89
Intervention (n = 360)	176 (48.9%)	15 (33%)	30 (66%)	45

The ADR rate in the control group was 23.9% compared to 12.5% (p<0.0001), representing an absolute ADR risk reduction of 11.4% and a number needed to treat of 9 after statistical adjustment for number of drugs, PIMs, renal failure, liver disease, heart failure, age, dementia and falls.

In relation to older patients with psychiatric morbidity, there are several instances where STOPP criteria are relevant (Box 21.1). These include the potential adverse drug–disease interactions between adverse tricyclic antidepressants (TCAs) and dementia, glaucoma, cardiac conductive abnormalities, chronic constipation, prostatism and prior history of urinary retention [39]. Long-term (i.e. >1 month), long-acting benzodiazepines, for example chlordiazepoxide, flurazepam, nitrazepam, chlorazepate, and benzodiazepines with long-acting metabolites such as diazepam may also be detrimental in susceptible older people, such as those prone to falls and fractures [40]. Long-term neuroleptics, particularly high-potency neuroleptics such as haloperidol, in older patients with Parkinsonism are particularly detrimental in terms of mobility and falls risk [41]. Neuroleptic antipsychotics that can lower seizure threshold are potentially dangerous in older patients with cerebrovascular epilepsy [42]. Anticholinergics, which are often used to counteract extra-pyramidal side effects of neuroleptic drugs, carry a higher risk of drug-induced morbidity in patients with dementia or cognitive impairment, by worsening cognitive function [43]. Selective serotonin re-uptake inhibitors, which are now the most commonly prescribed antidepressant class worldwide, may cause or exacerbate hyponatraemia and should, therefore, be avoided or used with great caution in patients with a history of clinically significant hyponatraemia [44].

There is evidence that older nursing home residents are overprescribed antidepressants [45]. Similarly, there is evidence of overprescribing of psychotropic drugs in older residents of dementia units. One recent large-scale study found psychotropic prescription therapy in 85% of patients [46]. A recent study in Geneva detected PIMs in 77% of a cohort of older patients with known chronic psychiatric morbidity admitted to an acute geriatric unit; in the same cohort, PPOs were detected in 65% of patients [47]. In the same study, living in institutional care was an independent predictor of PIMs and PPOs.

Other methods of detection and prevention of IP in older people

A number of other methods for detection and prevention of IP have been described, including Comprehensive Geriatric Assessment, medication use review, prescriber education/audit/feedback and computerized order entry with clinical decision support.

Comprehensive Geriatric Assessment (CGA)

The overall clinical and functional benefits of CGA have been well documented for many years [48, 49]. CGA encompasses careful medication review and optimization. A number of controlled clinical trials have shown improved prescribing appropriateness as a result of CGA-based assessment and optimization of pharmacotherapy. Crotty *et al.* showed that CGA applied to nursing home residents at two time points, that is six weeks and 12 weeks post-randomization, led to significant improvement in mean MAI score compared to control patients who did not receive CGA [50]. Schmader *et al.* also showed highly significant improvement in mean MAI score in intervention patients versus control patients in the outpatient setting [51]. Strandberg *et al.* found significant improvement in uptake of evidence-based pharmacotherapy aimed at cardiovascular prevention in patients aged over 75 as a result of a CGA-type intervention [52]. However, none of these three studies showed clinical benefit in terms of ADR prevention or enhanced survival. Also, CGA is limited in its widespread applicability because it is relatively expensive and time consuming.

Pharmacist review and intervention

A structured medication review by a trained pharmacist is another way of minimizing IP in older people. Spinewine *et al.* [53] have developed a pharmaceutical care pathway for older hospitalized patients that encompasses pharmacist review of medication from admission to discharge, participation by the pharmacist in routine ward rounds with feedback and discussion with attending doctors and formulation of detailed pharmaceutical care for each patient, which is discussed in detail with the patient and/carer prior to discharge. Almost 88% of prescription changes recommended by the pharmacist in the system were accepted by the prescribing physicians and 84% of treatment changes were still in place three months after hospital discharge. Although tested by randomized clinical trial, it was a single centre study with a relatively small number of patients (n = 109).

Medication Use Review (MUR) has been in common practice in the United Kingdom for over 10 years, since it was included in the National Service Framework for Older People in 2001 [54]. MUR involves a consultation with a clinical pharmacist in the community, detailed medication review, identification of potential and actual drug-related problems and feedback to the patient or carer. Regrettably, there are no published randomized trials involving MUR as an intervention to establish its efficacy in terms of medication appropriateness or ADR incidence.

Prescriber education, audit and feedback

Several studies of prescriber education interventions show efficacy in relation to improved prescribing quality of specific drug classes, such as antibiotics, analgesics and psychotropics. Studies involving multimorbid older people taking multiple medications are, however, lacking. One recent randomized controlled study by Trivalle *et al.* [55] showed that a structured education programme for staff in a cluster of geriatric rehabilitation units in Paris significantly reduced the rate of adverse drug events. However, this was an open-label, single centre trial involving less than 600 patients; the findings, whilst encouraging, have not been replicated elsewhere.

Computerized provider order entry with clinical decision support

There is conflicting evidence regarding the benefit of computerized provider order entry with clinical decision support (CPOE/CDS) in terms of IP prevention. Application of CPOE/CDS is based on the consistent observation that prescribing errors are more likely as new drugs are initiated and at points of transition of care (e.g. admission and discharge from hospital([56]. A systematic review in 2003 concluded that use of CPOE/CDS can improve prescribing behaviour and reduce medication error rates, although most studies had insufficient statistical power to detect differences in adverse drug event occurrence in patients whose medications were subjected to CPOE/CDS compared to standard pharmaceutical care [57]. A more recent cluster-randomized controlled clinical trial of CPOE/CDS in over 1100 nursing home residents in the USA concluded that CPOE/CDS as an intervention did not reduce the adverse drug event rate or preventable adverse drug event rate in the long-term care setting [58].

Conclusions

Inappropriate prescribing (IP) is prevalent in the general elderly population, in particular among frailer older people with multimorbid chronic illness and associated polypharmacy [22]. This is particularly problematic if, for example, there are associated pain, sleep, behavioural or anxiety problems for which older people are concurrently taking opioid analgesics, antipsychotics or sedative hypnotics. This may result in misuse or abuse of these medications, and/or interactions with other prescription drugs, leading to acute and chronic adverse effects and other health problems. The intoxicating effects of tranquillizing drugs and opioids in combination may heighten the risk of falls and injury. Concurrent alcohol abuse is likely to heighten this risk. There is also clear evidence that IP is common among older residents of long-term care facilities, where overuse of neuroleptic tranquillizers has been well documented [59, 60]. Older people with chronic psychiatric morbidity are at greater risk of IP compared to other older people and early and consistent review of these patients by a physician and a psychiatrist can greatly reduce the rate of IP [61]. When defined by STOPP/START criteria, IP is clearly and significantly associated with ADRs and ADEs; the relationship between Beers IP criteria and ADRs/ADEs is less clear. Recent evidence indicates that application of STOPP/START criteria and structured pharmacist review of medication facilitated by clinical decision support software represent two viable interventions for attenuation of IP and related hospital-acquired ADRs in older hospitalized patients with acute illness, although these findings have not yet been replicated in other centres. Comprehensive geriatric assessment (CGA), expert pharmacist medication review and prescriber education, audit and feedback may also reduce the rate of ADRs/ADEs in older people in hospital, although cost may be a limiting factor. The evidence for effective optimization of older people's medication appropriateness and ADR/ADE prevention through routine medication use review (MUR) and scrutiny with computerized provider order entry with clinical decision support (CPOE/CDS) systems is lacking.

There is a distinct lack of high quality research-based data on the prevalence and nature of IP among older substance abusers which needs to be addressed. As regards IP prevention, future research must focus on more sophisticated and more user-friendly software systems designed to detect and correct inappropriate prescribing in older people, particularly frailer, sicker patients with chronic multimorbid illness, patients with alcohol dependency and patients who are on long-term psychotropics, particularly benzodiazepines. Closer collaboration between physicians, pharmacists and those involved in treating people with substance problems will also be necessary for more effective IP prevention. In particular, there is an increasingly obvious need for more clinical pharmacists who are highly trained and specialized in geriatric pharmacotherapy.

References

1. Gallagher, P. and O'Mahony, D. (2008) Inappropriate prescribing in older people. *Rev Clin Gerontol*, **18**, 1–12.
2. O'Mahony, D., Gallagher, P., Ryan, C. *et al.* (2010) STOPP & START criteria: a new approach to detecting potentially inappropriate prescribing in old age. *Eur Geriatr Med*, **1**, 45–51.
3. Hamilton, H., Gallagher, P., Ryan, C. *et al.* (2011) Potentially inappropriate medications defined by STOPP criteria and the risk of adverse drug events in older hospitalized patients. *Arch Intern Med*, **171**(11), 1013–1019.
4. Lord, S.R., Sherrington, C. and Menz, H.B. (2001) *Falls in Older People. Risk factors and strategies for prevention.* Cambridge University Press, pp. 112–113.
5. Campbell, A.J., Robertson, M.C., Gardner, M.M. *et al.* (1999) Psychotropic medication withdrawal and a home-based exercise program to prevent falls: a randomized, controlled trial. *J Am Geriatr Soc*, **47**(7), 850–853.
6. Leipzig, R.M., Cumming, R.G. and Tinetti, M.E. (1999) Drugs and falls in older people: a systematic review and meta-analysis: I. Psychotropic drugs. *J Am Geriatr Soc*, **47**(1), 30–39.
7. Montastruc, F., Gardette, V., Cantet, C. *et al.* (2013) Potentially inappropriate medication use among patients with Alzheimer disease in the REAL.FR cohort: be aware of atropinic and benzodiazepine drugs! *Eur J Clin Pharmacol*, **69**(8), 1589–1597.
8. Gustafsson, M., Karlsson, S., Gustafson, Y. and Lövheim, H. (2013) Psychotropic drug use among people with dementia – a six-month follow-up study. *BMC Pharmacol Toxicol*, **14**(1), 56.
9. Manthey, L., van Veen, T., Giltay, E.J. *et al.* (2011) Correlates of (inappropriate) benzodiazepine use: the Netherlands Study of Depression and Anxiety (NESDA). *Br J Clin Pharmacol*, **71**(2), 263–172.
10. Berger, A., Mychaskiw, M., Dukes, E. *et al.* (2009) Magnitude of potentially inappropriate prescribing in Germany among older patients with generalized anxiety disorder. *BMC Geriatr*, **9**, 31. doi: 10.1186/1471-2318-9-31.
11. Katona, C.L.E., Watkin, V. and Livingston, G. (2003) Functional psychiatric illness in old age. In: *Brocklehurst's Textbook of Geriatric Medicine and Gerontology*, 6th edn (eds R.C. Tallis and H.M. Fillit). Churchill Livingstone, pp. 847–848.

12. Phillips, D.P., Barker, G.E. and Eguchi, M..M. (2008) A steep increase in domestic fatal medication errors with use of alcohol and/or street drugs. *Arch Intern Med*, **168**(14), 1561–1566.

13. Brower, K.J., Mudd, S., Blow, F.C. *et al.* (1994) Severity and treatment of alcohol withdrawal in elderly versus younger patients. *Alcohol Clin Exp Res*, **18**(1), 196–201.

14. Liskow, B.I., Rinck, C., Campbell, J. and DeSouza, C. (1989) Alcohol withdrawal in the elderly. *J Stud Alcohol*, **50**(5), 414–421.

15. Auret, K. and Schug, S.A. (2005) Underutilisation of opioids in elderly patients with chronic pain: approaches to correcting the problem. *Drugs Aging*, **22**(8), 641–654.

16. Crome I. (2008) Pain and addiction. In: *Pain and Older People* (eds P. Crome, C.J. Main and F. Lally). Oxford University Press, Oxford, pp. 89–108.

17. Manchikanti, L., Helm, S., 2nd, Fellows, B. *et al.* (2012) Opioid epidemic in the United States. *Pain Physician*, **15**(3 Suppl), E39–38.

18. Hanlon, J.T., Schmader, K.E., Samsa, G.P. *et al.* (1992) A method for assessing drug therapy appropriateness. *J Clin Epidemiol*, **45**(10), 1045–1051.

19. Jeffry, S., Ruby, C.M., Twersky, J. *et al.* (1999) Effect of an inter-disciplinary team on suboptimal prescribing in a long-term care facility. *Consult Pharm*, **14**, 957–963.

20. Wenger, N.S. and Shekelle, P.G. (2001) Assessing care of vulnerable elders: ACOVE project overview. *Ann Intern Med*, **135**, 642–646.

21. Shekelle, P.G., MacLean, C.H., Morton, S.C. and Wenger, N.S. (2001) Assessing care of vulnerable elders: methods for developing quality indicators. *Ann Intern Med*, **135**: 647–652.

22. O'Connor, M.N., Gallagher, P. and O'Mahony, D. (2012) Inappropriate prescribing: criteria, detection and prevention. *Drugs Aging*, **29**(6), 437–452.

23. Beers, M.H., Ouslander, J.G., Rollingher, I. *et al.* (1991) Explicit criteria for determining inappropriate medication use in nursing home residents. UCLA Division of Geriatric Medicine. *Arch Intern Med*, **151**(9), 1825–1832.

24. Beers, M.H. (1997) Explicit criteria for determining potentially inappropriate medication use by the elderly. An update. *Arch Intern Med*, **157**(14), 1531–1536.

25. Fick, D.M., Cooper, J.W., Wade, W.E. *et al.* (2003) Updating the Beers criteria for potentially inappropriate medication use in older adults: results of a US consensus panel of experts. *Arch Intern Med*, **163**(22), 2716–2724; Erratum in **164**(3), 298.

26. American Geriatrics Society 2012 Beers Criteria Update Expert Panel (2012) American Geriatrics Society updated Beers Criteria for potentially inappropriate medication use in older adults. *J Am Geriatr Soc, 2012; **60**(4), 616–361.

27. Levy, H.B., Marcus, E.L. and Christen, C. (2010) Beyond the Beers criteria: A comparative overview of explicit criteria. *Ann Pharmacother*, **44**(12), 1968–1975.

28. Laroche, M.L., Charmes, J.P. and Merle, L. (2007) Potentially inappropriate medications in the elderly: a French consensus panel list. *Eur J Clin Pharmacol*, **63**(8), 725–731.

29. Barry, P.J., Gallagher, P., Ryan, C. and O'Mahony, D. (2007) START (screening tool to alert doctors to the right treatment) – an evidence-based screening tool to detect prescribing omissions in elderly patients. *Age Ageing*, **36**(6), 632–638.

30. Basger, B.J., Chen, T.F. and Moles, R.J. (2008) Inappropriate medication use and prescribing indicators in elderly Australians: development of a prescribing indicators tool. *Drugs Aging*, **25**(9), 777–793.

31. Rognstad, S., Brekke, M., Fetveit, A. *et al.* (2009) The Norwegian General Practice (NORGEP) criteria for assessing potentially inappropriate prescriptions to elderly patients. A modified Delphi study. *Scand J Prim Health Care*, **27**(3), 153–159.

32. Corsonello, A., Onder, G., Abbatecola, A.M. *et al.* (2012) Explicit criteria for potentially inappropriate medications to reduce the risk of adverse drug reactions in elderly people: from Beers to STOPP/START criteria. *Drug Saf*, **35**(Suppl 1), 21–28.

33. Hamilton, H., Gallagher, P., Ryan, C. *et al.* (2011) Potentially inappropriate medications defined by STOPP criteria and the risk of adverse drug events in older hospitalized patients. *Arch Intern Med*, **171**(11), 1013–1019.

34. Onder, G., Landi, F., Liperoti, R. *et al.* (2005) Impact of inappropriate drug use among hospitalized older adults, *Eur J Clin Pharmacol*, **61**(5–6), 453–459.

35. Laroche, M.L., Charmes, J.P., Nouaille, Y. *et al.* (2007) Is inappropriate medication use a major cause of adverse drug reactions in the elderly? *Br J Clin Pharmacol*, **63**(2), 177–186.

36. Gallagher, P., Ryan, C., Byrne, S. *et al.* (2008) STOPP (Screening Tool of Older Person's Prescriptions) and START (Screening Tool to Alert doctors to Right Treatment). Consensus validation. *Int J Clin Pharmacol Ther*, **46**(2), 72–83.

37. Gallagher, P.F., O'Connor, M.N. and O'Mahony, D. (2011) Prevention of potentially inappropriate prescribing for elderly patients: a randomized controlled trial using STOPP/START criteria. *Clin Pharmacol Ther*, **89**(6), 845–854.

38. O'Connor, M.N., O'Sullivan, D., Gallagher, P. *et al.* (2012) Prospective application of Screening Tool of Older Persons' Prescriptions/Screening Tool to Alert to Right Treatment criteria and its effects on Adverse Drug Events in Hospitalised Older People: a randomised controlled trial. *Eur Geriatr Med*, **3**(Suppl 1), S132.

39. Mintzer, J. and Burns, A. (2000) Anticholinergic side-effects of drugs in elderly people. *J R Soc Med*, **93**, 457–462.

40. Madhusoodanan, S. and Bogunovic, O.J. (2004) Safety of benzodiazepines in the geriatric population. *Expert Opin Drug Saf*, **3**(5), 485–493.

41. Mena, M.A. and de Yébenes, J.G. (2006) Drug-induced parkinsonism. *Expert Opin Drug Saf*, **5**(6), 759–771.

42. Alexopoulos, G.S., Streim, J., Carpenter, D. *et al.* (2004) Using antipsychotic agents in older patients. *J Clin Psychiatry*, **65**(Suppl 2), 5–99.

43. Drimer, T., Shahal, B. and Barak, Y. (2004) Effects of discontinuation of long-term anticholinergic treatment in elderly schizophrenia patients. *Int Clin Psychopharmacol*, **19**(1), 27–29.

44. Jacob, S. and Spinler, S.A. (2006) Hyponatremia associated with selective serotonin-reuptake inhibitors in older adults. *Ann Pharmacother*, **40**(9), 1618–1622.

45. Hanlon, J.T., Wang, X., Castle, N.G. *et al.* (2011) Potential underuse, overuse, and inappropriate use of antidepressants in older veteran nursing home residents. *J Am Geriatr Soc*, **59**(8), 1412–1420.

46. Olsson, J., Bergman, A., Carlsten, A. *et al.* (2010) Quality of drug prescribing in elderly people in nursing homes and special care units for dementia: a cross-sectional computerized pharmacy register analysis. *Clin Drug Investig*, **30**(5), 289–300.

47. Lang, P.O., Hasso, Y., Dramé, M. *et al.* (2010) Potentially inappropriate prescribing including under-use amongst older patients with cognitive or psychiatric co-morbidities. *Age Ageing*, **39**(3), 373–381.

48. Stuck, A.E., Siu, A.L., Wieland, G.D. *et al.* (1993) Comprehensive geriatric assessment: a meta-analysis of controlled trials. *Lancet*, **342**(8878), 1032–1036.

49. Ellis, G., Whitehead, M.A., O'Neill, D. *et al.* (2011) Comprehensive geriatric assessment for older adults admitted to hospital. *Cochrane Database Syst Rev* 7 (Art. No.: CD006211). doi: 10.1002/14651858.CD006211.pub2.

50. Crotty, M., Halbert, J., Rowett, D. *et al.* (2004) An outreach geriatric medication advisory service in residential aged care: a randomised controlled trial of case conferencing. *Age Ageing*, **33**(6), 612–617.

51. Schmader, K.E., Hanlon, J.T., Pieper, C.F. *et al.* (2004) Effects of geriatric evaluation and management on adverse drug reactions and suboptimal prescribing in the frail elderly. *Am J Med*, **116**(6), 394–401.

52. Strandberg, T.E., Pitkala, K.H., Berglind, S. *et al.* (2006) Multifactorial intervention to prevent recurrent cardiovascular events in patients 75 years or older: the Drugs and Evidence-Based Medicine in the Elderly (DEBATE) study: a randomized, controlled trial. *Am Heart J*, **152**(3), 585–592.
53. Spinewine, A., Swine, C., Dhillon, S. *et al.* (2007) Effect of a collaborative approach on the quality of prescribing for geriatric inpatients: a randomized, controlled trial. *J Am Geriatr Soc*, **55**(5), 658–665.
54. National Service Framework for Older People (2001) Medicines and older people – implementing medications-related aspects of the NSF for older people. Department of Health, HMSO, London.
55. Trivalle, C., Cartier, T., Verny, C. *et al.* (2010) Identifying and preventing adverse drug events in elderly hospitalised patients: a randomised trial of a program to reduce adverse drug effects. *J Nutr Health Aging*, **14**(1), 57–61.
56. Kuperman, G.J. and Gibson, R.F. (2003) Computer physician order entry: benefits, costs, and issues. *Ann Intern Med*, **139**(1), 31–39.
57. Kaushal, R., Shojania, K.G. and Bates, D.W. (2003) Effects of computerized physician order entry and clinical decision support systems on medication safety: a systematic review. *Arch Intern Med*, **163**(12), 1409–1416.
58. Gurwitz, J.H., Field, T.S., Rochon, P. *et al.* (2008) Effect of computerized provider order entry with clinical decision support on adverse drug events in the long-term care setting. *J Am Geriatr Soc*, **56**(12), 2225–2233.
59. Gallagher, P., Barry, P. and O'Mahony, D. (2007) Inappropriate prescribing in the elderly. *J Clin Pharm Ther*, **32**(2), 113–121.
60. Hughes, C.M. and Lapane, K.L. (2005) Administrative initiatives for reducing inappropriate prescribing of psychotropic drugs in nursing homes: how successful have they been? *Drugs Aging*, **22**(4), 339–351.
61. Lang, P.O., Vogt-Ferrier, N., Hasso, Y. *et al.* (2012) Interdisciplinary geriatric and psychiatric care reduces potentially inappropriate prescribing in the hospital: interventional study in 150 acutely ill elderly patients with mental and somatic comorbid conditions. *J Am Med Dir Assoc*, **13**(4), 406.e1–7.

Chapter 22

AGE-SENSITIVE PSYCHOSOCIAL TREATMENT FOR OLDER ADULTS WITH SUBSTANCE ABUSE

Kathleen Schutte[1], Sonne Lemke[2], Rudolf H. Moos[3] and Penny L. Brennan[1]

[1] Center for Health Care Evaluation, Veterans Affairs Palo Alto Health Care System, USA
[2] Program Evaluation and Resource Center, Department of Veteran Affairs, USA
[3] Stanford University/Center for Health Care Evaluation, Veterans Affairs Palo Alto Health Care System, USA

Introduction

It has been estimated that by 2020, the number of adults in the United States with a substance use disorder who are over the age of 50 will have more than doubled since the beginning of the century (an annual average of 1.7 million for 2002–2006 vs 4.4 million in 2020) [1]. Among adults aged 60–69, the number is expected to triple (annual average of 0.6 million for 2002–2006 vs 1.9 million in 2020) [1]. The anticipated increase in late-life substance abuse is largely due to the aging of the post-World War II 'baby boom' birth cohort. In addition, acceptance of psychosocial treatment is increasing [2, 3] and the rate of late-life drug abuse is expected to rise [4, 5]. Consistent with the latter, the reason for admission to US substance use disorder treatment by older adults is changing: among all substance use disorder treatment admissions for adults aged 55 or older, those for alcohol abuse declined from 89.4% in 1992 to 69.0% in 2005 while drug abuse admissions increased between 1992 and 2005, including those for heroin (5.9 to 14.1%), cocaine (2.0 to 8.5%) and prescription opioid medications (0.7 to 2.8%), respectively [6]. Furthermore, between 1992 and 2009, the proportion of admissions for older adults with co-occurring alcohol and drug abuse increased from 12.4 to 42.0% [7].

Baby boomers have begun to turn age 65 and interest in how to most effectively and efficiently provide substance abuse treatment to older adults is growing [8]. As compared to most younger adults with substance abuse, older adults are likely to have more complicated patterns of health-related problems, including multiple chronic illnesses, disability and functional, mobility, sensory and cognitive limitations [9].

Guidance regarding how to modify existing treatment methods to meet the needs of older adults with substance abuse has been enhanced by clinician-scientists who have worked extensively with this population. In 1998, the Substance Abuse and Mental Health Services Administration (SAMHSA) asked a group of such experts to identify consensus recommendations about age-sensitive treatment [10]. For this chapter, information from that consensus report is combined with more recent recommendations and research findings to highlight seven characteristics and six major components of age-sensitive treatment. Also described are several recommended psychotherapeutic approaches. Firstly, however, the use of primary terms in this chapter is clarified.

Substances: The focus is mainly on alcohol use and abuse. Alcohol is the most frequently abused substance among older adults and the one for which treatment is most often sought [5, 11, 12]. Furthermore, research and treatment efforts have focused primarily on alcohol abuse; therefore, descriptions are based largely on alcohol abuse. (Treatment for nicotine dependence is considered elsewhere in this book).

Late-life: Different definitions of 'late life' abound. Defining late-life by a single age is somewhat arbitrary since people age at different rates: For example, some 50 year old adults suffer more chronic illness and disability than those aged 70. The focus is primarily on adults aged 65 years or older; however, some cited research included individuals as young as 50.

Substance abuse: Use of the term 'substance abuse' is not directly tied to a diagnostic system or category: formal diagnostic criteria do not apply as well to older as to younger adults [5, 10, 13]. Substance abuse is viewed as occurring when substance use results in significant distress or impaired medical, mental health or social functioning, regardless of the amount of substance consumed or whether formal diagnostic criteria for a substance use disorder are met. Substance use or misuse without distress or impaired functioning is not included as abuse.

Psychosocial treatment: Psychosocial treatments for substance abuse are regarded as comprising formal interventions that aim to reduce substance use and substance-related problems and that include multiple meetings between a client and a healthcare provider who is formally trained to address psychological, psychiatric or substance-related problems. This definition of psychosocial treatment includes interventions that may be delivered in mental health or nonmental health inpatient, outpatient or residential treatment settings. Although important, the definition of psychosocial treatment used here does not include pharmacological treatments, detoxification services, mutual self-help group participation (e.g. in Alcohol Anonymous) or counselling received by a potential client's concerned loved ones. In this chapter the focus is on individuals who have entered treatment. This includes those who may be ambivalent about treatment entry but have done so on their own or due to the influence of others (e.g. court, significant others, employers, healthcare providers).

> **Box 22.1 Characteristics of age-sensitive treatment**
>
> Supportive and Nonconfrontational
> Flexible
> Sensitive to Gender Differences
> Sensitive to Cultural Differences
> Sensitive to Client Functioning
> Holistic
> Focused on Coping and Social Skills
>
> Listed characteristics were among those described in the 1998 SAMSHSA/CSAT Treatment Improvement Protocol (TIP) addressing substance abuse among older adults [10].

Seven characteristics of age-sensitive treatment

Features in Box 22.1 were first described by a SAMHSA expert panel [10].

1 – Supportive and nonconfrontational

A supportive, respectful and positive therapeutic style is considered key to psychosocial treatment success [14–16]. This is consistent with a long line of research indicating that nonspecific factors, especially establishment of a positive therapeutic alliance, are often more predictive of good treatment outcomes than the specific empirically-supported treatment approach used [17]. Confrontational approaches should be avoided: they commonly evoke anger, alienation and resistance and are associated with worse treatment outcomes among younger adults [18–20]. They are expected to do so with older adults, too. Treatment staff with training in empirically-supported interventions that enjoy working with older adults and who have the capacity to access and evaluate their own feelings and expectations about ageing and late life can help ensure that a supportive therapeutic climate is maintained [10, 21, 22].

2 – Flexible

Flexibility regarding treatment goals, approach, location, mode and duration is necessary to address older adults' changing problems, needs and functional limitations [10]. Flexibility might comprise being open to providing treatment in different locations (e.g. in a nursing or client's home) or in different ways (e.g. over the phone). Flexibility of treatment goals might mean postponing focus on substance use to initially address basic, practical needs such as finding safe, drug-free housing and obtaining food. Alternatively, it could comprise accommodating a clients' improving mental status, such as can occur after detoxification and with continued abstinence. For the latter, individual treatment using behavioural techniques (e.g. replacing substance-using activities with other rewarding activities) and a highly structured approach might initially provide a good match to clients' needs and capacities. As functioning improves, relying more on cognitive interventions or adding group-based treatment might be appropriate [23].

3 – Sensitive to gender differences

There are physiological gender differences in the metabolism of alcohol, and the course of alcohol-related problems, co-morbidities and barriers to treatment retention differ for women and men [10, 24, 25]. The need to attend to such differences is heightened by the increasing number of older women among alcohol abuse admissions to substance abuse treatment programmes. Among all older (50 years or older) alcohol admissions, the proportion of females increased from 16.9% in 1992 to 22.2% in 2009. Additional increases are expected [7].

Older women are less likely than older men to have drinking problems and, when problems do occur, women tend to experience later problem onset [26]. However, women often exhibit more rapid progression from regular intoxication to alcohol dependence [27] and from onset of alcohol dependence to negative health consequences (e.g. liver damage) [27, 28]. In addition, compared to older men, older women are at higher risk for co-occurring mental health conditions and social isolation: two factors that are associated with alcohol and prescription drug abuse [29–32]. (Please note that the terms co-occurring conditions and co-morbid conditions are used here interchangeably).

Whereas older men are more likely than older women to abuse alcohol, older women appear more likely to abuse prescription drugs. This finding seems closely tied to the fact that women are more likely to be prescribed psychoactive medications than are men (e.g. narcotic analgesics, sedatives, tranquilizers and anti-anxiety medications) and for longer periods of time [32–34]. Abuse of psychoactive prescription medications frequently occurs concurrently with alcohol use or abuse [35, 36]. Mixing medication and alcohol is dangerous and can contribute to injury, falls, accidents and death [29, 37–39], and should be addressed with clients. Resources for doing so with older female and male clients include a toolkit available from SAMHSA (http://www.samhsa.gov/aging/docs/GetConnectedToolkit.pdf).

Older women with drinking problems tend to face more barriers to treatment entry and retention than do their male counterparts. Compared to older men, older women have lower income, less insurance coverage and are more likely to live in poverty. In addition, older women are more likely to continue to hold major care-giving roles into late life (e.g. for parents, partner, grandchildren) [40, 41]. They are also more likely than men to seek mental health rather than specialized alcohol treatment [8, 32, 35, 42] and are overrepresented in late-life alcohol abuse treatment programme admissions [5].

4 – Sensitive to cultural differences

The sociocultural context in which we mature influences our world view, value system and expectations – including those regarding the nature of substance abuse [10, 43, 44] and acceptability of seeking psychosocial treatment. Understanding clients' current and past life context can facilitate empathy and strengthen the therapeutic alliance which, in turn, is associated with better treatment outcomes

[10, 43]. Clients who see their beliefs or expectations as incompatible with those of the treatment provider are at risk of discontinuing treatment [45].

It is estimated that, by 2030, 25% of older adults in the United States will be from an ethnic minority group [45], heightening the need for healthcare providers to understand cultural differences associated with ethnicity and common variations in the process of acculturation [45]. Treatment providers need to be aware of how the individual client identifies with the majority, minority and/or both cultures. It is important to determine the client's primary language and whether they are comfortable using spoken or written English [45, 46]. When available, using print materials developed in the client's primary language is recommended if doing so is consistent with clients' preferences and language skills [45]. In addition to individual differences related to ethnic and cultural identity, awareness of differences associated with birth cohort [43, 44], religion, sexual orientation and geographic area (urban or rural, within or outside of the United States) are likewise important [47]. It is useful to engage clients in discussion about their culture, world views and values [10]

5 – Focus on client functioning

There is much heterogeneity among older adults in substance abuse treatment; however, many older adults experience sensory, mobility or cognitive limitations or disabilities. Treatment providers should understand the potential psychological and emotional impact of such limitations and recognize that older adults may require special help or assistance [10, 44]. Treatment delivery should be adjusted to accommodate clients' needs. Recommendations include: slowing the general pace of treatment; speaking slowly and clearly; using shorter treatment sessions; making use of multiple modalities to present information (e.g. through speech, written material and role playing); increasing structure (e.g. providing a written agenda for treatment sessions); repeating and reviewing key treatment ideas and content frequently; and asking clients to summarize what they have understood [48].

Regardless of age, communication with clients is enhanced by sidestepping any limitations and taking advantage of existing information-processing strengths. Understanding common age-related changes in cognitive functioning can help the treatment provider anticipate needed adaptations [43, 44]. Although there is wide variability in memory and learning among older individuals, information processing generally slows with increasing age, and our ability to recognize is better maintained than our ability to recall information. Encouraging note-taking during sessions or providing a written or recorded summary of key concepts takes advantage of recognition skills and provides clients a valuable resource to which they can refer between sessions [44].

As we age, learning new skills tends to become more challenging than building upon existing ones [43, 44]. Encouraging older clients to reminisce takes advantage of this developmental change. In addition, incorporating reminiscences or life review focused specifically on coping strategies used earlier in life may increase self-esteem as clients recall prior successes [41, 49, 50]. Providing a structure for treatment sessions can help guide clients away from reminiscence back to the present. Despite some changes in memory function [51, 52], there is evidence that, when material is meaningful and relevant to individuals, memory differences between older and younger adults shrink [53, 54].

6 – Holistic

An holistic approach to substance abuse treatment considers the roles of physical, medical and mental health conditions, disabilities, cognitive, sensory or functional limitations; and psychological (e.g. depressive symptoms, anxiety, loneliness), social (e.g., practical problems, multiple losses and changes in a number of life domains, and social isolation), vocational and legal factors in explaining treatment retention, engagement, remission and relapse [10]. The client's resources (e.g. financial security, social support, personal resilience) as well as stressors are key. Addressing issues contributing to problematic substance use is expected to facilitate long-term maintenance of remission as well as short-term behaviour change.

7 – Focus on coping and social skills

In addition to facilitating remission, treatment seeks to teach clients skills and different ways of adapting to their environment. Using substances to cope can be replaced with other behaviours that have fewer negative consequences and help clients develop a life context supportive of sobriety. Treatment can guide clients towards identification of the circumstances, events or situations that prompt their substance use. Once these antecedents are identified, the treatment provider can then help clients develop coping and problem-solving strategies and social skills that help them manage situations differently [10, 17].

One alternative to drinking to cope is seeking help or support from loved ones. However, adoption of this coping strategy may be more challenging for older adults whose drinking-related problems began early in life. It is estimated that about two-thirds of older adults with alcohol abuse first developed problems prior to late-middle age, for example, before age 50 [10, 55, 56]. Compared to individuals with late-onset problems (e.g. older adults whose first drinking problems occurred after the age of 50), those with early-onset problems are more likely to have alcohol-related medical, mental health and cognitive problems, disrupted interpersonal relationships, legal problems and a family history of alcohol dependence [21, 55]. Older adults with early-onset problems are also more likely to have strained interpersonal relationships and alienated family and friends. For such clients, treatment goals should include helping to rebuild relationships and find new sources of support.

As is the case among adolescents and younger adults, friends' attitudes towards drinking influence older adults' drinking behaviour. Having friends who do not drink heavily nor approve of heavy drinking is a strong and consistent predictor of obtaining and sustaining remission [17, 57]. Treatment may need to focus on helping clients shape their social network so that exposure to individuals who drink or use drugs is minimized and contact with abstinent individuals and those supportive of sobriety is increased. Treatment providers can help clients develop interpersonal skills necessary to identify groups or organizations whose activities do not focus on drinking (e.g. AA, volunteer activities, institutionally- or community-sponsored education and recreation programmes).

Box 22.2 Components of age-sensitive treatment

Biopsychosocial Assessment

Treatment Plan

Attention to Co-occurring Conditions

Referrals and Care Coordination

Empirically-Supported Psychosocial Interventions

Treatment Adjuncts

Listed components were among those described in the 1998 SAMSHSA/CSAT Treatment Improvement Protocol (TIP) addressing substance abuse among older adults [10].

Six components of age-sensitive psychosocial treatment

Features in Box 22.2 were first described by a SAMHSA expert panel [10].

1 – Biopsychosocial assessment

Identification of the most appropriate, individual-specific treatment goals and plans requires completion of a comprehensive biopsychosocial assessment. Details regarding the recent and lifetime course, nature and severity of substance-related behaviour, along with information about the physical, psychological and social factors associated with the client's substance abuse, are used to plan treatment and identify important issues that, if unattended, might waylay treatment (e.g. a history of seizures when withdrawing from alcohol, self-harming behavior, physical or sexual abuse, legal problems) [43–45, 58].

It is essential to determine whether the client views his or her substance use as problematic and gauge the client's motivation and readiness to change. This information will help determine which treatment modality and intensity is most appropriate (e.g. focus on increasing motivation for change versus more intensive psychotherapy). Information obtained regarding the quantity and frequency of the client's substance use at the beginning of treatment can be compared to use throughout treatment to track changes and treatment progress. Some older adults over the course of their life or within late-life substitute use of one substance for another (e.g. alcohol use substituted with benzodiazepines, opioid medication or marijuana use) [26, 59–62]. Therefore, assessment of the client's use of alcohol, illegal substances and prescription drugs is recommended. It should not be assumed that the older adult client is not and has not ever used illicit drugs. The way in which illicit drug use is assessed can influence descriptions of it [61]. Compared to asking about use of illegal drugs overall (e.g. 'Have you ever used drugs?'), more complete information can be obtained when individuals are asked separately about their use each illicit drug, one at a time [61]. Some individuals will not view use of certain substances as comprising 'drug use' (e.g. marijuana use, other illicit drug use that occurred in the context of drug experimentation) and, therefore, might not report it [61]. In addition, embarrassment, stigma or fear of legal reprisals can prevent some individuals from describing current or past drug abuse. Such trepidations are likely to be eased by the treatment provider's successful communication of empathy, acceptance and a nonjudgmental, direct approach [61]. Regarding use of prescription or other psychoactive substances, a 'brown bag medication review'can be used. The client is asked to put into a brown (or other) bag all prescription and over-the-counter (OTC) medications, supplements, vitamins or herbs that he or she is taking and bring it to treatment [10].

Obtaining information about the nature, context, timing and helpfulness of prior treatment experiences, involvement in mutual self-help groups such as AA and informal efforts to change substance-related behaviour (e.g. prayer, consulting loved ones) allows the treatment provider to incorporate previously helpful strategies into the current treatment plan. For clients at risk of withdrawal symptoms (e.g. namely regarding alcohol, sedative-hypnotics, benzodiazepines and opioids), it is essential to obtain information about history of reactions to acute withdrawal [63, 64]. Prior alcohol withdrawals characterized by serious complications (e.g. seizures, delirium tremens, hallucinations, mental confusion, disorientation, delirium, chronic memory disorder) confers high risk for severe, life-threatening reactions to subsequent detoxification [65] and indicates a need for high intensity care [66].

Learning about the medical, psychological and social factors that act as antecedents, consequences or independent (but co-occurring) conditions will also facilitate treatment planning [67, 68]. Needed information can be obtained in various ways, for example clinical and psychiatric interview, psychological assessment, self-report questionnaires and surveys, and blood and urine tests. When possible, it is useful to obtain information from individuals familiar with the client's behaviour (e.g. family, close friends or caregivers).

The assessment process is likely to be more intensive for clients whose substance-related problems began prior to late-life (i.e. early-onset problems), are severe and chronic or accompanied by mental illness [55, 56]. In less severe cases, a briefer assessment combined with the use of reliable, validated screening instruments might be considered [20].

2 – Treatment planning

Problem list and integrated summary

Organizing and making sense of assessment information is facilitated by creating comprehensive lists of the client's problems and resources [67–69]. Such a list can help the care provider see the breadth of the client's health- and nonhealth-related problems and identify which problems may be interrelated [67, 69]. The lists can also facilitate efforts to identify factors that may be sustaining the client's substance abuse, anticipate likely barriers to remission and identify potential types and sources of support [67, 68]. An integrated summary comprises the compilation of these issues and should provide insight into how to motivate the client to stay in treatment, help him or her obtain remission and improve his or her psychosocial functioning or social environment as needed to support sustained remission.

Treatment goals

Collaborative development of treatment goals by the provider and client facilitates good treatment outcomes [10]. Some clients may not want to set abstinence as their substance-related goal. Harm-reduction goals are consistent with age-sensitive treatment [10]. Some clients may decide to set reduction in substance-use as an intermediary goal and abstinence as the ultimate one. Others might not want to focus on substance-related behaviour and prefer instead to address other issues related to substance abuse (e.g. reducing depression or obtaining safe drug-free housing). In such cases, in addition to working toward the agreed-upon treatment goal, it is important to engage the client in a collaborative process that examines how changes in drinking behaviour could facilitate attainment of the client's desired goals [70].

Treatment intensity, unit of treatment and duration

Clients should be offered the least intensive treatment needed to address their substance abuse [8, 10, 66]. Selection of treatment setting can be broadly guided by the American Society of Addiction Medicines' (ASAM) Client Placement Criteria [66]. ASAM criteria consider six major dimensions: withdrawal potential, medical conditions and complications, emotional and behavioural conditions and complications, treatment acceptance, relapse potential, and recovery environment.

The selected unit of treatment (e.g. individual, group, couple or family) will depend on client preferences and needs, treatment provider recommendations and the availability and willingness of relevant others to participate. In regards to treatment duration, it appears that duration of treatment is more closely associated with improved treatment outcomes than is treatment intensity [17, 20, 71–73].

Treatment goals, priorities and intensity of care needed can change throughout treatment. The treatment practitioner must frequently reassess clients' needs and behaviour to determine if modifications are indicated. Whatever the goals, the treatment provider should decide how treatment progress and success should be assessed.

3 – Attention to co-occurring conditions

Chronic, co-occurring medical or mental health conditions that contribute to, exacerbate or complicate the course and outcomes of substance abuse treatment should be addressed during substance abuse treatment [74]. Decisions regarding how to address them will be influenced by several factors, including the nature, severity and urgency of each condition or problem, client preferences, consultation and coordination with other healthcare providers and availability of services [10, 75]. For example, it may be deemed desirable to provide psychosocial treatment for co-occurring substance abuse and mental health conditions concurrently. This might be done within the same treatment, especially if the selected treatment approach has been validated for use of both conditions. Alternatively, if co-occurring conditions cannot be addressed concurrently within substance abuse treatment, then linkages with other services should be accessed and referrals made and followed-up to ensure that clients received proper concurrent care [76]. It should be noted that empirical evidence has not clearly indicated if concurrent or sequential psychosocial treatment may be superior [77]. If it is not possible to concurrently address factors that appear to be contributing to the client's substance use, or if a sequential approach to addressing co-morbid conditions is preferred, an important element of the treatment plan is to reassess such decisions at a later, specified date. Four conditions that often co-occur with late-life substance abuse are considered in more detail here: chronic pain, depression, dementia and concurrent use of multiple substances.

Chronic pain

Pain can complicate treatment of individuals in substance abuse treatment [78] and increases risk for late-life alcohol and prescription medication abuse [32, 79, 80]. For clients whose alcohol or drug use appears to be associated with chronic pain, treatment can introduce empirically-supported nonpharmacological options for controlling it. These include cognitive behavioural therapy, relaxation training, biofeedback, exercise and physical therapy. These interventions are most effective for older adults who do not have significant cognitive or physical impairment; however, for more impaired clients, a modified cognitive behavioural treatment (CBT) approach has been developed [81]. In addition, collaboration with the client's physician(s) regarding the client's pharmacologic pain management and monitoring is indicated.

Depression

The percentage of older adults entering alcohol-related treatment with a co-occurring psychiatric condition is increasing: from 10.5% in 1992 to 31.4% in 2009 [82, 83]. Depression is one of the most common mental health issues among older adults with substance abuse. It is imperative to note that there is little empirical support for the belief that treatment of depression will resolve alcohol dependence in the absence of substance abuse treatment [20]. On the other hand, even modest reductions in alcohol consumption can benefit older adults with depression [84], and prolonged abstinence from alcohol (a central nervous system depressant) can reduce or relieve depression. However, prolonged abstinence is not always achieved and health risks of not treating depression are considerable. Furthermore, some clients are less likely to obtain alleviation of depressive symptoms, regardless of whether prolonged abstinence is achieved. This includes individuals that experienced their first episode of depression prior to their first episode of alcohol abuse or, alternatively, ever experienced a depressive episode during a long period of abstinence from alcohol. The latter has been referred to as alcohol-independent depression. Individuals who have experienced depression only during periods of alcohol use are described as having alcohol-dependent depression.

It is estimated that, for up to 30% of older adults with co-occurring depression and alcohol abuse, depression is substance independent [85, 86]. Clients whose depression appears to be substance independent might be good candidates to receive intensive psychosocial interventions and earlier psychopharmacological treatment of depression. However, depression is painful and should be addressed, regardless of whether criteria for a depressive diagnosis are met and apart from whether the depression is believed to be substance independent or dependent [76].

The risk of suicide among older adults who use substances is higher than in the general population [87, 88]. When substance use occurs in the context of co-occurring depression, suicide risk is further heightened [87, 88]. In the general population, the rate of suicide for older men, especially those 85 years and older, is among the highest for any demographic group [89]. Compared to younger adults and older women, older men are much more likely to select highly lethal suicide methods and die on their first suicide attempt [8, 58, 89]. Whereas the rate of suicide by firearms for adults of all ages was 11.2 per 100 000 deaths in 2010 (the most recent year for which data were available), the rate among men aged 65 and older was 22.6/100 000. The rate increased with age: among men aged 85 or older, the rate was 36.3/100 000 [90, 91]. The risk of suicide by firearms, combined with the high rate of gun ownership among older adults in the United States [92], is particularly alarming and highlights the need to assess and address older adult clients' suicidal thoughts, plans and means. Older clients' access to lethal methods (e.g. a firearm or stockpile of psychoactive medications) should be assessed and addressed in the presence of suicidal thoughts or behaviour.

Significant cognitive impairment or dementia

If cognitive impairment exceeds normal age-expected changes and dementia is suspected, additional evaluation is warranted. Vision and hearing loss can be mistaken for dementia and should be ruled out as contributing factors. Sometimes a potentially treatable underlying condition is found to be contributing to cognitive impairment (e.g. depression, delirium, Korsakoff syndrome and Wernicke's encephalopathy) [36]. Improvements in cognitive functioning can sometimes – but not always – be obtained with treatment of the underlying condition and abstinence. In addition, alcohol-induced dementias sometimes resolve with time and abstinence. However, persistent alcohol-induced dementias are estimated to afflict 12–25% of older adults in treatment [93].

The presence of significant cognitive deficits or dementia will have implications for identification of obtainable treatment goals and selection of a treatment plan. Providing emotional support and using behavioural interventions is likely to be more effective in such situations than cognitive therapy. On the other hand, interventions that appeal to the client's long-term values may help motivate him or her complete structured behavioural interventions [81, 93]. The treatment provider might also coordinate care with the client's loved ones, caregivers or long-term care staff to implement structured behavioural and environmental interventions. Individuals with more severe dementia who continue to drink are unlikely to benefit from treatment and, with continued alcohol consumption, can experience additional alcohol-related cognitive decline and other negative health consequences. In such cases, adult foster or day care might be helpful. If not, closed residential facilities with no-alcohol policies might be considered [94].

Substance-related disorders

As noted earlier, older adult (aged 50 and older) admissions to US substance abuse treatment programmes that are due solely to alcohol abuse are decreasing while admissions for co-occurring alcohol and drug abuse increase [7]. Treatment of co-occurring alcohol and drug abuse will depend upon the client's unique problems and situation and should consider psychopharmacological treatment when indicated and available. Tobacco use, which frequently co-occurs with alcohol abuse, contributes to relapse of alcohol abuse [95] and should be addressed in substance abuse treatment. It has been shown among younger adults that smoking cessation interventions provided during addiction treatment increase the likelihood of longer-term abstinence from alcohol and illicit drugs and improve mortality outcomes [96]. Empirical evaluation is needed to confirm if this is likewise the case among older adults.

4 – Referrals and care coordination

It is unlikely that one treatment provider will possess all the expertise needed to address the full spectrum of older adults' substance abuse, medical, psychological and social service needs [8]. However, traditional healthcare systems are generally not organized to support coordination of older clients' multiple and varied treatment needs [8, 97]. Treatment providers should be prepared to coordinate treatment with other treatment providers and furnish referrals as needed to medical, mental health and social agency resources [8, 97]. Appropriate and successful referrals could be facilitated by the treatment provider's development of linkages to relevant helpful services [8, 10, 97]. When a referral is made, the treatment provider should follow-up with the client to determine if the referral was successful or if a different referral is needed. SAMHSA [98] has made available suggestions for developing referral resources at http://www.samhsa.gov/aging/docs/GetConnectedToolkit.pdf.

5 – Empirically-supported psychosocial interventions

It is established that older adults with substance use disorders can benefit from empirically-supported psychosocial interventions that were originally developed for and tested among mixed-aged adult samples [20, 72, 73]. However, not all modalities with demonstrated efficacy among younger adults have been evaluated for an older audience. Furthermore, among assessed treatments, there has been insufficient research to indicate if one treatment is more effective than another among older adults. Few studies have compared treatment modalities and none have compared treatment modalities to no treatment with older adult samples [62]. Until empirical data become available, it seems reasonable to expect older adults to respond similarly to treatments designed for and tested with younger adults. Four psychosocial interventions being used to address late-life alcohol abuse are described here: brief intervention, motivational enhancement therapy, cognitive behavioural therapy and relapse prevention therapy for older adults.

Brief intervention (BI)

BI was designed to address at-risk or hazardous drinking. However, some work has demonstrated that it can be used successfully to treat mild to moderate alcohol abuse and abuse of some other substances [99–102]. For individuals with more severe alcohol abuse, it has been clinically noted that BI can be helpful in reducing alcohol consumption and facilitate entry into more intensive psychosocial treatment. In BI, setting achievable goals is considered essential in keeping clients engaged and motivated to address other goals. Six elements believed to be active ingredients of BI are summarized by the acronym FRAMES [101]: *FEEDBACK* of personal risk or impairment; *RESPONSIBILITY* for change lies within the client; *ADVICE* regarding changing behaviour; *MENU* of alternative change options; *EMPATHY* on the part of the treatment provider; and *SELF-EFFICACY* or optimism on the part of the client, facilitated by the treatment provider.

Several variations of BI are available. A BI called BRief Intervention and Treatment for Elders (BRITE) [103] was designed specifically for older adults and follows recommendations for treatment of late-life substance abuse [10]. Treatment comprises a limited number of one-on-one sessions – usually fewer than five – and is considered finished when the BRITE Health Promotion Workbook (http://brite. fmhi.usf.edu/Files/BRITEWorkbook-English.pdf) is complete and the treatment provider believes that the client has retained presented information. BRITE comprises multiple steps that are described in the BRITE Health Promotion Workbook [104].

It is recommended that a *Motivational Interviewing (MI) style* be used alongside BRITE [103]. MI is an empathic, supportive yet directive counselling style that views ambivalence towards behaviour change as normal but also the key barrier to behaviour change [105, 106]. Reducing ambivalence relies on the client's recognition and acknowledgment of discrepancy between his or her values or goals and current drinking-related behaviour. The treatment provider's role is to create a collaborative partnership and guide – not actively lead – the client to the realization that attainment of goals requires behaviour change. MI uses reflective listening rather than asking for information and avoids confrontation and argumentation. Key elements of MI include expressing empathy, developing discrepancy, avoiding argumentation, rolling with resistance and supporting self-efficacy. Five useful MI strategies are: (i) use open-ended questions that cannot be answered with a single word or phrase; (ii) demonstrate understanding by reflecting what the client said; (iii) periodically summarize what has transpired in the treatment session; (iv) support and comment on the client's strengths, motivation, intentions and progress; (v) have the client voice personal concerns and intentions, rather than trying to persuade him or her that change is necessary [107].

Motivational enhancement therapy (MET)

MET is an active, goal-oriented, manual-based brief treatment developed for use in Project MATCH [108]. Like BRITE, MET combines MI's supportive, empathetic, nonconfrontational counselling style with BI's individual-specific feedback. MET accepts the client where he or she is in the stage of change process [109] then helps him or her progress through the stages of behaviour change: pre-contemplation, contemplation, preparation, action and maintenance [109]. Treatment is tailored to the client's current stage of change. Consistent with MI, MET tries to evoke internal motivation for change rather than directing or guiding the client through a stepwise recovery process.

MET comprises four planned but individualized treatment sessions and clients are encouraged to bring a supportive significant other to one or two sessions. The four sessions are aligned with treatment goals that include strengthening the client's internal motivation for change and working with the client to develop a plan to do so. The therapist encourages the client's efforts to change and discusses possible coping strategies for managing high risk situations with the client.

Cognitive behavioural therapy (CBT)

CBT approaches have strong empirical support and demonstrated efficacy and effectiveness for treating alcohol abuse as well as conditions that often accompany late-life substance abuse (e.g. depression, anxiety, pain, insomnia, disability, other substance abuse) [110–112]. CBT has an active, goal focused, problem solving, skill building focus, and usually incorporates homework into treatment to reinforce concepts that the treatment provider and client discuss during treatment sessions. Like other approaches, CBT relies on the establishment of a collaborative relationship between the treatment provider and client.

An 'ABC' approach is commonly used to explain problematic alcohol use wherein Antecedent events or situations (A) lead to Beliefs (B) (thoughts, interpretations, attitudes, opinions) about the antecedent event. In turn, beliefs about the antecedent event are conceptualized as leading to a particular emotional or behavioural Consequence (C) [113, 114]. Each ABC combination is called a behavioural chain. The CBT treatment provider helps the client identify, then dismantle, the multiple behavioural chains involved in explaining his or her drinking behaviour.

CBT assumes that behavioural problems and distressing emotions can be altered by learning to identify, challenge and change cognitions or thoughts that are distorted or maladaptive. Therefore, in CBT, the client learns to identify situations, thoughts, feelings, drinking cues and urges that precede and initiate their alcohol use; the client then learns skills and adaptive coping strategies that help him or her to avoid or otherwise manage high-risk situations.

Relapse prevention therapy (RPT)

RPT is a manual-driven, CBT-based group therapy designed specifically for older adults [115, 116]. It is designed to last 16 weeks and includes identification of individual-specific behavioural chains that describe the client's high-risk situations for substance abuse. Treatment includes nine pre-specified, structured modules that can be repeated as needed and that address factors commonly related to relapse, including managing social pressure, situations at home and alone, negative thoughts and emotions associated with substance abuse (especially anxiety, tension, anger and frustration), controlling substance abuse cues, coping with urges, and preventing a slip from becoming a relapse [116].

6 – Adjuncts to psychosocial interventions

Common adjuncts to psychosocial treatment include psychopharmacological treatment (discussed elsewhere in this book), psychoeducation, screening for infectious diseases and mutual self-help group participation. Each is briefly addressed here.

Psychoeducation

The content of information shared with the client will depend upon his or her current concerns and needs. Psychoeducation might comprise explaining to a client's family members and caregivers the harmful effects of drinking on cognitive functioning, incontinence, depression, gait disturbance and so on. For other clients, it might be more helpful to provide information about the size of a standard drink – older adults overestimate the size [117] – risks associated with binge drinking and normative information about what amount of alcohol is considered moderate, the effect of alcohol on sleep and description of good sleep hygiene and risks of serious injury, disability or death associated with combining consumption and alcohol and psychoactive and other medication. Regarding the latter, consumer-friendly information about potentially harmful alcohol-drug interactions is available from a variety of organizations [38, 75, 118] and at http://pubs.niaaa.nih.gov/publications/Medicine/Harmful_Interactions.pdf.

Screening for infectious diseases

It is estimated that by 2020, 50% of individuals in the United States with the Human Immunodeficiency Virus (HIV) will be 50 and older [119]. Although the Center for Disease Control (CDC) does not at this time recommend routine HIV/AIDS testing for individuals 65 and older, treatment providers should understand their clients' risks for HIV/AIDS and deliver HIV prevention messages as needed [120, 121]. Guidance on how to do so with older adults is helpfully described by Brooks and colleagues [119], who provide links to existing HIV prevention and related programmes designed specifically for older adults (e.g. http://www.aoa.gov/AoARoot/AoA_Programs/HPW/HIV_AIDS/index.aspx). The CDC *does* recommend that all baby boomers (regardless of substance abuse status) be tested for the Hepatitis C Virus (HCV), as they are at high risk of having the virus and undiscovered HCV-related liver disease [122].

Mutual self-help group participation

Groups such as AA, Smart Recovery and Moderation Management (MM) support sobriety and can be useful adjuncts to treatment by helping older adults achieve, and then sustain, remission [123, 124]. Greater AA attendance has been shown to predict better drinking outcomes among older adults and, once in AA, older adults' attendance is comparable to that of younger members [123–125]. Nevertheless, there is some evidence that older adults who attend AA are less engaged than younger members (e.g. being less likely to consider themselves as AA members or to have contacted an AA sponsor for help) [124]. To facilitate AA membership, the treatment provider can introduce the client to an AA sponsor or recovery guide; follow up with the client on agreements made to attend AA and encourage further engagement (e.g. doing service or becoming a sponsor) [126].

Older adults can face barriers to self-help group meeting attendance, including transport-related problems, disabilities that preclude attendance or risk injury, reluctance to go out in the evening, discomfort being among younger adults and those who have abused illicit drugs as well as alcohol [47, 124, 127]. Attending age-specific groups (e.g. Seniors in Sobriety) may help overcome some of these barriers. The number of such groups is reported to be limited but growing [36].

Age-segregated or mixed-age treatment

There has been debate about whether treatment should be age-segregated as well as age-sensitive [5, 10, 36]. Research has demonstrated that age-segregated treatment is associated with good outcomes [128] *and* that older adults who receive mixed-aged treatment can benefit from it at least as much as do younger adults [20, 123, 129–131]. However, these conclusions are based on the results of a small handful of studies. It seems likely that there are subgroups of older adults who could obtain good treatment retention and outcomes regardless of whether they receive mixed- or age-segregated treatment (all other factors being equal).

However, for others, being in an age-segregated group may be essential for treatment retention. For example, older adults who are more advanced in years (e.g. aged 75–84 rather than aged 65–74) generally have more co-occurring chronic health problems and functional limitations than do younger adults: They may prefer and be more likely to complete age-segregated rather than mixed-aged treatment. For older adults with certain medical problems (e.g. those with HCV) or mental health conditions (e.g. bipolar disorder), it is unclear when being among similarly-aged adults may become more important for treatment retention and outcomes than receiving mixed-age care that addresses their co-occurring conditions. Until more data are available on the matter, healthcare systems might consider providing special groups or services that address the particular needs of older clients who share a specific type of co-occurring condition [35].

Future directions

As previously noted, evidence does not favour one empirically-validated psychosocial treatment strategy over another when addressing late-life alcohol abuse. One approach that has received little attention is Twelve-Step Facilitation (TSF) treatment [132]. Results from one study that included older men aged 55–77 being treated in inpatient alcohol treatment programmes suggested no differences in outcomes for those who received CBT or TSF [130]. Replication and confirmation of this finding among older adults receiving outpatient care is indicated. However, it seems likely that, as was found for mixed-aged adults in Project MATCH [133], TSF is as effective as CBT among older adults. This may be surprising given major differences between the two approaches: Whereas CBT focuses on the influence of malleable factors in explaining and changing behaviour (e.g. thoughts and attitudes, environmental features), TSF emphasizes clients' acceptance of an alcoholic identity and powerlessness over alcohol. However, as outlined by Moos[17, 19], the two approaches share important characteristics common to effective treatments: They provide support, structure and goal-direction, highlight the value of life-style change and finding nonpharmacological substitutes for substance use, and provide opportunities to develop adaptive coping skills and a social network that values sobriety [17, 19].

The focus in this chapter has been mostly on alcohol abuse. More information is needed about the effectiveness of psychosocial treatment for illicit and prescription drug abuse [5, 32]. For example, it would be useful to find out the extent to which empirically supported treatments are efficacious among older adults with illicit and prescription drug abuse. Moreover, additional information is needed regarding the characteristics, predictors, course and untreated outcomes of late-life illicit and prescription medication abuse. Such knowledge will have implications for the identification and design of effective and efficient treatment for older adults. For prescription drug abuse, it has been noted that development and comparison of psychosocial interventions is currently hindered by the absence of commonly-accepted definitions and measures of intentional misuse, unintentional misuse and abuse of prescription medications [134].

For all types of late-life substance abuse, recommendations for age-sensitive treatment include working with clients' other care providers. Such coordination can be complicated and difficult. There is general consensus that systematic improvements in care coordination are needed to provide the most efficient and effective care for older adults who have complex combinations of chronic medical, mental health and substance abuse conditions. More than one agency has discussed the need for infrastructure changes to healthcare systems to facilitate and enhance care coordination [97, 125]. General recommendations for infrastructure changes have included alteration of service reimbursement structures; improved interdisciplinary communication and development of information technology (IT) systems to facilitate record keeping and communication among practitioners [8, 97]. Efforts to address limitations in healthcare delivery also include development of alternative models of care. The Patient-Centered Medical Home (PCMH) healthcare delivery model is focused on designing primary care services that can better provide comprehensive, coordinated, patient-centred care to clients who have multiple chronic health conditions [135]. The model specifies use of a multidisciplinary team that includes mental health and substance abuse treatment.

There is also general consensus that treatment should be stepped. In stepped care, the least intensive treatment that meets the individual client's needs is used before more intensive treatment is implemented. For example, BI offered in a primary care setting is less intensive than treatment provided in a substance abuse specialty setting yet retains the opportunity to refer clients to higher intensity care as needed [102]. Individuals who are likely to need higher-intensity treatment (e.g. longer-term specialty substance abuse treatment services) include older adults with polysubstance abuse or mental health co-morbidity.

A promising area of research is the identification of effective treatment approaches that are less intense than BI. These could include use of interactive telehealth and web-based brief interventions [73, 102]. These have already demonstrated utility and efficacy among younger adults with low-severity problems [136–138]. Their use among older adults seems feasible: late–middle aged and older adults are increasingly becoming comfortable using interactive technologies [138]. Such low-intensity, nontraditional models for treatment delivery might be particularly useful to older adults unwilling or unable to access traditional treatment and for those concerned with the stigma of seeing a substance abuse specialty provider. If telephone and web-based interventions are found to be safe and cost effective among older adults, these methods could help address increasing demand and limited resources for treating late-life substance abuse while at the same time providing an attractive treatment option for many older adults.

Although more definitive information is needed, the current state of research indicates that treatment providers are likely to help older adults with substance abuse if they are guided by the seven characteristics of age-sensitive psychosocial treatment and apply its main components, are knowledgeable about the issues and conditions that affect older adults and develop expertise in and use empirically-supported psychosocial interventions.

Acknowledgements

Department of Veterans Affairs Health Services Research and Development Service funds and National Institutes of Alcoholism and Alcohol Abuse grants AA06699 Moos (PI); AA15685 Moos (PI); AA017477 Brennan (PI) supported preparation of this chapter. *The views expressed here are the authors' and do not necessarily reflect the views of the Department of Veterans Affairs.*

References

1. Han, B., Groerer, J.C., Colliver, J.D. and Penne, M.A. (2009) Substance use disorder among older adults in the United States in 2020. *Addiction*, **104**(1), 88–96.
2. Arean, P.A., Alvidrez, J., Barrera, A. *et al.* (2002) Would older medical patients use psychological services? *Gerontologist*, **42**(3), 392–398.
3. Mackenzie, C.S., Scott, T., Mather, A. and Sareen, J. (2008) Older adults' help-seeking attitudes and treatment beliefs concerning mental health problems. *Am J Geriatr Psychiatry*, **16**(12), 1010–1019.
4. Gfroerer, J.C. and Epstein J.F. (1999) Marijuana initiates and their impact on future drug abuse treatment need. *Drug Alcohol Depend*, **54**(3), 229–237.
5. Wu, L.-T. and Blazer, D.G. (2011) Illicit and nonmedical drug use among older adults: A review. *J Aging Health*, **23**(3), 481–504.
6. Lofwall, M.R., Schuster, A. and Strain, E.C. (2008) Changing profile of abused substances by older persons entering treatment. *J Nerv Ment Dis*, **196**(12), 898–905.
7. SAMHSA (2011) *Older Adult Admissions Reporting Alcohol as a Substance of Abuse*: 1992 and 2009. The TEDS Report, Center for Behavioral Health Statistics and Quality, Substance Abuse and Mental Health Services Administration (SAMHSA), Rockville, MD.
8. Institute of Medicine (IOM) (2009) *The Mental Health and Substance Use Workforce for Older Adults: In Whose Hands?* The National Academies Press, Washington, DC. 2012.
9. Blow, F.C., Barry, K.L., Fuller, B.E. and Booth, B.M. (2002) Analysis of the National Health and Nutrition Examination Survey (NHANES): Longitudinal analysis of drinking over the lifespan. In: *Substance Use by Older Adults: Estimates of Future Impact on the Treatment System* (eds S.P. Korper and C.L. Council). OAS Analytic Series #A-21, DHHS Publication No. (SMA) 03-3763, Substance Office of Applied Studies; Abuse and Mental Health Services Administration, Rockville, MD, pp. 107–123.
10. Center for Substance Abuse Treatment (CSAT) (1998) *Substance Abuse Among Older Adults*. Treatment Improvement Protocol (TIP) 26, HHS Publication No. (SMA) 12-3918, Substance Abuse and Mental Health Services Administration, Rockville, MD.
11. SAMHSA (2010) *Changing Substance Abuse Patterns Among Older Admissions: 1992 and 2008*. The Treatment Episode Data Set (TEDS) Report, Substance Abuse and Mental Health Services Administration (SAMHSA), Rockville, MD.
12. SAMHSA (2013) *National Admissions to Substance Abuse Treatment Services*. Treatment Episode Data Set (TEDS): 2001–2011, BHSIS Series S-65, HHS Publication No. (SMA) 13-4772, Center for Behavioral Health Statistics and Quality, Substance Abuse and Mental Health Services Administration (SAMHSA), Rockville, MD.
13. Patterson, T.L. and Jeste, D.V. (1999) The potential impact of the baby-boom generation on substance abuse among elderly persons. *Psychiatr Serv*, **50**(9), 1184–1188.
14. Finney, J.W. and Moos, R.H. (2002) Psychosocial treatments for alcohol use disorders. In: *A Guide to Treatments that Work*, 2nd edn (eds P.E. Nathan and J.M. Gorman JM.). Oxford University Press, New York, pp. 157–168.
15. Najavits, L.M. and Weiss, R.D. (1994) Variations in therapist effectiveness in the treatment of patients with substance use disorders. An empirical review. *Addiction*, **89**(6), 679–688.
16. Patterson, C.H. (1984) Empathy, warmth, and genuineness in psychotherapy: A review of reviews. *Psychotherapy*, **21**(4), 431–438.
17. Moos, RH. (2003) Addictive disorders in context: Principles and puzzles of effective treatment and recovery. *Psychol Addict Behav*, **17**(1), 3–12.
18. Miller, W.R., Benefield, R.G. and Tonigan, J.S. (1993) Enhancing motivation to change in problem drinking: a controlled comparison of two therapist styles. *J Consult Clin Psychol*, **61**(3), 455–461.

19. Moos, R.H. (2005) Iatrogenic effects of psychosocial interventions for substance use disorders: Prevalence, predictors, prevention. *Addiction*, **100**(5), 595–604.
20. Department of Veteran Affairs (VA), Department of Defense (DoD). (2009) *VA/DoD Clinical Practice Guideline for the Management of Substance Use Disorders (SUD)*, Version 2.0. VA and DoD, Washington, DC.
21. Atkinson, R.M. (2002) Scourge, solace, or safeguard of health? *Am J Geriatr Psychiatry*, **10**(6), 649–652.
22. Garner, J. (2003) Psychotherapies and older adults. *Aust NZ J Psychiatry*, **37**(5), 537–548.
23. Knight, B.G. and Satre, D.D. (1999) Cognitive-behavioral psychotherapy with older adults. *Clinical Psychology: Science and Practice*, **6**(1999), 188–203.
24. Brady, T.M. and Ashley, O.S. (2005) *Women in Substance Abuse Treatment: Results from the Alcohol and Drug Services Study*. DHHS Publication No. SMA 04-3968, Analytic Series A-26, Substance Abuse and Mental Health Services Administration, Office of Applied Studies, Rockville MD.
25. Center for Substance Abuse Treatment (CSAT). (2009) *Substance Abuse Treatment: Addressing the Specific Needs of Women*. Treatment Improvement Protocol (TIP) Series 51, HHS Publication No. (SMA) 09-4426, Substance Abuse and Mental Health Services Administration, Rockville, MD.
26. Bucholz, K.K., Sheline, Y. and Helzer, J.E. (2013) The epidemiology of alcohol use, problems, and dependence in elders: A review. In: *Alcohol and Aging* (eds T.P. Beresford and E. Gomberg). Oxford University Press, New York, pp. 19–41.
27. Gilbertson, R., Prather, R. and Nixon, S.J. (2008) The Role of selected factors in the development and consequences of alcohol dependence. *Alcohol Res Health*, **31**(4), 389–399.
28. NIAAA (2001) *Alcohol: An important Women's Health Issue*. Alcohol alert no. 62, National Institute on Alcohol Abuse and Alcoholism (NIAAA), Bethesda, MD.
29. National Institute of Health (NIH) (2007) *Harmful Interactions: Mixing Alcohol with Medications*. NIH Publication No. 03-5329. http://pubs.niaaa.nih.gov/publications/Medicine/Harmful_Interactions.pdf (last accessed 16 April 2014).
30. Blow, F.C. (2000) Treatment of older women with alcohol problems: Meeting the challenge for a special population. *Alcohol Clin Exp Res*, **24**(8), 1257–1266.
31. SAMHSA (2010) *Gender Differences Among Older Black Admissions to Treatment*. The TEDS Report, Office of Applied Studies, Substance Abuse and Mental Health Services Administration (SAMHSA), Rockville, MD.
32. Simoni-Wastila, L. and Yang, H.K. (2006) Psychoactive drug abuse in older adults. *Am J Geriatr Pharmacother*, **4**(4), 380–394.
33. Blazer, D.G. and Wu, L.-T. (2009) Nonprescription use of pain relievers by middle-age and elderly community-living adults: National Survey on Drug Use and Health. *J Am Geriatr Society*, **57**(7), 1252–1257.
34. Gomberg, E.S. (1995) Older women and alcohol. Use and abuse. *Recent Dev Alcohol*, **2**, 61–79.
35. Grella, C.E. (2009) *Older Adults and Co-occurring Disorders*. Alcohol and Drug Policy Institute, Sacramento, CA. http://aodpolicy.org/Docs/Older_Adults_COD.pdf (last accessed 16 April 2014).
36. Taylor, M.H. and Grossberg, G.T. (2012) The growing problem of illicit substance abuse in the elderly: A review. *Prim Care Companion CNS Disord*, **14**(4). http://www.ncbi.nlm.nih.gov/pmc/articles/PMC3505129/?report=printable (last accessed 17 April 2014).
37. Moore, A.A., Whiteman, E.J. and Ward, K.T. (2007) Risks of combined alcohol/medication use in older adults. *Am J Geriatr Pharmacother*, **5**(1), 64–74.

38. SAMHSA (2012) Older America's Behavior Health Issue Brief 5: Prescription medication misuse and abuse among older adults. Administration on Aging (AoA), Substance Abuse and Mental Health Service Administration. http://www.aoa.gov/AoARoot/AoA_Programs/HPW/Behavioral/docs2/Issue%20Brief%205%20Prescription%20Med%20Misuse%20Abuse.pdf (last accessed 17 April 2014).

39. Weathermon, R. and Crabb, D.W. (1999) Alcohol and medication interactions. *Alcohol Res Health*, **23**(1), 40–54.

40. Antonucci, T.C., Ajrouch, K.J. and Birditt, K.S. (2006) Social relations in the third age: Assessing strengths and challenges using the Convoy Model. In: *Annual Review of Gerontology and Geriatrics: Vol. 26. The Crown of Life Dynamics of the Early Postretirement Period* (eds J.B. James, P. Wink and K.W. Schaie). Springer Publishing, New York, pp. 193–209.

41. Berk, L.E. (2010) Emotional and social development in late adulthood. In: *Development Through the Lifespan*, 5th edn (ed. L.E. Berk). Allyn & Bacon, Boston, pp. 473–499.

42. Brennan, P.L., Moos, R.H. and Kim, Y.J. (1993) Gender differences in the individual characteristics and life contexts of late middle-aged and older problem drinkers. *Addiction*, **88**(6), 781–790.

43. Knight, B.G. and Robinson, G.S. (2002) *Cognitive-Behavioral Therapy*. [Online] Encyclopedia of Aging. http://www.encyclopedia.com (last accessed 17 April 2014).

44. Satre, D.D., Knight, B.G. and David, S. (2006) Cognitive-behavioral interventions with older adults: integrating clinic and gerontological research. *Prof Psychol Res Pr*, **37**(5), 489–498.

45. Lau, A.W. and Kinoshita, L.M. (2013) Cognitive-behavioral therapy with culturally diverse older adults. In: *Culturally Responsive Cognitive-Behavioral Therapy* (eds P.A. Hayes and G.Y. Iwamasa). American Psychological Association, Washington, DC, pp. 179–197.

46. Center for Substance Abuse Treatment (CSAT) (2006) *Substance Abuse: Administrative Issues in Outpatient Treatment*. Treatment Improvement Protocol (TIP) Series 46, DHHS Publication No. (SMA) 06-4151, Substance Abuse and Mental Health Services Administration, Rockville, MD.

47. Timko, C. (2008) Outcomes of AA for special populations. In: Research on Alcoholics Anonymous and Spirituality. *Recent developments in alcoholism*, Volume **XVIII** (eds M. Galanter and L. Kaskutas). Springer Publishing, New York, pp. 373–392.

48. Karlin, B.E. (2011) Cognitive Behavioral Therapy with older adults. In: *Cognitive Behavior Therapy with Older Adults. Innovations Across Care Settings* (eds K.H. Sorocco and S. Lauderdale). Springer Publishing, New York, pp. 1–28.

49. Bohlmeijer, E., Roemer, M., Cuijpers, P. and Smit, F. (2007) The effects of reminiscence on psychological well-being in older adults: A meta-analysis. *Aging Ment Health*, **11**(3), 291–300.

50. Watt, L.M. and Cappeliez, P. (2000) Integrative and instrumental reminiscence therapies for depression in older adults: Intervention strategies and treatment effectiveness. *Aging Ment Health*, **4**(2), 166–177.

51. Zelinski, E.M. and Steward, S.T. (1998) Individual differences in 16-year memory changes. *Psychol Aging*, **13**(4), 622–630.

52. Zelinski, E.M., Dalton, S.E. and Hindin, S.B. (2011) Cognitive changes in healthy older adults. *Generations*, **35**(2), 13–20.

53. Mcgaugh, J.L. (2013) Making lasting memories: Remembering the significant. *Proc Natl Acad Sci USA*, **110**(Suppl 2), 10402–10407.

54. Small, B.J., Hultsch, D.F. and Masson, M.E. (1995) Adult age differences in perceptually based, but not conceptually based implicit tests of memory. *J Gerontol B Psychol Sci Soc Sci*, **50**(3), 162–170.

55. Brennan, P.B. and Moos, R.H. (1991) Functioning, life context, and help-seeking among late-onset problem drinkers: Comparisons with nonproblem and early-onset problem drinkers. *Br J Addict*, **86**(9), 1139–1150.
56. Liberto, J.G. and Oslin, D.W. (1995) Early versus late onset of alcoholism in the elderly. *Int J Addict*, **30**(13–14), 1799–1818.
57. Satre, D.D., Blow, F.C., Chi, F.W. and Weisner, C. (2007) Gender differences in seven year alcohol and drug treatment outcomes among older adults. *Am J Addict*, **16**(3), 216–221.
58. APA (2006) Practice guideline for the treatment of patients with substance use disorders, 2nd edition. In: *American Psychiatric Association Practice Guidelines for the Treatment of Psychiatric Disorders: Compendium 2006*, 314–339. American Psychiatric Association (APA), Arlington, VA. 2006.
59. Gomberg, ES. (1995) Older women and alcohol. Use and abuse. *Recent Dev Alcohol*, **12**, 61–79.
60. Zarba, A., Storr, C. and Wagner, F. (2005) Carrying habits into old age: Prescription drug use without medical advice by older American adults. Letter to the Editor. *J Am Geriatr Soc*, **53**(1), 170–171.
61. Arnaout, B. and Petrakis, I.L. (2008) Diagnosing co-morbid drug use in patients with alcohol use disorders. *Alcohol Res Health*, **31**(2), 148–154.
62. Royal College of Psychiatrists, Older People's Substance Misuse Working Group (2011) *Our Invisible Addicts*. College Report CR165. http://www.thementalelf.net/wp-content/uploads/2011/06/CR165-Our-Invisible-Addicts.pdf (last accessed 17 April 2014).
63. Center for Substance Abuse Treatment (CSAT) (2006) *Detoxification and Substance Abuse Treatment*. Treatment Improvement Protocol (TIP) Series 45, DHHS Publication No. (SMA) 06-4131, Substance Abuse and Mental Health Services Administration, Rockville, MD.
64. Sullivan, L.E., Fiellin, D.A. and O'Connor, P.G. (2005) The prevalence and impact of alcohol problems in major depression: A systematic review. *Am J Med*, **118**(4), 330–341.
65. Tevisan, L., Boutros, N., Petrakis, I. and Krystal, J.H. (1998) Complications from alcohol withdrawal. *Alcohol Health Res World*, **22**(1), 61–66.
66. ASAM (2001) *Patient Placement Criteria for the Treatment of Substance-Related Disorders*, 2nd edn, Revised (ASAM PPC-2R). American Society of Addiction Medicine (ASAM), Chevy Chase, MD.
67. Persons, J.B. and Tompkins, M.A. (2007) Cognitive-behavioral case formulation. In: *Handbook of Psychotherapy Case Formulation*, 2nd edn (ed. T.D. Eells). Guilford Press, New York, pp. 290–316.
68. Teachman, B. and Clerkin, E. (2010) A case formulation approach to resolve treatment complications. In: *Avoiding Treatment Failures in the Anxiety Disorders* (eds M. Otto and S. Hoffmann S). Springer Publishing, New York, pp. 7–30.
69. Persons, J.B. (2008) *A Case Formulation Approach to Cognitive Behavioral Therapy*. Guilford Press, New York.
70. Davis, A.K. and Rosenberg, H. (2012) Acceptance of non-abstinence goals by addiction professionals in the United States. *Psychol Addict Behav*, **27**(4), 1102–1109.
71. Moos, R.H. (2007) Theory-based active ingredients of effective treatments for substance use disorders. *Drug Alcohol Depend*, **88**(2–3), 109–121.
72. Moy, I., Crome, P., Crome, I. and Fisher, M. (2011) Systematic and narrative review of treatment of older people with substance problems. *Eur Geriatr Med*, **2**(4), 212–236.
73. Kuerbis, A. and Sacco, P. (2013) A review of existing treatments for substance abuse among the elderly and recommendations for future directions. *Subst Abuse*, **7**, 13–37.

74. Center for Substance Abuse Treatment (CSAT. (2008) *Managing Depressive Symptoms in Substance Abuse Clients During Early Recovery*. Treatment Improvement Protocol (TIP) Series 48, DHHS Publication No. (SMA) 08-4353, Substance Abuse and Mental Health Services Administration, Rockville, MD.

75. National Institute on Drug Abuse (NIDA) (2012) *Principles of Drug Addiction Treatment. A Research-Based Guide*, 3rd edn (Revised December 2012). National Institutes of Health Publication No. 12–4180. http://www.drugabuse.gov/sites/default/files/podat_1.pdf (last accessed 17 April 2014).

76. Center for Substance Abuse Treatment (CSAT) (2005) *Substance Abuse Treatment for Persons with Co-Occurring Disorders*. Treatment Improvement Protocol (TIP) Series 42, DHHS Publication No. (SMA) 05-3992, Substance Abuse and Mental Health Services Administration, Rockville, MD.

77. Tiet, Q.Q. and Mausbach, B. (2007) Treatments for patients with dual diagnosis: A review. *Alcohol Clin Exp Res*, **31**(4), 513–536.

78. Trafton, J.A., Oliva, EM., Horst, D.A. *et al.* (2004) Treatment needs associated with pain in substance use disorder patients: Implications for concurrent treatment. *Drug Alcohol Depend*, **73**(71), 2023–2031.

79. Brennan, P.L., Schutte, K.K., Soohoo, S. and Moos, R.H. (2011) Painful medical conditions and alcohol use in later life. *Pain Med*, **12**(7), 1049–1059.

80. Brennan, P.L. and Soohoo S. (2013) Pain and use of alcohol later in life. Prospective evidence from the Health and Retirement Study. *J Aging Health*, **25**(4), 656–677.

81. Clifford, P.A., Cipher, D.J., Roper, K.D. *et al.* (2008) Cognitive-behavioral pain management interventions for long-term care residents with physical and cognitive disabilities. In: *Handbook of Behavioral and Cognitive Therapies with Older Adults* (eds D. Gallagher-Thompson, A.M. Steffen and L.W. Thompson). Springer Science and Business Media, LLC, New York, pp. 76–101.

82. Dodge, R., Sindelar, J. and Sinha, R. (2005) The role of depression symptoms in predicting drug abstinence in outpatient substance abuse treatment. *J Subst Abuse Treat*, **28**, 189–196.

83. SAMHSA (2011) *Older Adult Admissions Reporting Alcohol as a Substance of Abuse*: 1992 and 2009. The TEDS Report. 2011. Center for Behavioral Health Statistics and Quality, Substance Abuse and Mental Health Services Administration (SAMHSA), Rockville, MD.

84. Oslin, D.W., Katz, I.R., Edell, W.S. and Ten Have, T.R. (2000) Effects of alcohol consumption on the treatment of depression among elderly patients. *Am J Geriatr Psychiatry*, **8**(3), 215–220.

85. Finlayson, R., Hurt, R., Davis, L. and Morse, R. (1988) Alcoholism in elderly persons: A study of the psychiatric and psychosocial features of 216 inpatients. *Mayo Clin Proc*, **63**, 761–768.

86. Koenig, H.G. and Blazer, D.G. II. (1996) Depression. In: *Encyclopedia of Gerontology: Age, Aging, and the Aged*. Vol. I (ed. J.E. Birren). Academic Press, San Diego, CA, pp. 415–428.

87. Blow, F.C., Brockmann, L.M. and Barry, K.L. (2004) Role of alcohol in late-life suicide. *Alcohol Clin Exp Res*, **28**(5 Suppl), 48S–56S.

88. Bartels, S.J., Coakley, E., Oxman, T.E. *et al.* (2002) Suicidal and death ideation in older primary care patients with depression, anxiety, and at-risk alcohol use. *Am J Geriatr Psychiatry*, **10**(4), 417–427.

89. Center for Substance Abuse Treatment (CSAT) (2009) *Addressing Suicidal Thoughts and Behaviors in Substance Abuse Treatment*. Treatment Improvement Protocol (TIP) Series 50, HHS Publication No. (SMA) 09-4381, Substance Abuse and Mental Health Services Administration, Rockville, MD.

90. Centers for Disease Control and Prevention (2013) Suicide among adults aged 35–64 years – United States, 1999–2010. *MMWR*, **62**(17), 321–342.
91. Centers for Disease Control and Prevention (2005) Web-based Injury Statistics Query and Reporting System (WISQARS) [online]. http://www.cdc.gov/injury/wisqars/index. html (last accessed 17 April 2014).
92. Mertens, B. and Sorenson, S.B. (2012) Current considerations about the elderly and firearms. *Am J Public Health*, **102**(3), 396–400.
93. Atkinson, R.M. and Misra, S. (2002) Further strategies in the treatment of aging alcoholics. In: *Treating Alcohol and Drug Abuse in the Elderly* (eds A.M. Gurnack, R.M. Atkinson and N.J. Osgood). Springer Publishing Company, New York, pp. 131–154.
94. Atkinson, R.M. and Misra, S. (2002) Mental disorders and symptoms in older alcoholics. In: *Treating Alcohol and Drug Abuse in the Elderly* (eds A.M. Gurnack, R.M. Atkinson and N.J. Osgood). Springer Publishing Company, New York, pp. 32–49.
95. NIAAA (2001) *Alcohol and Tobacco*: Alcohol alert no. 71, National Institute on Alcohol Abuse and Alcoholism (NIAAA), Bethesda, MD.
96. Prochaska, J.J., Delucchi, K. and Hall, S.M. (2004) A meta-analysis of smoking cessation interventions with individuals in substance abuse treatment or recovery. *J Consult Clin Psychol*, **72**(6), 1144–1156.
97. American Geriatrics Society Expert Panel on the Care of Older Adults with Multi-morbidity (2012) Patient-centered care for older adults with multiple chronic conditions: A stepwise approach from the American Geriatrics Society. *J Am Geriatr Soc*, **60**(10), 1957–1968.
98. Substance Abuse and Mental Health Services Administration (SAMHSA) (2009) *Get Connected! Toolkit: Linking Older Adults with Medication, Alcohol, and Mental Health Resources*. http://www.samhsa.gov/aging/docs/GetConnectedToolkit.pdf (last accessed 17 April 2014).
99. Fleming, M.F., Manwell, L.B., Barry, K.L. *et al.* (2013) Brief physician advice for alcohol problems in older adults: A randomized community based trial. *J Fam Pract*, **48**(5), 378–384.
100. Kaner, E.F.S., Dickinson, H.O., Beyer, F. *et al.* (2007) Effectiveness of brief alcohol intervention in primary care populations. *Cochrane Database of Systematic Reviews* **2** (Art. No.: CD004148). doi: 10.1002/14651858.CD004148.pub3.
101. Center for Substance Abuse Treatment (CSAT) (1999) *Brief Interventions and Brief Therapies for Substance Abuse*. Treatment Improvement Protocol (TIP) Series 34, HHS Publication No. (SMA) 09-3952, Substance Abuse and Mental Health Services Administration, Rockville, MD.
102. McKellar, J., Austin, J. and Moos, R. (2012) Building the first step: A review of low-intensity interventions for stepped care. *Addict Sci Clin Pract*, **7**, 26. http://www. ncbi.nlm.nih.gov/pmc/articles/PMC3554471/pdf/1940-0640-7-26.pdf (last accessed 17 April 2014).
103. Schonfeld, L., Kin-Kallimanis, B.L., Duchene, D.M. *et al.* (2010) Screening and brief intervention for substance misuse among older adults: The Florida BRITE Project. *Am J Public Health*, **100**(1), 108–114.
104. Florida BRief Intervention and Treatment for Elder (BRITE) Project Health Promotion Workbook; Version1-4-06. http://brite.fmhi.usf.edu/Files/BRITEWorkbook-English. pdf (last accessed 17 April 2014).
105. Miller, W. and Rollnick, S.S. (1991) *Motivational Interviewing: Preparing People to Change Addictive Behavior*. The Guilford Press, New York.
106. Smedslund, G., Berg, R.C., Hammerstrøm, K.T. *et al.* (2011) Motivational interviewing for substance abuse. *Cochrane Database Syst Rev* **5** (Art.No.:CD008063). doi: 10.1002/14651858.CD008063.pub2.

107. Center for Substance Abuse Treatment (CSAT) (1999) *Brief Interventions and Brief Therapies for Substance Abuse.* Treatment Improvement Protocol (TIP) 34, HHS Publication No. (SMA) 09-3952, Substance Abuse and Mental Health Services Administration, Rockville, MD.

108. Miller, W.R., Zweben, A., DiClemente, C.C. and Rychtarik, R.G. (1999) Motivational enhancement therapy manual: A clinical research guide for therapists treating individuals with alcohol abuse and dependence. Project MATCH Monograph Series, Vol. 2 (reprinted), DHHS Publication No. 94-3723, National Institute on Alcohol Abuse and Alcoholism (NIAAA), Rockville, MD.

109. Prochaska, J.O. and DiClemente, C.C. (1986) Toward a comprehensive model of change. In: *Addictive Behaviors: Processes of Change* (eds W. Miller and N. Heather). Plenum Press, New York, pp. 3–28.

110. Wang, D.S. (2011) Interdisciplinary methods of treatment of depression in older adults: A primer for practitioners. *Act Adapt Aging*, **35**(4), 298–314.

111. Gallagher-Thompson, D., Steffen, A.M. and Thompson, L.W. (eds) (2008) *Handbook of Behavioral and Cognitive Therapies with Older Adults.* Springer Science and Business Media, LLC, New York.

112. Gurnack, A. (2002) Introduction and overview. In: *Treating Alcohol and Drug Abuse in the Elderly* (eds A.M. Gurnack, R.M. Atkinson and N.J. Osgood). Springer Publishing Company, New York, pp. 1–8.

113. Kadden, R., Carroll, K.M., Donovan, D. *et al.* (1994) *Cognitive-Behavioral Coping Skills Therapy Manual: A Clinical Research Guide for Therapists Treating Individuals with Alcohol Abuse and Dependence.* Project MATCH Monograph Series, Vol. 3, DHHS Publication No. 94-3724, National Institute on Alcohol Abuse and Alcoholism (NIAAA), Rockville, MD.

114. Westbrook, D., Kennerley, H. and Kirk, J. (2011) *An Introduction to Cognitive Behaviour Therapy.* Sage Publications Ltd, London.

115. Dupree, L.W., Schonfeld, L., Dearborn-Harshman, K.O. and Lynn, N. (2008) A relapse-prevention model for older alcohol abusers. In: *Handbook of Behavioral and Cognitive Therapies with Older Adults* (eds D. Gallagher-Thompson, A.M. Steffen and L.W. Thompson). Springer Science and Business Media, LLC, New York, pp.76–101.

116. Dupree, L.W. and Schonfeld, L. (1998) *Substance Abuse Relapse Prevention for Older Adults: A Group Treatment Approach.* Center for Substance Abuse Treatment, Rockville, MD.

117. Wilkinson, C., Allsop, S. and Chikritzhs, T. (2011) Alcohol pouring practices among 65- to 74-year-olds in Western Australia. *Drug Alcohol Rev*, **30**(2), 200–206.

118. Adams, W.L. (2002) The effects of alcohol on medical illnesses and medication interactions. In: *Treating Alcohol and Drug Abuse in the Elderly* (eds A.M. Gurnack, R.M. Atkinson and N.J. Osgood). Springer Publishing Company, New York, pp. 32–49.

119. Brooks, J.T., Buchacz, K., Gebo, K.A. and Mermin, J. (2012) HIV infection and older Americans: The public health perspective. *Am J Public Health*, **102**(8), 1516–1526.

120. Centers for Disease Control and Prevention (CDC) (2013) *Diagnoses Of HIV Infection Among Adults Aged 50 Years And Older In The United States And Dependent Areas, 2007–2010. HIV Surveillance Supplemental Report*, **18**(No. 3). http://www.cdc.gov/hiv/topics/surveillance/resources/reports/#supplemental (last accessed 16 April 2014).

121. Centers for Disease Control and Prevention (CDC) (2008) *HIV/AIDS Among Persons Aged 50 and Older: CDC HIV/AIDS Facts.* US Department of Health and Human Services, Washington, DC.

122. Center for Disease Control and Prevention (CDC) (2012) Recommendations for the identification of chronic hepatitis C virus infection among persons born during 1945–1965. *MMWR*, **61**(4), 1–32.

123. Lemke, S. and Moos, R.H. (2003) Outcomes at 1 and 5 years for older patients with alcohol use disorders. *J Subst Abuse Treat*, **24**(1), 43–50.
124. Satre, D.D., Mertens, J.R., Arean, P. and Weisner, C. (2004) Five-year alcohol and drug treatment outcomes of older adults versus middle-aged and younger adults in a managed care program. *Addiction*, **99**(10), 1286–1297.
125. Institute of Medicine (IOM) (2012) *The Mental Health and Substance Use Workforce for Older Adults: In Whose Hands?* The National Academies Press, Washington, DC.
126. Timko, C. and DeBenedetti, A. (2007) A randomized controlled trial of intensive referral to 12-step self-help groups: One-year outcomes. *Drug Alcohol Depend*, **90**(2–3), 270–279.
127. Timko, C. (2008) Research on Alcoholics Anonymous and spirituality. In: *Recent Developments in Alcoholism*, Vol. **XVIII** (M. Galanter and L. Kaskutas). Springer Publishing, New York, pp. 373–392.
128. Blow, F.C., Walton, M.A., Chermack, S.T. *et al.* (2000) Older adult treatment outcome following elder-specific inpatient alcoholism treatment. *J Subst Abuse Treat*, **19**(1), 67–75.
129. Brennan, P.L., Nichol, A.C. and Moos, R.H. (2003) Older and younger patients with substance use disorders: Outpatient mental health service use and functioning over a 12-month interval. *Psychol Addict Behav*, **17**(1), 42–48.
130. Lemke, S. and Moos, R. (2002) Prognosis of older patients in mixed-age alcoholism treatment programs. *J Subst Abuse Treat*, **22**(1), 33–43.
131. Oslin, D., Pettinati, H. and Volpicelli, J. (2002) Alcoholism treatment adherence: older age predicts better adherence and drinking outcomes. *Am J Geriatr Psychiatry*, **10**(6), 740–747.
132. Nowinski, J., Baker, S. and Carroll, K. (1999) *Twelve Step Facilitation Therapy Manual. A Clinical Research Guide for Therapists Treating Individuals with Alcohol Abuse And Dependence*. Project MATCH Monograph Series, Vol. 1 (reprinted), DHHS/NIH Publication No. 94-3722, National Institute on Alcohol Abuse and Alcoholism (NIAAA), Rockville, MD.
133. Longabaugh, R.H. and Wirtz, P.W. (2001) *Project MATCH Hypotheses, Results and Causal Chain Analyses*. Project MATCH Monograph Series, Vol. 8, DHHS Publication No. 01-4238, National Institute on Alcohol Abuse and Alcoholism (NIAAA), Rockville, MD.
134. Isaacson, J.H., Hopper, J.A., Alford, D.P. and Parran, T. (2005) Prescription drug use and abuse. Risk factors, red flags, and prevention strategies. *Postgrad Med*, **118**(1), 19–26.
135. Agency for Healthcare Research and Quality (AHRQ) Patient Centered Medical Home Resource Center. http://pcmh.ahrq.gov (last accessed 17 April 2014).
136. Brown, R.L., Saunders, L.A., Bobula, J.A. *et al.* (2007) Randomized controlled trial of a telephone and mail intervention for alcohol use disorders: three-month drinking outcomes. *Alcohol Clin Exp Res*, **31**: 1372–1379.
137. Kypri, K., Hallett, J., Howat, P. *et al.* (2009) Randomized controlled trial of proactive web-based alcohol screening and brief intervention for university students. *Arch Intern Med*, **169**(16), 1508–1514.
138. White, A., Kavanagh, D., Stallman, H. *et al.* (2010) Online alcohol interventions: a systematic review *J Med Internet Res*, **12**(5), e62

Chapter 23
INTEGRATED TREATMENT MODELS FOR CO-MORBID DISORDERS

Rahul (Tony) Rao

Institute of Psychiatry/Dual Diagnosis, Mental Health of Older Adults and Dementia Clinical Academic Group, South London and Maudsley NHS Foundation Trust, UK

Introduction

The presence of psychiatric co-morbidity in older people with substance misuse usually raises additional challenges for the delivery of safe and clinically effective services to meet the needs of both substance misuse (including those taking one or more substance) and one or more mental disorders. In this chapter, the term Substance Misuse and Co-morbid Mental Disorder (SMCD) will be used to describe this group. Co-morbid mental disorders (termed 'co-occurring disorders' or 'dual diagnosis') in older people refer to any accompanying mental disorder, but most often depression and cognitive impairment; with the latter mostly referring to alcohol-related brain injury.

In community settings, the highest level of co-morbidity in older people is most common in the 75–84 age group and is largely attributable to dependence and delirium associated with benzodiazepine use and withdrawal [1]. There is also a range of co-morbidities associated with intoxication and withdrawal from drugs and alcohol, such sedation, agitation, suicidal ideation, delirium and psychotic symptoms [2]. SMCD ranges from 21–66%, with higher rates seen across inpatient settings for those with more severe mental health problems [3]. Older adults with depression are three to four times more likely to have alcohol-related problems than those without [4], with higher risk of suicide and social/functional impairment [5].

Older people with SMCD show greater service use in both inpatient and outpatient samples compared with those without co-occurring disorders [6]. This observation has been replicated within the national Veterans Affairs (VA) Network, which provides substance abuse, detoxification services and continuing care across the United States. In a study of more than 21 000 patients aged 55 and above in the VA system, 28% were diagnosed with both substance use and psychiatric disorders at the time of admission to treatment [7]. Patients with SMCD had more outpatient mental health visits prior to admission for substance abuse treatment, and were more likely to be readmitted for treatment at one-year and four-year follow-up,

Substance Use and Older People, First Edition.
Edited by Ilana B. Crome, Li-Tzy Wu, Rahul (Tony) Rao and Peter Crome.
© 2015 John Wiley & Sons, Ltd. Published 2015 by John Wiley & Sons, Ltd.

compared to those without co-occurring disorders [8]. The four-year follow up study also found a higher death rate in SMCD compared with the general population matched for age, race and gender compared with general population rates [9]. The death rate was higher still for those older people with organic brain injury. Reduced mortality rates at a three-year follow up were seen for people who survived for one year after discharge from the index episode and had between one and five outpatient mental health visits, as compared to those who received no mental health follow-up.

In spite of a growing body of evidence for the need to provide services for this 'invisible' group, there has been no cohesive global strategy to address this need. In the United Kingdom, The National Service Framework for Older People [10] makes no mention of service planning for older people with SMCD. Policy documents for geriatric medicine mention substance misuse only in relation to delirium or falls [11, 12]. Although some progress has been made in *Alcohol Use Disorders: Diagnosis, Assessment and Management of Harmful Drinking and Alcohol Dependence* [13], there is only fleeting reference to the needs of older people, again with no mention of SMCD. Guidelines for the management of drug dependence [14] devote just one page to older people. The most significant advance has been the publication of the second report of the UK Enquiry into Mental Health and Wellbeing in Later Life [15], which briefly details epidemiology and psychosocial risk factors in the context of SMCD. United Kingdom policy on SMCD in older people is considerably overshadowed by similar policy strategies in the USA, which has produced a specific treatment intervention protocol guide for the implementation of substance misuse services for older people [16]. This has been further developed into a coordinated approach to address medication, alcohol and mental health problems [17].

Methodological approach to examining SMCD in older people

A. Current systems of care for substance misuse and mental disorders

Service configuration for substance misuse and mental disorders has often meant either sequential or parallel treatment, with the potential for an un-coordinated approach to treatment [18]. Sequential treatment approaches result in patients receiving treatment for one problem at a time, with treatment for the other problem being deferred until the first is resolved or improved. The only contact between the two services is when the patient transfers between them. In parallel treatment, approaches involve different providers from different services system treating the two disorders simultaneously.

Integrated treatment models offer comprehensive services for both mental illness and substance misuse from a multidisciplinary treatment team, thereby overcoming barriers to care and debate over which disorder is primary. Both disorders are case managed to improve health and social function within a single care plan.

B.   Service implications

Targeting service delivery for SMCD in older people with dual diagnosis requires a different focus, with particular consideration given to those at highest risk. Such groups include those older people at risk as a consequence of previous history of mental illness or bereavement, retirement, social isolation and physical problems, as well as those with depression, anxiety and cognitive impairment [19]. Integrated approaches to treatment cannot be achieved unless there is an approach addressing all these areas of need. For example, in the United States, only 12% of older adults who are in need of substance abuse treatment actually receive substance abuse treatment [20]. There may be a multitude of reasons for this, including perceived cost of treatment, stigma around labelling as an 'addict', unwillingness to give up substance use and a false sense of autonomy in believing that they can give up substance misuse without additional help [21]. Cultural competence is also a core component of service for older people with SMCD. There remain significant barriers to providing culturally appropriate services. For example, in the United Kingdom, older Irish people living in England have particular problems in accessing mental health services and such services are not sufficiently equipped to meet their needs [22]. There is also a higher rate of co-morbid depression in older compared with younger people in this ethnic group [23]. Creating a culturally competent workforce is, therefore, central to providing a needs-led service for older people with substance misuse and co-morbid mental disorders. The level of unmet need in service provision for older people with substance misuse remains unknown.

C.   Principles underlying integrated treatment models for SMCD in older people

At the heart of integrated treatment is shared decision making based on a common vision. This is best exemplified by discussions around treatment by a range of disciplines [24–27] These disciplines comprise addiction psychiatrists, old age psychiatrists, mental health nurses, psychologists, social workers, occupational therapists and support workers. Each team member has a unique perspective around medical, cognitive/behavioural, social and functional aspects of lifestyle and illness. Integrated treatment has core components, the most pertinent of which are comprehensiveness, assertiveness, reduction of negative consequences, a long-term perspective, motivation-based treatment and the availability of multiple psychotherapeutic modalities [28]. A comprehensive assessment should cover both substance misuse and age-related aspects that are relevant to management (Box 23.1).

Another component is an 'assertive' approach that involves the use of outreach models, such as the home-based model adopted in the United Kingdom approach (see below), particularly for housebound older people who cannot access traditional substance misuse services. Such an approach is key to success in engaging older people with SMCD and incorporates crisis intervention, practical support (monitoring safety, food intake, medication management, benefits, arranging transport), monitoring of mental disorders, a review of treatment, social engagement

Box 23.1 Comprehensive assessment of SMCD in older people

- Demographics age/sex/ethnicity/living arrangements/living environment
- Presenting problem (may be masked and requires a flexible approach)
- Discuss substances separately (alcohol/nicotine/OTC/prescribed/illicit)
  - Age at first use, weekend, weekly and daily use
  - Age of dependence syndrome
  - Maximum use and when/how long
  - Pattern (quantity/frequency) over day/week
  - Route
  - Cost/funding
  - Abstinence/relapse and link to stability/life events
  - Preferred substance
- Treatment (dates, service, intervention, outcome)
- Past and family psychiatric history
- Occupational and psychosexual history
- Medical history (especially known complications form substance and effects on existing age-related impairment)
- Forensic history (especially public order and acquisitive offences)
- Social vulnerability – risk of falls, social/cultural isolation, financial abuse
- Social function – activities of daily living, statutory/voluntary/private care
- Social support – informal carers and friends
- Social pressures – debt, substance using 'carers', open drug dealing
- Mental state (including evidence of mental disorder)
- Consent and capacity
- Insight and motivation to change substance misuse behaviour
- Collateral information from:
  - Relatives
  - GP consultations
  - Hospital discharge summaries
  - Home carers
  - Day centres
  - Housing officers/wardens of supported housing
  - Criminal justice agencies
  - Investigations (including cognitive testing and neuroimaging)

and family support. The final component is the largest in terms of time and resource allocation; this covers harm reduction and relapse prevention. Harm reduction differs from approaches involving abstinence in that it seeks to improve quality of life through minimizing the risks associated with substance misuse. For example, in older people with alcohol misuse, this involves interventions such as motivational interviewing to address ambivalence over changing drinking behaviour, limiting access to alcohol and monitoring the physical effects of alcohol-related liver disease.

Approaches to harm reduction will involve substituting substance use with alternative activities such as improving social networks, improving physical function and reducing risks such as adverse drug interactions, delirium and falls, encouraging new hobbies, brief intervention and brief advice, supportive psychotherapy, cognitive behavioural therapy, social skills training around refusal of substance use, psychoeducation (including family education), pharmacological treatment (e.g. anti-craving medication, methadone maintenance, nicotine replacement treatment), detoxification and consideration of alternative housing [29–31].

Once harm reduction has been implemented, relapse prevention will involve a longer term perspective and involves expanding opportunities for social integration, such as attending self-help groups (e.g. Alcoholics Anonymous), increasing family support, maintaining healthy lifestyles and living environments and encouraging volunteering activities.

D. Developing integrated treatment models for older people with substance misuse and co-morbid psychiatric disorders

In the United States, the Treatment Improvement Protocol Consensus Panel (US Department of Health and Human Services, 1998) recommended incorporating the following features into substance abuse treatment for older adults:

- Age-specific group treatment that is supportive and nonconfrontational to improve self-esteem.
- Coping with depression, loneliness and loss.
- Rebuilding support networks.
- Age-appropriate pace and content.
- Appropriately trained staff who are interested in working with older people.
- Links with medical and social services, as well as institutional settings.
- Clinical case management for co-occurring disorders.

Several areas of best practice exist in the United States, particularly in Florida, where a screening and intervention programme has been evaluated to address the underuse of substance abuse treatment for older adults [32]. The programme provided relapse prevention and social skills training, identifying high-risk situations for relapse. By developing coping skills for dealing with social pressure, social isolation, feelings of depression and anxiety, those who completed the programme demonstrated higher rates of abstinence compared to the noncompleters. However, there was a 50% drop-out rate for programme completion.

Key to this service model was integrated assessment and treatment for SMCD, comprising:

- Awareness raising.
- Outreach, screening, and intervention by generalists (e.g. general practitioners, geriatricians and practitioners working in preventative medicine), addiction specialists, nurses, social workers and mental health counsellors.

- Specific settings targeted to the elderly, including health fairs, day centres, retirement communities and housing sites.
- Working with community agencies to develop referral networks, such as primary care, social, ageing and other service providers.
- Screening protocols for misuse of alcohol, prescription medications, over-the-counter medications and illegal drugs, as well as depression and risk of suicide.

The same study found that of the 3300 adults referred for screening, approximately 60% screened positive for at least one problem. Half of those screening positive for alcohol misuse also screened positive for depression.

In England, London currently has the highest prevalence of alcohol-related mortality in people aged 75 and over, with an average of 25.7 per 100 000 deaths between 1998 and 2004 [33]. Within Southwark (a London borough), this mortality rate is two and a half times that of London as a whole. For North Southwark Community Mental Health Team (CMHT), between 10 and 20% of referrals at weekly multidisciplinary meetings in the late 1990s and between 2000 and 2001 were for SMCD and between 10 and 50% of admissions to the local catchment area acute mental health unit for older people had SMCD. These figures were based on annual clinical audit of community mental health team caseloads. A clinical audit of this CMHT referrals was therefore undertaken between January and December 2000. It demonstrated that nearly 15% of referrals for depression were accompanied by alcohol misuse.

After a senior member medical staff acquired clinical and research expertise in addictions, a service to meet the needs of older people with SMCD was developed in London over the following years [34]. The service was and continues to be located within the existing generic mainstream community mental health team. This generic team is based on the 'Guy's model' of care, which was the first open-access service in the United Kingdom for older people's mental health, accepting referrals from any source (including self-referrals) and offering a system of multi-disciplinary assessment and case management across the range of specialties. This service model is now termed 'New Ways of Working' [35], although the service was set up in 1981, long before this UK government initiative was launched. It remains one of the few services in the country that has doctors as care coordinators/key workers, thereby allowing a 'hands-on' approach to care and an in-depth experience of day-to-day management problems. This has been particularly advantageous in the area of SMCD involving alcohol misuse, where the consultant psychiatrist (referred to above with experience in addiction) is care coordinator for older people with complex problems relating to alcohol misuse, sharing expertise and seeking help from other specialties when required. Between 2005 and 2009, this model of service provision was associated with a fall in the percentage of alcohol-related admissions with dual diagnosis from up to 50% to fewer than 5%. However, the problem of alcohol misuse in the area has increased further, with an 80% increase in the number of older people with dual diagnosis on the team caseload between 2003 and 2009. This is likely to be a reflection of an improvement in the clinical effectiveness of community-based approaches to alcohol misuse, even in the face of rising numbers of older people with alcohol misuse.

In 2009, a strategic vision was introduced for all clinical services within the South London and Maudsley NHS Foundation Trust, with the main aim of improving the detection, treatment and health outcomes for older people with SMCD. The following objectives were identified:

- Building on existing good practice improving access to services.
- Creating new service options where possible.
- Developing clinically effective care pathways.
- Promoting robust partnerships with key stakeholders (including working with service users and carers).
- Building a skilled workforce skilled to address unmet need.
- Promoting health education/prevention/early intervention.

The SMCD strategy is currently being evaluated, with key performance indicators being training in core SMCD for at least 80% of all clinical staff, audit of drug (including cigarettes, illicit, prescribed and over-the-counter medication) and alcohol screening from electronic patient records and identifying 'champions' within each clinical multidisciplinary team who undergo advanced SMCD training and offer supervision to clinical staff. There has also been considerable progress in raising awareness of SMCD and formal teaching in this area to care of the elderly medicine services, social services, day centres and voluntary organisations such as Age Concern and Alcohol Concern.

A recent study of this service has shown that 40% of older people with SMCD referred from medical inpatient settings achieved either abstinence or controlled drinking within the Mental Health of Older Adults Clinical Academic Group [36]. Although there was no control group, this outcome is similar to outcomes in younger people [37].

E. Research evidence for integrated treatment models

Controlled studies of integrated treatment models have shown that long-term, motivation-based integrated treatment models have significantly better outcomes than those using standard, nonintegrated approaches, such as those using parallel or sequential approaches [38–41]. A more recent study [42, 43] provides sound evidence (based on a methodologically robust study design) for global improvements in outcomes such as social functioning and reduction in use of secondary substances. However, none of these controlled studies included older people and studies in this age group that include a range of health and social outcomes are still awaited.

United Kingdom guidance on the treatment of psychosis with co-existing substance misuse [44] offers an integrated approach to managing SMCD, outlining general approaches to forging a therapeutic relationship (e.g. being nonjudgemental and flexible), detecting substance use from a variety of sources, including people with SMCD within both mental health and substance misuse services, joint working between services (including staff competency in carrying out a complete needs assessment) and policies that promote a safe and therapeutic inpatient environment for people with SMCD. Although the guidance refers to 'age-appropriate' service provision, this refers to younger rather than older people.

Future direction and challenges

The development of an integrated approach to care from a workforce that has competencies in the assessment and treatment of older people with substance misuse and co-occurring mental disorders remains the most pressing challenge for the twenty-first century [45]. Older people with SMCD require a considerably different approach to younger people, focusing more on chronic physical disorders, depression and organic brain disorders, as well as social aspects such as social isolation, bereavement, activities of daily living, mental capacity, safeguarding and carer support. Challenges also lie within the prevention of hospital admission and institutionalization through the delivery of home-based services, as well as the detection of SMCD by geriatricians within inpatient settings.

In the United Kingdom, the development of the first training course for health professionals in improving knowledge skills and attitudes around older people with SMCD marks a turning point for developing a competent workforce [46]. However, true integration will also mean engaging physicians, social care agencies and the voluntary sector in improving the quality of life for older people with SMCD. The demand for SMCD services is likely to increase over the coming decades [47], with alcohol-related brain injury likely to comprise a large part of this demand, yet even integrated treatment approaches find it problematic to alter substance use behaviour in this patient group [36]. In developing countries, services for SMCD in older people are still in their infancy. To develop and ensure that they are sustained will mean a coordinated approach from clinicians, academics, care staff and voluntary sector in driving policy change at a national level.

References

1. Frisher, M., Crome, I., Macleod, J. *et al.* (2005) Substance misuse and psychiatric illness: a prospective observation study. *Journal of Epidemiology and Community Health*, 58, 847–850.
2. Crome, I.B. and Day, E. (2002) Substance misuse. In: *Mental Health in Primary Care* (eds. A. Elder and J. Holmes). Oxford University Press, pp. 221–240.
3. Bartels, S.J., Blow, F.C., Van Citters, A.D. and Brockmann, L.M. (2006) Dual diagnosis among older adults: Co-occurring substance abuse and psychiatric illness. *Journal of Dual Diagnosis*, 2(3), 9–30.
4. Devanand, D.P. (2002) Comorbid psychiatric disorders in late life depression. *Biological Psychiatry*, 52(3), 236–242.
5. Davis, L., Uezato, A., Newell, J.M. *et al.* (2008) Major depression and comorbid substance use disorders. *Current Opinion in Psychiatry*, 21, 14–18.

6. Bartels, S.J., Coakley, E., Zubritsky, C. *et al.* (2004) Improving access to geriatric mental health services: a randomized trial comparing treatment engagement in integrated and enhanced referral care for depression, anxiety, and at-risk alcohol use. *American Journal of Psychiatry* **161**, 1455–1462.

7. Moos, R.H., Brennan, P.L. and Mertens, J.R. (1994) Diagnostic subgroups and predictors of one-year re-admission among late-middle-aged and older substance abuse patients. *Journal of Studies on Alcohol*, **55**, 173–183.

8. Moos, R.H., Mertens, J.R. and Brennan, P.L. (1994) Rates and predictors of four-year readmission among late-middle-aged and older substance abuse patients. *Journal of Studies on Alcohol*, **55**, 561–570.

9. Moos, R.H., Brennan, P.L. and Mertens, J.R. (1994) Mortality rates and predictors of mortality among late-middle-aged and older substance abuse patients. *Alcoholism, Clinical and Experimental Research*, **18**, 187–195.

10. UK Department of Health (2001) *National Service Framework for Older People*. Department of Health, London.

11. British Geriatrics Society (2006) *Guidelines for the Prevention, Diagnosis and Management of Delirium in Older People in Hospital*. Royal College of Physicians, London.

12. British Geriatrics Society (2007) *Best Practice Guide 4.5, Falls*. Royal College of Physicians, London.

13. NICE (2010) *Alcohol Use Disorders: Diagnosis, Assessment and Management of Harmful Drinking and Alcohol Dependence*. Clinical Guideline 115, National Institute of Clinical Excellence (NICE), London.

14. Department of Health, London (United Kingdom); Scottish Office Dept. of Health, Edinburgh (United Kingdom); Department of Health and Social Services for Northern Ireland, Belfast (United Kingdom) (2007) *Drug Misuse and Dependence Guidelines on Clinical Management*. The Stationery Office, London.

15. Age Concern (2007) *Improving Services and Support to Older People with Mental Health Problems–Second Report from the UK Enquiry into Mental Health and Wellbeing in Later Life*. Age Concern, London.

16. US Department of Health and Human Services (1998) *Substance Abuse Among Older Adults*. Treatment Improvement Protocol (TIP) #26, Center for Substance Abuse Treatment, Substance Abuse and Mental Health Services Administration, Rockville, MD.

17. US Department of Health and Human Services (2002) *Promoting Older Adult Health*. Pub. No. 02-3628, Substance Abuse and Mental Health Services Administration (SAMHSA), Rockville, MD.

18. Torrens, M., Rossi, P.C., Martinez-Riera, R. *et al.* (2012) Psychiatric co-morbidity and substance use disorders: treatment in parallel systems or in one integrated system? *Substance Use and Misuse*, **47**, 1005–1014.

19. Rao, R. (2006) Alcohol misuse and ethnicity. Hidden populations with growing problems need specific services – and more research. *British Medical Journal*, **332**, 682.

20. Gfroerer J., Penne M., Pemberton M. *et al.* (2003) Substance abuse treatment need among older adults in 2020: the impact of the aging baby-boom cohort. *Drug and Alcohol Dependence*, **69**, 127–135.

21. US Department of Health and Human Services (2013) *Results from the 2012 National Survey on Drug Use and Health: Summary of National Findings*. NSDUH Series H-46, HHS Publication No. (SMA) 13-4795, Substance Abuse and Mental Health Services Administration, Rockville, MD.

22. Rao, R., Wolff, K. and Marshall E.J. (2008) Alcohol use and misuse in older people: a local prevalence study comparing English and Irish inner-city residents living in the UK. *Journal of Substance Use*, **13**, 17–26.

23. Atkinson, R. (1999) Depression, alcoholism and ageing: a brief review. *International Journal of Geriatric Psychiatry* , **14**, 905–910.
24. Oslin, D.W. (2004) Late-life alcoholism: Issues relevant to the geriatric psychiatrist. *American Journal of Geriatric Psychiatry*, **12**(6), 571–583.
25. Dawes, E. and Murphy, B. (2011) *Older Adults and Alcohol: Visioning a Service Delivery Network*. University of Pittsburgh School of Social Work, Pittsburgh, PA.
26. Satre, D.D., Sterling, S.A., Mackin, R.S. and Weisner, C. (2011) Patterns of alcohol and drug use among depressed older adults seeking outpatient psychiatric services. *The American journal of geriatric psychiatry: official journal of the American Association for Geriatric Psychiatry*, **19**(8), 695.
27. Christie, M.M., Bamber, D., Powell, C. *et al*. (2013). Older adult problem drinkers: Who presents for alcohol treatment? *Aging & Mental Health*, **17**(1), 24–32.
28. Mueser, K.T., Noordsy, D.L., Drake, R.E. *et al*. (2003) *Integrated Treatment for Dual Disorders: A Guide to Effective Practice*. Guilford Press, New York, NY.
29. Marlatt, G.A. and Witkiewitz, K. (2002) Harm reduction approaches to alcohol use: Health promotion, prevention, and treatment. *Addictive Behaviors*, **27**(6), 867–886.
30. Bean, K.F., Shafer, M.S. and Glennon, M. (2013) The impact of housing first and peer support on people who are medically vulnerable and homeless. *Psychiatric Rehabilitation Journal*, **36**(1), 48.
31. Ligon, J. (2013) When older adult substance abuse affects others: What helps and what doesn't? *Journal of Social Work Practice in the Addictions*, **13**(2), 223–226.
32. Schonfeld, S., King-Kallimanis, B.L., Duchene, D.M. *et al*. (2010) Screening and Brief Intervention for Substance Misuse Among Older Adults: The Florida BRITE Project. *American Journal of Public Health*, **100**(1),108–114.
33. ICHSC (2006) *Statistics on Alcohol, England 2006*. Information Centre for Health & Social Care (ICHSC), London.
34. Rao, R. and Shanks, A. (2011) Development and implementation of a dual diagnosis strategy for older people in south east London. *Advances in Dual Diagnosis*, **4**, 28–35.
35. Care Services Improvement Partnership, National Institute for Mental Health in England (2007) *Mental Health: New Ways of Working for Everyone: Developing and Sustaining a Flexible and Capable Workforce*. UK Department of Health, London.
36. Rao, R. (2013) Outcomes from liaison psychiatry referrals for older people with alcohol use disorders in the UK. *Mental Health and Substance Use*, **6**(4), 362–368.
37. Adamson, S.J., Heather, N., Morton, V. and Raistrick, D. (2010) Initial preference for drinking goal in the treatment of alcohol problems: II. Treatment outcomes. *Alcohol and Alcoholism*, **45**(2),136–142.
38. Carmichael, D., Tackett-Gibson, M., O'Dell, L. *et al*. (1998) *The Texas Dual Diagnosis Project Evaluation Report, 1997–1998*. Public Policy Institute, Texas A&M University, College Station, TX.
39. Drake, R.E., Yovetich, N.A., Bebout, R.R. *et al*. (1997) Integrated treatment for dually diagnosed homeless adults. *Journal of Nervous & Mental Disease*, **185**, 298–305.
40. Godley, S.H., Hoewing-Roberson, R. and Godley, M.D. (1994) *Final MISA Report*. Lighthouse Institute, Bloomington, IL.
41. Herman, S.E., Frank, K.A., Mowbray, C.T. *et al*. (2000) Longitudinal effects of integrated treatment on alcohol use for persons with serious mental illness and substance use disorders. *Journal of Behavioral Health Services & Research*, **27**, 286–302.
42. Barrowclough, C., Haddock, G., Tarrier, N. *et al*. (2001) Randomized controlled trial of motivational interviewing, cognitive behavior therapy, and family intervention for patients with comorbid schizophrenia and substance use disorders. *American Journal of Psychiatry*, **158**(10),1706–1713.

43. Barrowclough, C., Haddock, G., Wykes, T. *et al.* (2010) Integrated motivational interviewing and cognitive behavioural therapy for people with psychosis and comorbid substance misuse: randomised controlled trial substance misuse: randomised controlled trial. *British Medical Journal*, **341**, 1204–1206.

44. NICE (2011) *Psychosis with Coexisting Substance Misuse: Assessment and Management in Adults and Young People*. Clinical Guideline 120, National Institute for Health and Clinical Excellence (NICE), London.

45. Academy of Medical Royal Colleges (2012) *Alcohol and Other Drugs: Core Medical Competencies*. Royal College of Psychiatrists, London.

46. Saxton, L., Lancashire, S. and Kipping, C. (2011) Meeting the training needs of staff working with older people with dual diagnosis. *Advances in Dual Diagnosis*, **4**, 36–46.

47. Crome, I., Dar, K., Jankiewicz, S. *et al.* (2011) *Our Invisible Addicts. First Report of the Older Persons' Substance Misuse Working Group of the Royal College of Psychiatrists*. The Royal College of Psychiatrists, London.

POLICY: PROPOSALS FOR DEVELOPMENT

Chapter 24

PROPOSALS FOR POLICY DEVELOPMENT: DRUGS

Susanne MacGregor

London School of Hygiene and Tropical Medicine, University of London, UK

Introduction

Drug use among older people is a neglected topic [1, 2]. Need remains hidden and policy documents are largely silent on the issue [1, 3]. Since the 1960s, debates have focused on the young [4] and use of drugs is not even recorded for some age groups [5].

Increasingly, however, influential voices have mobilized evidence and called for more attention to the issue [1, 2, 6–10]. In Europe, ageing was first highlighted by the Amsterdam cohort study, which followed 899 chronic drug users from 1985 to 2002. The findings challenged the idea that the majority of drug users would 'mature out' to a drug-free state [11]. The issue was recognized earlier in the USA, where guidelines were developed in 1998 [12]. However, even there, much still remains to be done [1, 13, 14]. Policy responses have to adapt to the constantly changing shape of epidemics and changing profiles of drug users, which vary over time and across different countries.

Policies centred on the assumption that drug use is entirely a young people's issue are increasingly inappropriate. However, it would be wrong to replace them simply by a focus on 'older drug users'. Like drug users in general, older drug users are a mixed bag – in different situations, with different health statuses and needs, each requiring a different response [15]. Not all drug users pose a social problem [16].

Policy (as distinct from wider public discussion) primarily focuses on 'problem drug users' (users of 'hard' drugs like heroin or cocaine), and often on the socially excluded, poor or criminal. To adapt policies to both a changing reality and altered perceptions of the problem, a series of linked activities would need to be initiated:

- recognition of the need or problem, supported by collecting evidence;
- articulation of a justification for the development of policy, citing values or pragmatism;
- identification of policy options;

Substance Use and Older People, First Edition.
Edited by Ilana B. Crome, Li-Tzy Wu, Rahul (Tony) Rao and Peter Crome.
© 2015 John Wiley & Sons, Ltd. Published 2015 by John Wiley & Sons, Ltd.

- formal adoption of policy recommendations and acceptance of responsibility;
- detailed policy design;
- implementation and evaluation.

This chapter reviews the development of policy through each phase of this process.

Recognition of a need or problem and arguments made to justify the development of policy

Arguments for a new policy response often refer to 'need', assuming that pointing out a growing problem and the existence of need are in themselves enough to justify the development of services [1, 2]. These claims rest on concepts of human rights, ethics and values, or social justice. Others refer more pragmatically to the consequences of failing to respond, citing evidence of effects and costs: for example, the misuse of expensive resources in hospital emergency departments or prisons if drug dependence is not dealt with in more appropriate locations [17]; or the cost effectiveness of early interventions that can prevent more complex conditions, which would cost more to treat. Or they refer to social disorder, citing behaviours such as prostitution, homelessness or criminality among unsupported drug dependents and the ineffectiveness of criminal justice interventions [18].

Growing awareness among front-line staff, with evidence from epidemiological studies, has charted a looming public health problem, an estimated more than doubling in the numbers of older illicit drug users between 2001 and 2020 [1, 10, 13, 14, 19]. Drug treatment services will need to adapt [2, 20]. Mainstream clinical services specializing in the care of older people may also have to adapt and the general treatment infrastructure become sensitive to the problems of older illicit drug users [1, 10]. At present, there is a high level of unmet need with underidentification and undertreatment for substance abuse. In addition, there is higher prevalence of prescription use and misuse and age-related changes in metabolism can increase the potential for negative effects [1, 2]. There is a need to look for early warning signs and develop and test screening instruments specific to this population [1, 18]. Where these are used, the finding is often one of co-morbidity [2]. Older drug users suffer from accumulated physical handicaps or impairments and have higher levels of both physical and mental health problems [7].

Studies in the United States have noted increased need for hospitalization or nursing home placement and a lack of substance abuse treatment facilities with programmes or groups designed specifically for seniors [14, 21]. Others have noted the value of community-based services [1, 22]. Han and colleagues concluded there is an urgent need to expand treatment services for older patients and to integrate primary care with substance abuse treatment programmes [14]. They emphasized the value of providing substance misuse services in primary care settings, offering screening, identification and brief interventions. There is potential to take this forward, as in the United Kingdom, by developing a group of primary care physicians with specialist expertise in substance dependence.

Not all drug users need treatment [16]. Recreational drug users, such as long-term cannabis users, should, however, have their drug use recognized when their general health is being assessed. But disclosure may be hindered by the illegal status of some substance use. Primary care physicians and other specialists should be prepared to ask about use of substances, both legal and illegal, as a routine matter. All practitioners should be aware of the possible existence of psychotropic drug use among older people [1].

Much of the evidence on drug dependence is drawn from treatment populations, which can distort understanding. Studies of other groups, such as those out of treatment, in prison, the homeless, those living in the community and employed, give a different profile and understanding of need, implying different policy responses [23]. Older women may have specific needs, as would those who use prescription and over-the-counter (OTC) drugs [24, 25]. In surveys of populations currently not in treatment, a lack of education regarding hepatitis C has been found, including among middle and upper middle class respondents. In one survey of sexual minorities in the United States, high rates of health insurance coverage were found but low use of substance abuse treatment, thought to be explained by age discrimination and fear of rejection [26]. These authors called for screening and services sensitive to the needs of lesbian, gay and bisexual older people. Other specific groups have been studied (e.g. long-term injecting, heroin using, ageing, Mexican American men) indicating needs specific to each [27]. It would, however, be impossible and even undesirable to provide separate services for each finely differentiated subgroup. What is needed is for all services to be sensitive to the wide range of lifestyles and needs that may be found among older clients and patients and training to include cultural competence [1]. Local needs assessments are important when planning services and appropriate training and recruitment of staff.

Studies of socially excluded and marginalized groups, especially of the homeless, find high levels of need. Evidence from studies of homeless, uninsured or socially isolated groups has led to calls for an expansion of services, especially harm reduction programmes, focused on older adult drug users. Dietz concluded in 2009 from a detailed study in the USA that 'there is a need for more pointed efforts in addressing substance misuse among the homeless and marginally housed' [23]. Street level sex work may continue and jails and prisons are high-risk environments for infectious diseases. Other studies have identified specific needs among older veterans [21] and new AIDS cases [30]. The needs of injection drug users (IDUs) require an urgent response, as IDU remains one of the most frequently cited modes of HIV transmission worldwide, contributing to epidemics in Russia, India and other countries. Researchers have demonstrated the value of community-based services for these groups, such as nonprofit organizations operating in open drug markets. They have concluded that older drug users are vulnerable to contracting infectious diseases and more needs to be done to reach this ageing population [28]. Those working with older drug users, such as prison officials, social workers and public health workers, could help to reduce transmission of infectious diseases by incorporating harm reduction strategies into their policies.

Policy options

How a problem is defined shapes the proposed policy response and the way a problem is perceived is influenced by both values and evidence. The shape of the evidence reflects the way data are gathered, especially what subpopulations are observed. Research evidence is also supplemented by evidence gained from experience.

In looking at how the problem is defined, the first question is whether drug users are seen as a 'problem' or as 'normal' people? Related to this is the general question of whether opioid addiction is seen as a chronic relapsing condition [7, 29, 30], requiring perhaps decades of maintenance treatment, together with relapse prevention and other psychosocial supports, or whether a more assertive and optimistic focus on recovery, abstinence and mutual aid could work wonders [31]. In the USA, there have been successful innovations like GET SMART in Los Angeles, which started in 1991 and provided weekly support groups to veterans aged 60 and older with problems including use of illicit drugs [21]. While arguments about the potential for recovery are well made and it is important not to write people off, especially simply because they are older, at the same time, it is sensible to be realistic about the likelihood of relapse and be aware of the danger of overdose as a consequence [32].

Secondly, what is 'old'? The literature shows a variety of age categories from 37–55, to 40+, 45+, 50+, 65+ and 50–74 [1, 2, 7, 9, 14, 18, 19, 21, 22, 23, 24, 30]. As a start, there is a clear need to develop common agreement about the ages policy would be interested in. It should be required to record the age of older users and distinguish specific ages more finely. The issue is the degree of fit between chronological, physical and mental age and the early ageing of drug users' bodies. At the age of 40, drug users may need a level of care corresponding to that required by nonsubstance using elderly people [33]. The policy question then is how to respond to 'older' rather than 'old' drug users. Many people feel increasingly invisible and marginalized as they get old and social isolation is linked to a decline in well-being, so older drug users are doubly disadvantaged [34]. Polydrug use, including a mixture of drugs prescribed for different conditions, often has deleterious side effects, only increased by illicit drug use, along with tobacco and alcohol [1].

As well as expanding and adapting to the needs of older service users, through improved training of staff, ensuring the age of staff better match the age of service users and paying attention to medication management [1, 2], it has been argued that clinical services should engage in outreach and active engagement [1, 35, 36], use peer educators [4] and make better links to other services, specialized and mainstream, including geriatric services [1, 36]. A comprehensive approach, multiagency and multidisciplinary, is favoured – encouraging that much desired but often elusive 'joined up' system (Box 24.1) [1, 7].

Advocates for reform point to the need to rethink drugs-related support and rehabilitation services. The European Monitoring Centre for Drugs and Drug Addiction (EMCDDA) has commented that 'alternative social reintegration policies and options may have to be developed' for older problem drug users [7]. The relevance of job training programmes has been questioned for people who are unlikely to be classified as employable [37]. Debates about reintegration into society and

Box 24.1 Examples of policy recommendations and guidelines

UK Royal College of Psychiatrists Report [2]	Scottish Drugs Forum [36]

UK Royal College of Psychiatrists Report [2]

- Close liaison between professionals
- Clinical guidelines with care pathways addressing the various needs of older substance misusers
- Specific local policies
- Access on the basis of need
- Elimination of age barriers
- Easy transfer between services
- Joint working and decisions regarding the lead service
- Protocols
- Training of health professionals
- Improved attitudes – address stigma, therapeutic nihilism and social exclusion
- Service models with a particular focus on long-term outcome

Scottish Drugs Forum [36]

- Assertive outreach for those dropping out of services
- Meeting general health care needs effectively
- Community services that plan for the care of problem drug users who are unable to leave their home
- Good therapeutic relationships
- Age-specific services and better match of ages of staff and service users
- Good interagency work
- Practice which is nonjudgemental
- Harm reduction information
- Services which act as advocates
- Service user involvement
- Home support
- Recovery
- Training
- Supported accommodation
- Screening
- Pain management

employment presuppose that drug users are of working age and are healthy enough to work. In England and in Scotland, for example, greater emphasis than ever is being placed on facilitating the reintegration of drug users into society through employment and to incentivise engagement with drug treatment services for those claiming financial benefits paid to those not in work [9]. In the context of increased healthy life-expectancy, many countries propose to raise the retirement age. For those who are unhealthy, this implies an even longer period of time in long-term unemployment, and consequent poverty and 'welfare dependency'. The intermediary years between becoming an adult, when one is expected to be self-supporting, and reaching an age when eligibility for pension, income support and other services is reached are the crucial ones for policy to deal with.

The early ageing of very unhealthy and disadvantaged groups is the key factor. For whatever cause (lifestyle choice, effect of some earlier trauma or response to environmental constraints), such people constitute a significant group in many post-industrial societies and they cannot match up to the demands of the contemporary work environment. They are one group among the long-term unemployed, some-times perceived as chronically sick and disabled or incapacitated but sometimes as an underclass and 'work-shy' [38–44]. They form a distinctive group among the users of health and social services, where such exist, or form an outsider excluded group, living in the margins of society geographically and socially, where such supports are not available. Their situation varies across different soci-eties, depending on the general health, social services and social security policy framework and generosity of benefits in each country. Whether they are classed as 'mad, bad or sad', their health and income status reflects the income level of the society and the way it chooses to allocate resources. Ideally, if full rehabilita-tion is not possible, policy would provide sheltered housing and employment. However, provision of facilities for drug users, unlike, for example, people with learning disabilities, lacks public support, especially in an era of fiscal austerity. Even 'deserving' groups, such as the physically disabled, are unsupported in some welfare regimes. There is a need to devise imaginative ways to encourage less employable groups to make a social contribution, thus reducing moral condem-nation. The dilemma is how to provide needed services without too great a public subsidy. One radical proposal that might meet the needs of older problem drug users as well as other disadvantaged groups would involve a basic citizen's income provided to all adults on condition of 'participation' possibly through volunteer-ing with an NGO.

In the United States, eligibility for many social benefits is based on concepts of normal ageing. The drug user exhibiting early onset physical and mental ageing can become part of a homeless population, excluded from support, whose only recourse to assistance is through use of emergency rooms. A similar situation is found in Poland [45]. In Warsaw, homeless drug addicts have only limited access to therapy, including antiretroviral treatment. In richer societies such as Germany, the Netherlands or Sweden, with well- established welfare systems, the situation of the ageing drug dependent is better [33, 46, 47].

This links most poignantly to debates about palliative and end-of-life care. Illicit drug use poses a challenge to these services [48]. For the most disadvantaged, homeless, illicit drug users, policy decisions surround questions of access and service delivery, the role of harm reduction and pain management. Drug users are likely to be excluded from mainstream end-of-life care services, such as community hospices and hospitals, because of differences in lifestyles, behavioural problems or complaints from other residents. Balancing the wishes and needs of different client groups is a challenge to managers of services. From a study in Canada, McNeil and Guirguis-Younger suggest alternatives might include low-barrier, shelter-located palliative care based on a harm reduction model [48]. A few countries, such as Denmark, Germany and the Netherlands, have developed specialized nursing homes and accommodation services for older problem drug users with multiple health and social needs but these are few and far between [7].

There is a need for research on the application of harm reduction models to end-of-life care settings, including the question of the suitability of supervised drug injection. The European Commission Public Health Executive Agency has partially funded a project SDDCARE (Senior Drug Dependents and Care Structure Project) that made recommendations at the European Union level for services and responses [49]. This project compiled information on provision in Germany, Scotland, the Netherlands and Poland [50]. It recommended experimenting at national levels with both separate services for older drug users and integrated settings (perhaps involving young and old drug users, old drug users and old nondrug users).

Two innovations highlighted by the Scottish Drugs Forum are the Housing First Model (based on a model from New York providing secure tenancy irrespective of social issues and drug use) and heroin prescribing. They note that complex, older, chronic drug users require accommodation with a tenure that is not threatened by their continued drug use. But workers have noted that the use of generic services can be limited by deviant behaviour and/or stigma and they conclude there is a need for individual, person-centred decisions to find the most suitable provision. However, implementing this is hampered by a general lack of choice [51, 52].

For any of these policy proposals to be taken forward, government must accept responsibility and institutionalize principles in funding and action [1, 2]. Before government feels a need to know and act, there has to be pressure from stakeholders, along with awareness by policy makers at national and local levels that the efficient functioning of services requires adapting to the new demands.

Policy design and implementation

There remains a need for more research on the service needs of these groups and acceptance of the fact that the task of caring for them is complex [1]. In general, in many countries, policies need to pay more attention to chronic conditions, clarify statutory responsibilities and revise funding arrangements [1, 53]. The specific way in which policy on older drug users would be designed at any national or local level would have to reflect their general framework of health, social and criminal justice policies, as well as link to their wider drug strategy [7]. The process would involve developing strategies and action plans, policy and practice briefings and guidelines, training, policy instruments and networks of concerned agencies and individuals to build support. There is a need for more training opportunities, guidance, mentorship, and financial incentives to develop both generic and specialist workforces appropriately [1]. Forums for stakeholders with a series of workshops could discuss developments and encourage learning from experience. There would be advantage in establishing a high-level national steering group as well as at local levels to maintain priority attention to the issue [1]. Evaluation and monitoring of initiatives, together with dialogue, feedback and redesign in the light of experience, would help to improve the policy response.

Conclusion

Underlying proposals for policy development is the question of whose responsibility it is to deal with the problem of older illicit drug users and to pay for services for them. The European Union recognizes a need to balance human rights with wider community interests [7]. With a stigmatized and often excluded group, whose choices are exacerbated by the illegal nature of their drug use, public attitudes will be hostile and there will be resistance to paying for services for groups who are thought to have brought their misfortune on themselves. Older people in general are more likely to need long-term care and experience financial pressures related to paying for care [34, 54]. A key question is whether to provide targeted or mainstream services. Adequate mainstream services are a prerequisite: selective services specific to minority needs and interests can only be provided adequately as extensions to an adequate level of provision for mainstream service users, currently often lacking. This applies especially to personal and nursing care for those in their own homes, in retirement communities and in care homes. And there is a general need to value more highly and better train those who provide care for older people and encourage inter-professional collaboration [1].

What emerges is the value of policy development being led by health professionals and agencies, mainly because of their expertise, experience and adherence to ethical practices. In addition, the more that decisions are taken on a pragmatic and technical basis and do not become fodder for media and political exploitation, the more likely it is that sensitive and effective policies will emerge.

In many countries, the situation is one of endemic rather than epidemic drug use [55]. In the end, however, the problem will only be fully addressed through prevention and promotion of healthy living [56]. These goals must be rediscovered as a priority, since for ageing post-industrial societies the health care burden of a range of unhealthy life styles – not only illicit drug use – is becoming increasingly unsustainable.

References

1. IOM (2012) *The Mental Health and Substance Use Workforce for Older Adults: In Whose Hands?* The National Academies Press, Washington, DC.
2. Royal College of Psychiatrists (2011) *Our Invisible Addicts. First Report of the Older Persons Substance Misuse Working Group of the Royal College of Psychiatrists.* Royal College of Psychiatrists, London.
3. Feidler, K., Leary, S., Pertica, S. and Strohl, J. (2002) *Substance Abuse among Aging Adults: A Literature Review.* NEDS, CSAT, Washington, DC.
4. Levy, J.A. (1998) AIDS and injecting drug use in later life. *Research on Aging,* **20:** 776–797.
5. The Information Centre for Health and Social Care (2012) *Statistics on Drug Misuse: England 2012.* NHS, England.
6. EMCDDA (2008) *Substance use among older adults: a neglected problem.* Drugs in Focus, European Monitoring Centre for Drugs and Drug Addiction (EMCDDA), Lisbon, Portugal.

7. EMCDDA (2010) *Treatment and Care for Older Drug Users*, European Monitoring Centre for Drugs and Drug Addiction (EMCDDA), Lisbon, Portugal.

8. Beynon, C.M. (2009) Drug use and ageing: older people do take drugs. *Age and Ageing*, **38**, 8–10.

9. Beynon, C., McVeigh, J., Hurst, A. and Marr, A. (2010) Older and sicker: changing mortality of drug users in treatment in the North West of England. *International Journal of Drug Policy*, **21**, 429–431.

10. Fahmy, V., Hatch, S.L., Hotopf, M. and Stewart, R. (2012) Prevalence of illicit drug use in people aged 50 years and over from two surveys. *Age and Ageing*, **241**(4), 553–556.

11. Termorshuizen, F., Krol, A., Prins, M. and van Ameijden, E.J.C. (2005) Long-term outcome of chronic drug use. The Amsterdam Cohort Study among drug users. *American Journal of Epidemiology*, **161**, 271–279.

12. US Department of Health and Human Services (1998) *Substance Abuse among Older Adults*. Treatment Improvement Protocol (TIP) Series No. 26, US Department of Health and Human Services, Washington, DC.

13. Gfroerer, J., Penne, M., Pemberton, M. and Folsom, R. (2003) Substance abuse treatment need among older adults in 2020: the impact of the aging baby-boom cohort. *Drug and Alcohol Dependence*, **69**, 127–135.

14. Han, B., Gfroerer, J.C., Colliver, J.D. and Penne, M.A. (2009) Substance use disorder among older adults in the United States in 2020. *Addiction*, **104**, 88–96.

15. Olszewski, D., Hedrich, D. and Montanari, L. (2012) *Users' Voices. Experiences and Perceptions of European Drug Users on Controlling Their Drug Consumption*. European Monitoring Centre for Drugs and Drug Addiction (EMCDDA), Lisbon, Portugal.

16. Waters, J. and Moxon, D. (2011) The illegal leisure of hidden older illicit drug users. *Crime Talk* (3 August 2011). www.crimetalk.org.uk (last accessed 17 April 2014).

17. Kerridge, B.T. (2009) Sociological, social psychological and psychopathological correlates of substance use disorder in the US jail population. *International Journal of Offender Therapy and Comparative Criminology*, **53/52**, 168–190.

18. Beynon, C.M., McVeigh, J. and Roe, B. (2007) Problematic drug user, ageing and older people: trends in the age of drug users in northwest England. *Ageing and Society*, **27**, 799–810.

19. Wu, L.-T. and Blazer, D.G. (2011) Illicit and nonmedical drug use among older adults: a review. *Journal of Aging and Health*, **223**, 481–504.

20. Moy, I., Crome, P., Crome, I. and Fisher, M. (2011) Systematic and narrative review of treatment for older people with substance problems *European Geriatric Medicine*, **2**, 212–236.

21. Schonfield, L., Dupree, LW., Dickson-Fuhrmann, E. *et al.* (2000) Cognitive behavioural treatment of older veterans with substance abuse problems. *Journal of Geriatric Psychiatry and Neurology*, **13**, 124–129.

22. Outlaw, F.H., Marquart, J.M., Roy, A. *et al.* (2012) Treatment outcomes for older adults who abuse substances. *Journal of Applied Gerontology*, **31**(1), 78–100.

23. Dietz, T.L. (2008) Drug and alcohol use among homeless older adults: predictors of reported current and lifetime substance misuse problems in a national sample. *Journal of Applied Gerontology*, **28**, 235–255.

24. Raffoul, P.R., Cooper, J.K. and Low, D.W. (1981) Drug misuse in older people. *The Gerontologist*, **21**(2), 146–150.

25. Boeri, M.W. and Tyndall, B.D. (2012) A contextual comparison of risk behaviours among older adult drug users and harm reduction in suburban versus inner city social environments. *Journal of Applied Social Science*, **6**, 72–91.

26. Jessup, M.A. and Dibble, S.L. (2012) Unmet mental health and substance abuse treatment needs of sexual minority elders. *Journal of Homosexuality*, **59**(5), 656–674.

27. Torres, L.R., Kaplan, C. and Valdez, A. (2011) Health consequences of long-term injection heroin use among aging Mexican American men. *Journal of Aging and Health,* **23**, 912–932.

28. Johnson, S.D., Striley, C. and Cottler, L.B. (2007) Comorbid substance use and HIV risk in older African American drug users. *Journal of Aging and Health,* **19**(4), 646–658.

29. Bevan, G. (2009) Problem drug use, the public health imperative: what some of the literature says. *Substance Abuse Treatment, Prevention and Policy,* **4**, 21. www.substanceabusepolicy.com/content/4/1/21 (last accessed 17 April 2014).

30. Boeri, M., Whalen, T., Tyndall, B. and Ballard, E. (2011) Drug use trajectory patterns among older drug users. *Substance Abuse and Rehabilitation,* **2**, 89–102.

31. Humphreys, K. (2004) *Circles of Recovery. Self Help Organisations for Addictions.* Cambridge University Press, Cambridge.

32. WHO (2009) *Guidelines for the Psychosocially Assisted Pharmacological Treatment of Opioid Dependence.* World Health Organization (WHO), Geneva, Switzerland.

33. Vogt, I., Simmedinger, R. and Kuplewatzky, N. (2009) *SDDCARE. Re-analysis of selected German national and local data.* Institut für Suchtforschung an der Fachhochschule Frankfurt am Main (ISFF), Germany.

34. House of Lords Select Committee on Public Services and Demographic Change (2013) *Ready for Ageing?* Report of Session 2012–2013, HL Paper 140.

35. Rush, B.R., Dennis, M.L., Scott, C.K. *et al.* (2008) The interaction of co-occurring mental disorders and recovery management check-ups on substance abuse treatment participation and recovery. *Evaluation Review,* **32**(1), 7–38.

36. Scottish Drug Forum (2010) *Senior Drug Dependents and Care Structures. Scotland: Guidelines for Service Response.* Scottish Drug Forum, Glasgow.

37. Watson, D.P. (2010) The mental health of the older homeless population: provider-perceived issues related to service provision. *Journal of Applied Social Science,* **4**, 27–43.

38. Mead, L.M. (1992) *The New Politics of Poverty.* Basic Books, New York.

39. Mead, L.M., Field, F., Deacon, A. (ed.) *et al.* (1997) *From Welfare to Work: Lessons from America.* Health and Welfare Unit, Institute of Economic Affairs (IEA), London.

40. Schram, S.F. (1995) *Words of Welfare.* University of Minnesota Press, Minneapolis/London.

41. Spicker, P. (1993) *Poverty and Social Security.* Routledge, London/New York.

42. Gallie, D. and Paugam, S. (eds) (2000) *Welfare Regimes and the Experience of Unemployment in Europe.* Oxford University Press, Oxford.

43. NatCen Social Research (2013) *British Social Attitudes Survey 28.* NatCen Social Research, London.

44. Stanisland, L. (2011) *Public Perceptions of Disabled People.* Office for Disability Issues, HM Government, London.

45. Moskalewicz, J. and Zygadlo, M. (2009) *Legal and Financial Framework for Senior Drug Dependents in Poland.* SDDCARE Project Interim Report.

46. Lenski, R. and Wichelmann-Werth, B. (2009) *Legal and Financial Framework for the Care of Senior Drug Dependents in Germany.* SDDCARE Project Interim Report.

47. LADIS (2010) *Elderly (55 and older) in Addiction Care in The Netherlands (2000–2009).* LADIS Bulletin, Stichting IVZ, Houten, The Netherlands.

48. McNeil, R. and Guirguis-Younger, M. (2012) Illicit drug use as a challenge to the delivery of end-of-life care services to homeless persons: perceptions of health and social services professionals *Palliative Medicine,* **26**, 350–359.

49. Working Group of the Senior Drug Dependents and Care Structure Project (2010) *Recommendations at the EU Level for Services and Responses.* Executive Agency for Health and Consumers, Frankfurt, Germany.

50. SDDCare. Home page. www.SDDCare.eu (last accessed 17 April 2014).
51. Liddell, D. and Brand, B. (2009) *Legal and Financial Framework for Senior Drug Dependents in Scotland*. SDDCARE Project Interim Report.
52. Brand, B. (n.d.) *Older Drug Users in Scotland: Professionals' Views*. Scottish Drugs Forum, Glasgow.
53. Nolte, E. and McKee, M. (eds) (2008) *Caring for People with Chronic Conditions: A Health System Perspective*. Open University Press, Maidenhead.
54. Eurohealth (Special edition) (2011) Ageing and Long-Term Care. *Eurohealth*, 17(2–3).
55. Caulkins, J.P. and Reuter, P. (2006) Reorienting US drug policy. *Issues in Science and Technology*, Fall 2006. Online. www.issues.org/23.1/caulkins.html (last accessed 17 April 2014).
56. Naaldenberg, J., Vaandrager, L., Koelen, M. and Leeuwis, C. (2012) Aging populations' everyday perspectives on healthy aging: new insights for policy and strategies at local level. *Journal of Applied Gerontology*, 31(6), 711–733.

Chapter 25

PROPOSALS FOR ALCOHOL-RELATED POLICY DEVELOPMENT IN THE UNITED STATES

Ralph Hingson[1] and Ting-Kai Li[2]

[1]Division of Epidemiology and Prevention Research, National Institute on Alcohol Abuse and Alcoholism, USA
[2]Department of Psychiatry and Behavioral Sciences, School of Medicine, Duke University Medical Center, USA

Owing to a growing older population, concern has been raised about risk and protective factors among those entering old age, including alcohol and drug use. The baby boom generation comprises just under 30% of the US population [1] and, in 2011, the first cohort of this group reached the age of 65. By 2020, the prevalence rates of substance use disorders among the elderly are projected to increase dramatically [2]. Some have hypothesized that retirement may contribute to unhealthy drinking, although one recent literature review did not find a strong direct impact of retirement on drinking behaviours [3].

Recommended low-risk alcohol consumption levels

Given the unique effect of alcohol on the aging body, older adults are advised by the US National Institute on Alcohol Abuse and Alcoholism (NIAAA) [4] to consume no more than seven standard drinks per week and/or three drinks per day. In the 2002 National Epidemiologic Survey of Alcohol and Related Conditions (NESARC), 7.5% of adults aged 65 and older exceeded those daily limits and 9.4% exceeded weekly limits. Because the elderly are more likely to be prescribed medications for treatment of chronic illness and because alcohol pharmacologically interacts with many medications (increasing the risk of being sleepy, drowsy and light-headed, and reducing mechanical skills and concentration), combined use of alcohol and drugs can make driving more dangerous. NIAAA has published Harmful Interactions: Mixing Alcohol with Medicines (2007) [5], which noted the special alcohol and drug interactions and driving risks for the elderly.

Substance Use and Older People, First Edition.
Edited by Ilana B. Crome, Li-Tzy Wu, Rahul (Tony) Rao and Peter Crome.
© 2015 John Wiley & Sons, Ltd. Published 2015 by John Wiley & Sons, Ltd.

Traffic crash risks among the elderly

Research shows that driver age and road traffic crash involvement is best modelled as a U-shaped function with young drivers (below age 24) and oldest drivers (above age 75) at greatest risk [6]. Furthermore, drivers aged 65 and older have an increased risk of death and serious injury when they are involved in a crash [7]. This increased risk of injury is believed to be caused by greater frailty. A lowered tolerance to physical trauma may result in more serious injuries for older drivers, passengers and pedestrians than would be sustained by younger people in comparable crashes [8].

Certain roadway characteristics, particularly high speed limits, have been associated with elderly crash involvement and injury among elderly drivers [7]. Intersections feature prominently in crash statistics for older drivers. Specific problem areas include 'failure to yield', 'looked but failed to see' and 'inaccurate gap selection' [9].

Visual impairment among elderly drivers may also increase risk of crash. In the United States, cataracts are the leading cause of visual impairment in older adults [10]. Older people with cataracts who do not elect to undergo cataract surgery have been found to experience roughly twice the rate of motor vehicle collision per mile driven compared to those who undergo cataract extraction [11]. However, currently in the United States most insurers do not allow payment for cataract surgery based on a physical examination unless accompanied by an individual complaint of visual difficulties that seriously interfere with driving or other daily activities, and individuals themselves may be slow or reluctant to complain and seek relief [12].

Useful field of vision, a measure of visual attention and information processing speed, also predicts crash risk in the elderly [13]. Decrements in processing speed of multiple pieces of information, such as needed when turning at intersections, have also been cited as contributors to motor vehicle crash involvement [14–17].

Driving policy questions

In light of these driving risks for the elderly, particularly after alcohol use, some have proposed specific driving restrictions for the elderly or policies to reduce harmful alcohol in that age group, particularly relative to traffic safety. With regard to driving restrictions on the elderly, concerns about safety must be balanced against personal need for community mobility and negative consequences of driving cessation. Driving cessation in older adults is associated with depression, placement into long-term care and decreased physical activity and health status [16]. In addition, senior drivers can be active economic contributors, strengthening the importance of keeping older drivers doing so safely [6].

Factors to consider when contemplating legal policies

A number of factors should be taken into account when considering use of policy. They apply to considering policy to change behaviour, to promote health in general and to reduce harmful alcohol use among the elderly in specific. Firstly, for policy to be considered, the problems created by the behaviour in question must be important. In 2009, elderly persons aged 65 and older accounted for 12.9% of the US population (39 571 000 out of 307 000 000 people) [1]. Between 2001 and 2005 according to the US Centers for Disease Control and Prevention [18], the elderly were disproportionately more likely to experience an alcohol-attributable death. During those years, on average annually the elderly experienced 26.4% of the alcohol-attributable deaths (20 827/78 727). Of those deaths, 8047 were acute injury or poisoning deaths and 12 725 were chronic disease deaths. The elderly experienced 18.5% of the acute injury or poisoning deaths (8,047/43 731) and 36.4% of chronic disease deaths (12 725/34 996). Elderly people experienced the highest number of alcohol-attributable deaths of any age group from acute pancreatitis (439/695 deaths), chronic pancreatitis (111/229), oesophageal cancer (288/458), hypertension (949/1,264), liver cancer (148/239), liver cirrhosis (unspecified) (3360/7055), oropharyngeal cancer (197/364), portal hypertension (19/40), prostate cancer (males only) (272/297), haemorrhagic stroke (557/631), ischemic stroke (557/631) and subventricular cardiac dysrhythmia (136/141). Among acute injury and poisoning deaths, the elderly aged 65 and older experienced the most alcohol-attributable deaths from aspiration (121/204), falls (4407/5532), and fires (458/1158). The disproportionate rates of alcohol-attributable deaths among the elderly clearly indicate the scale of the problem.

However, an examination of the drinking practices of the elderly in the National Epidemiologic Survey on Alcohol and Related Conditions (NESARC) reveal that, compared to younger adults aged 18–64, persons aged 65 and older were less likely to exceed low-risk drinking weekly guidelines (9.4 vs 11.1%) or daily guidelines (7.5 vs 30.7%) for adults or meet alcohol dependence criteria (0.3 vs 4.5%) or alcohol abuse criteria (1.1 vs 5.3%) [19]. Further, in 2011 people aged 65 and older had the lowest percentage of drivers involved in fatal crashes with blood alcohol content of 0.08% or higher [6% (N = 348/5469) versus 23% (N = 8948/38 199) for all other drivers) [20].

The lower risky drinking and alcohol-related fatal crash rates among the elderly relative to other adults may limit the appeal, not only among the elderly themselves but also among adults of other ages, of advocating for and implementing alcohol policies specifically for the elderly to reduce alcohol misuse and driving after drinking.

Secondly, there should be evidence that policies will produce reductions in the targeted behaviours above and beyond those achievable by clinical and educational interventions alone. There is a substantial literature that indicates a variety of policy changes can reduce harmful alcohol use and related morbidity and mortality in the general adult population and among persons under age 21 [20, 21]. The US Centers for Disease Control and Prevention's Guide to Prevention Services [21] recommends the following evidence-based strategies to reduce alcohol misuse and related harms in the general population: maintaining limits on days and hours of sale, regulating outlet density, commercial liability for sales to minors or intoxicated persons and alcohol price increases. It also recommends against privatization of retail alcohol sales. However, little if any research has explored the impact of these policy changes on drinking and related health consequences, specifically in the elderly population.

Although the specific effects on the elderly of screening and brief motivational counselling have not been studied, literature reviews of these interventions in adult primary care settings have consistently found them to be effective in reducing risky drinking and related problems [22, 23]. However, despite recommendations for universal alcohol screening, it is not consistently undertaken, in part because of policies limiting reimbursement. The effects on alcohol screening frequency of changes in reimbursement, such as those that may result from the Affordable Care Act, warrant investigation.

The leading causes of alcohol-attributable death according to the US Centers for Disease Control and Prevention among persons 65 and older are liver cirrhosis (unspecified) (annual average N = 3360), alcoholic liver disease (N = 2648), fall injuries (N = 4407) and suicide (N = 1234). Two reviews [24, 25] regarding the effects of higher alcohol prices or taxes identified nine separate studies that found higher price related to lower death rates from cirrhosis, although the strength of the association varied.

Three reviews [25–27] reported inconsistent associations between alcohol price and suicide. One study [28] found no association between price and death from falls, burns, other nontraffic injuries or homicide. The review did not specifically assess these relations among persons aged 65 and older.

In general, older drivers reduce the amount of their driving, tend to drive at lower speeds and avoid driving situations such as driving in dark or slippery conditions, in rush hour, in dense traffic or on routes involving complex intersections, motorways, left turns (right turns when driving on the left), long distances or driving to unfamiliar areas [28].

In the United States, perhaps the greatest alcohol policy impact in the past 30 years has been observed on alcohol-attributable traffic deaths whose rates have been cut in half [29]. It has been estimated that over 300 000 deaths in the United States have been prevented since the early 1980s because of reductions in drinking and driving [30]. The reductions exceed those attributed to increases in safety belt use, airbags and motorcycle and bicycle helmet use combined [31].

Numerous laws, such as raising the drinking age to 21, lowering legal blood alcohol limits, passage of administrative license revocation and criminal laws *per se*, have occurred and been found in scientific studies to have reduced alcohol-related traffic deaths [32]. Three literature reviews reported numerous studies that observed significant associations between higher alcohol prices and reduced alcohol-related traffic death rates [25–27]. Alcohol-related traffic deaths also are the outcome for which there are the most accurate annual trend data over multiple decades according to age group. In 1982, when the US National Highway Traffic Safety Administration first released national estimates, of the 23 589 people who died in crashes involving drinking drivers, 3% (640) died in crashes involving a drinking driver aged 65 and older, 438 of whom were the drinking driver aged 65 and older [29]. That same year, a majority (705), 62% of people aged 65 and older who died in crashes involving drinking drivers, were fatally injured in a crash involving a drinking driver under the age of 65.

Between 1982 and 2009, passage of the various drinking and driving laws listed above reduced the number of drivers of all ages with positive blood alcohol levels in fatal crashes. However, the steepest proportional declines in fatalities involved drinking drivers under age 65, not drinking drivers aged 65 and older. The decline in fatalities involving drinking drivers under 65 was 47% (1216 to 648), whereas the decline in fatalities involving drinking drivers aged 65 and older was 35% (640 to 418). The steepest and largest decline in traffic deaths among persons aged 65 and older involving drinking drivers resulted in declines from crashes involving drinking drivers under age 65 of 59% (715 to 296), compared to 41% (501 to 352) involving drinking drivers aged 65 and older.

Thus, alcohol policies to reduce alcohol-related traffic deaths reduced deaths in all age groups, including the elderly. But, these resulted more from reductions in alcohol-impaired driving among persons under age 65 than 65 and older. More of these declines in deaths aged 65 and older from traffic crashes involving drinking drivers resulted from declines in drinking and driving by persons under age 65 than age 65 and older.

National roadside surveys tested night drivers' blood alcohol levels in 1973, 1986, 1996, and 2007 [33]. These data reveal trends consistent with the traffic fatality data. While the proportion of drivers aged 65 and older with blood alcohol content of 0.05% declined from 8.4% in 1973 to 4.5% in 2007, every other age group examined had larger and proportionately greater declines. The respective declines per age group were:

- Age <21: 10.9 to 1.9%
- Ages 21–34: 15.4 to 5.9%
- Ages 45–54: 15.9 to 3.9%
- Ages 55–64: 11 to 2.2%

Research is also needed to assess the impact of alcohol policies other than just drinking and driving laws, such as price increases or alterations in alcohol outlet density, specifically on people aged 65 and older, before policy recommendations can be made specifically for that age group.

Thirdly, policies should be minimally intrusive and there should be no equally effective, less intrusive alternative. In the absence of research about alcohol policy effects, specifically on the elderly, there is no way to establish whether alcohol policy changes targeting the elderly would be more effective than less intrusive initiatives such as education or expansion of screening, brief counselling intervention and alcohol treatment programmes. Nor can one establish whether alcohol policy changes targeting adults of all ages will be more effective in reducing harmful drinking among the elderly than less intrusive interventions.

Fourthly, the behaviour in question should harm other people. Most alcohol-attributable deaths among persons aged 65 and older are deaths from chronic diseases, which directly affect the elderly drinker not other people. Deaths from acute injuries (e.g. from assaults, falls and drownings) which more often involve younger people are much more likely to impact people other than the drinker, especially traffic deaths. For example, half the people who die in traffic crashes involving drinking drivers aged 25 and younger are persons other than the drinking driver. One-third of the deaths involving drinking drivers under age 65 are persons other than the drinking driver. In 2009, drivers aged 65 and older were the age group with the smallest percentage (23%, 95/418) who died who were other than the elderly drinking driver.

Fifthly, the public should support the law. As was seen with prohibition [34], if they do not, then the law will be less likely to be enforced, compliance will be lower and the beneficial effects of the law will to some degree be compromised. Because the elderly drink at lower levels than younger people, they are less likely to harm other people after drinking and drinking and driving, and have been able to legally drink all of their adult lives, it is doubtful that policies specifically targeted to reduce alcohol misuse in their age group will be supported by them. The elderly also are disproportionately likely to vote. Hence, if opposed to alcohol policy initiatives targeting restrictions specifically on their drinking, the elderly may exert disproportionate influence in opposing such legislation.

If, on the other hand, policies were proposed that the elderly perceived as protecting them from the behaviours of younger drinkers, such as drinking and driving laws or laws directed at reducing alcohol-related crimes and violence, they might be supportive. They might also support creation of accessible safe public transport in urban, suburban and rural areas. To date, there is an absence of research exploring the perceptions of the elderly about this. The elderly might also favour legislation or policies that make alcohol treatment or treatment of numerous diseases and injuries related to alcohol misuse more accessible and affordable. They might favour other policies that increase financial access to treatment for other illnesses that could increase traffic safety, such as cataract surgery or special programmes to improve visual information processing while driving. Again, however, while research indicates potential benefits to the elderly from these interventions, research concerning public opinion of the elderly on these topics is missing.

Summary and conclusions

In summary, considerable evidence demonstrates that several alcohol policies reduce alcohol misuse and related deaths, including traffic deaths, in the general population. However, while the elderly are disproportionately represented in a variety of alcohol-attributable deaths, there is a lack of research on policies that specifically target the elderly's alcohol use and potential related harm [35–37]. For a variety of reasons, the case for elderly-specific policies to reduce drinking and particularly driving after drinking is weak and research support insufficient. Research is needed to test whether laws that reduce alcohol misuse and related morbidity and mortality in the general population can protect the elderly from elder abuse, other forms of violence, car crashes and other types of injury and the level of support for such policies among the elderly.

References

1. US Census Bureau (2010) *Population Profile of the United States.* US Department of Commerce, Washington, DC.
2. Han, B., Gfroerer, J.C., Colliver, J.D. *et al.* (2009) Substance use disorder among older adults in the United States in 2020. *Addiction,* **104**(1), 88–96.
3. Kuerbis, A. and Sacco, P. (2012) The impact of retirement on the drinking patterns of older adults: a review. *Addictive Behaviors,* **37**(5), 587–595.
4. National Institute on Alcohol Abuse and Alcoholism (2007) *Helping Patients Who Drink Too Much: A Clinician's Guide* (updated 2005 edition) NIH Publication No. 07-3769, US Department of Health and Human Services, Bethesda, MD.
5. National Institute on Alcohol Abuse and Alcoholism (2007) *Harmful Interactions: Mixing Alcohol with Medications.* NIH Publication No. 03-5329, US Department of Health and Human Services, Bethesda, MD.
6. Viamonte, S.M., Ball, K.K. and Kilgore, M. (2006) A cost-benefit analysis of risk-reduction strategies targeted at older drivers. *Traffic Injury Prevention,* 7(4), 352–359.
7. Thompson, J.P., Baldock, M.R., Mathias, J.L. and Wundersitz, L.N. (2013) An examination of the environmental, driver and vehicle factors associated with the serious and fatal crashes of older rural drivers. *Accident Analysis and Prevention,* 50, 768–775.
8. Li, G., Braver, E.R. and Chen, L.H. (2003) Fragility versus excessive crash involvement as determinants of high death rates per vehicle-mile of travel among older drivers. *Accident Analysis and Prevention,* **35**(2), 227–235.
9. Charlton, J.L., Catchlove, M., Scully, M. *et al.* (2013) Older driver distraction: a naturalistic study of behaviour at intersections. *Accident Analysis and Prevention,* 58, 271–278.
10. Centers for Disease Control and Prevention (2011) Vision Health Initiative, Common Eye Disorders. http://www.cdc.gov/visionhealth/basic_information/eye_disorders.htm (last accessed 17 April 2014).
11. Owsley, C., McGwin, G., Jr, Sloane, M. *et al.* (2002) Impact of cataract surgery on motor vehicle crash involvement by older adults. *Journal of the American Medical Association,* **288**(7), 841–849.
12. Mennemeyer, S.T., Owsley, C. and McGwin, G., Jr. (2013) Reducing older driver motor vehicle collisions via earlier cataract surgery. *Accident Analysis and Prevention,* **61**, 203-211.
13. Cross, J.M., McGwin, G., Jr, Rubin, G.S. *et al.* (2009) Visual and medical risk factors for motor vehicle collision involvement among older drivers. *The British Journal of Ophthalmology,* 93(3), 400–404.
14. Okonkwo, O.C., Wadley, V.G., Crowe, M. *et al.* (2007) Self-regulation of driving in the context of impaired visual attention are there gender differences? *Rehabilitation Psychology,* 52(4), 421–428.
15. Clay, O.J., Wadley, V.G., Edwards, J.D. *et al.* (2005) Cumulative meta-analysis of the relationship between useful field of view and driving performance in older adults: current and future implications. *Optometry and Vision Science,* 82(8), 724–731.
16. Friedman, C., McGwin, G., Jr, Ball, K.K. *et al.* (2013) Association between higher order visual processing abilities and a history of motor vehicle collision involvement by drivers ages 70 and over. *Investigative Ophthalmology & Visual Science,* 54(1), 778–782.
17. Leversen, J.S., Hopkins, B. and Signundsson, H. (2013) Ageing and driving: Examining the effects of visual processing demands. *Transportation Research Part F: Traffic Psychology and Behaviour,* 17, 1–4.
18. Centers for Disease Control and Prevention. Alcohol-Related Disease Impact (ARDI). http://apps.nccd.cdc.gov/ardi/HomePage.aspx (last accessed 17 April 2014).

19. National Institute on Alcohol Abuse and Alcoholism. National Epidemiologic Survey on Alcohol and Related Conditions, Wave 2, 2004–2005. National Institutes of Health, National Institute on Alcohol Abuse and Alcoholism, Bethesda, MD.

20. Babor, T.F., Caetano, R., Casswell, S. *et al.* (2010) *Alcohol: No Ordinary Commodity: Research and Public Policy*, 2nd edn. Oxford University Press, New York.

21. Centers for Disease Control and Prevention. The Guide to Community Prevention Services, Preventing Excessive Alcohol Consumption. http://www.thecommunityguide. org/alcohol/index.html (last accessed 17 April 2014).

22. Jonas, D.E., Garbutt, J.C., Amick, H.R. *et al.* (2012) Behavioral counseling after screening for alcohol misuse in primary care: a systematic review and meta-analysis for the U.S. Preventive Services Task Force. *Annals of Internal Medicine*, **157**(9), 645–654.

23. Moyer, V.A., Preventive Services Task Force. (2013) Screening and behavioral counseling interventions in primary care to reduce alcohol misuse: U.S. preventive services task force recommendation statement. *Annals of Internal Medicine*, **159**(3), 210–218.

24. Elder, R.W., Lawrence, B., Ferguson, A. *et al.* (2010) The effectiveness of tax policy interventions for reducing excessive alcohol consumption and related harms. *American Journal of Preventive Medicine*, **38**(2),217–229.

25. Xu, X. and Chaloupka, F.J. (2011) The effects of prices on alcohol use and its consequences. *Alcohol: Research and Health*, **34**(2), 236–245.

26. Wagenaar, A.C., Tobler, A.L. and Komro, K.A. (2010) Effects of alcohol tax and price policies on morbidity and mortality: a systematic review. *American Journal of Public Health*, **100**(11), 2270–2278.

27. Sloan, F.A., Reilly, B.A. and Schenzler, C. (1994) Effects of prices, civil and criminal sanctions, and law enforcement on alcohol-related mortality. *Journal of Studies on Alcohol*, **55**(4), 454–465.

28. Siren, A. and Meng, A. (2013) Older drivers' self-assessed driving skills, driving-related stress and self-regulation in traffic. *Transportation Research Part F: Traffic Psychology and Behaviour*, **17**: 88–97.

29. National Highway Traffic Safety Administration. U.S. Fatality Analysis Reporting System, 2013. http://www-fars.nhtsa.dot.gov (last accessed 17 April 2014).

30. Fell, J.C. and Voas, R.B. (2006) Mothers Against Drunk Driving (MADD): the first 25 years. *Traffic Injury Prevention*, **7**(3), 195–212.

31. Cummings, P., Rivara, F.P., Olson, C.M. *et al.* (2006) Changes in traffic crash mortality rates attributed to use of alcohol, or lack of a seat belt, air bag, motorcycle helmet, or bicycle helmet, United States, 1982–2001. *Injury Prevention*, **12**, 148–154.

32. Ferguson, S.A. (2012) Alcohol-impaired driving in the United States: contributors to the problem and effective countermeasures. *Traffic Injury Prevention*, **13**, 427–441.

33. Lacey, J.H., Kelley-Baker, T., Furr-Holden, D. *et al.* (2009) *2007 National Roadside Survey of Alcohol and Drug Use by Drivers: Alcohol Results*. DOT HS 811 248, 2009, National Highway Traffic Safety Administration, Washington, DC.

34. O'Krent, D. (2010) *Last Call: The Rise and Fall of Prohibition*. Simon and Schuster, New York.

35. Pun, V.C., Lin, H., Kim, J.H. *et al.* (2013) Impacts of alcohol duty reductions on cardiovascular mortality among elderly Chinese: a 10-year time series analysis. *Journal of Epidemiology and Community Health*, **67**(6), 514–518.

36. Neufeld, M. and Rehm, J. (2013) Alcohol consumption and mortality in Russia since 2000: are there any changes following the alcohol policy changes starting in 2006? *Alcohol and Alcoholism*, **48**(2), 222–230.

37. Stockwell, T., Auld, M.C., Zhao, J. and Martin, G. (2012) Does minimum pricing reduce alcohol consumption? The experience of a Canadian province. *Addiction*, **107**(5), 912–920.

Chapter 26
PROPOSALS FOR POLICY DEVELOPMENT: TOBACCO

Michael Givel

Department of Political Science, The University of Oklahoma, USA

Introduction

This chapter provides an overview of past and present public health intervention trends to reduce tobacco use and provides the best scientific practices linked to policy proposals to further reduce tobacco use for older adults age 50 and above. In 2010, 19.3% of adults or 45.3 million people in the United States, 18 or older, were current smokers [1]. The smoking prevalence rate was higher for men (21.5%) than for woman (17.3%) [1]. Additionally, adults aged 45–64 had one of the highest prevalence rates of tobacco use of all adults at 21.1% [1].

About 443 000 Americans died in the United States in 2013 from cigarette smoking [2]. Of these, about 49 400 Americans die annually due to second-hand tobacco smoke [2]. Second-hand tobacco smoke is defined as tobacco smoke emitted by a burning tobacco product or exhaled by a smoker. Far fewer Americans die due to smokeless tobacco use but only about 3.5% of Americans use smokeless tobacco [3]. The primary causes of tobacco use-related mortalities include various forms of cancers, such as lung, oral, pancreatic, bladder and kidney, cardiovascular diseases and respiratory diseases [2]. People who stop tobacco use greatly reduce their risks of diseases and death although the benefits are greater for those who end smoking at earlier ages [4].

Past and present approaches to reduce tobacco consumption

The history of public health efforts to reduce tobacco use in the twentieth and twenty-first centuries in the United States has gone through four distinct phases (Table 26.1). These phases, which are not mutually exclusive, commenced with phase one lasting from 1950 to 1964 [5]. In this first phase, several social epidemiological studies concluded there was a link between cigarette smoking and cancer, particularly lung cancer [6–9]. These findings were bolstered, in particular, by the large 1958 Hammond–Horn study on 187 783 male smokers between 50

Substance Use and Older People, First Edition.
Edited by Ilana B. Crome, Li-Tzy Wu, Rahul (Tony) Rao and Peter Crome.
© 2015 John Wiley & Sons, Ltd. Published 2015 by John Wiley & Sons, Ltd.

Table 26.1 Overview of four phases of tobacco control in the United States from 1950 to 2013

Name	Period	Description
Phase 1: Growing health dangers	1950–1964	Growing number of scientific studies indicate link between smoking and disease and death including lung cancer
Phase 2: Initial federal regulation of tobacco use	1964–1984	Included enactment of federal cigarette warning label laws
Phase 3: Increased regulation of tobacco use	1984–2001	Increased litigation for tobacco death and disease, more vigorous tobacco control education and regulation, and de-normalization of tobacco industry and societal smoking
Phase 4: New mixture of tobacco control approaches	2001–2013	Includes product modification for 'safer' cigarettes, harm reduction, cigarette neo-prohibitionism and smoke-free movies

and 69, which significantly correlated lung, larynx and oesophagus cancers with smoking. During this period, Doll also published key research on the international impact of smoking on doctors [9–11]. However, in the United States no policy actions were taken on this growing research until after 1964.

From 1964 to 1984, in the second phase, the primary policy response to the 1964 US Surgeon's General landmark report that linked smoking with lung cancer, laryngeal cancer and chronic bronchitis included less than vigorous federal regulatory actions [5, 12]. The primary approach included the passage of the federal *Cigarette Labeling and Advertising Act* of 1965 and the *Public Health Cigarette Smoking Act* of 1969, which required all packages of cigarettes to contain small font warning labels in a conspicuous place on cigarette packs [13]. There was no evidence that the warning labels had any impact on reducing tobacco consumption [13, 14]. They were used as a legal defence by tobacco companies to pre-empt product liability lawsuits with the industry arguing that smokers assumed the risk for smoking due to the message on the warning labels [13].

Phase three anti-tobacco efforts

In phase three, from 1984 to 2001 [5], three primary approaches to counter tobacco use were used. These included legal, regulatory and de-normalization approaches.

Legal approach

The legal approach consisted of three waves (Table 26.2). The first wave, from 1954 to 1978, consisted of 125 individual personal injury lawsuits alleging negligence, misrepresentation and breach of warranty. Only a very small number of

Table 26.2 Phases of litigation against the tobacco industry from 1954 to 2013

Phase	Dates	Description
Initial personal injury lawsuits against tobacco industry	1954–1978	Small number of personal injury lawsuits with tobacco industry victorious in all cases
Continuing personal injury lawsuits against tobacco industry	1979–1993	Small number of personal injury and product liability lawsuits with tobacco industry victorious in all but one case
Public and private lawsuits against tobacco industry	1994–2013	Numerous public class action and individual personal injury and product liability private lawsuits filed. Tobacco industry lost or settled a number of cases

these cases went to trial and the tobacco industry lost none of the cases [15]. In the second wave, from 1979 to 1993, approximately 200 personal injury lawsuits were filed based on the legal theories of negligence, misrepresentation, breach of warranty, breach of product liability and negligent failure to inform [15, 16]. Only 18 of these cases were litigated and only one case, in 1983 in New Jersey, *Cipollone v. Liggett Group, Inc.,* was decided against Liggett Tobacco Company.

In the third wave, from 1994 to the present, several successful individual and private class action lawsuits were decided against the tobacco industry using the legal theories of torts, fraud, conspiracy, misrepresentation, breach of warranty, breach of product liability and negligent failure to inform [15, 16]. Legal theories in United States state class action suits included using statistics to determine if a percentage of Medicaid smokers contracted a disease from smoking, violation of state tort laws, consumer protection, anti-trust and racketeering laws. Using statistical trends provided a much easier form of proof than proving direct causation between tobacco consumption and disease [15, 16]. A successful US Justice Department suit, decided on appeal in 2012, also used the legal theories of conspiracy and misrepresentation [17, 18].

Regulatory and tobacco tax approaches

The third phase also included the initiation of anti-tobacco regulatory and tobacco tax requirements from 1984 to 2001. Key programme efforts of this approach included using higher tobacco taxes to reduce consumption, provisions prohibiting second-hand tobacco smoke in public areas, tobacco warning labels, anti-tobacco counter-marketing campaigns and tobacco cessation programmes. The efficacy of each of these programmatic anti-tobacco approaches is reviewed here.

Tobacco taxes

The World Health Organization regards tobacco tax increases as the most cost efficient approach for reducing tobacco consumption [19]. Since the mid-1990s, the federal government and numerous states have substantially raised tobacco taxes [20]. A variety of studies have concluded that tobacco tax and price increases have a direct impact on tobacco cessation and reducing the frequency of tobacco use for all age groups [19]. Additionally, the World Health Organization recommends that to effectively reduce tobacco use, tobacco taxes should be at least 70% of the retail price [19]. In higher income countries like the United States, most studies indicate that a 10% increase in cigarette prices decreases demand by 2.5–5.0% [19]. Additionally, several studies indicate that minors and young adults are 'two to three' times more receptive to decreasing frequency and use due to tobacco price increases than older adults [19, 21]. Until recently, the very few studies that have been conducted providing more detailed information for older adults have focused on indirect impacts or tobacco tax increases on demographics by age [22]. However, for older adults aged 45–59, one recent scholarly article has shown that a one dollar increase in tobacco taxes will cause around 7% of these daily smokers to quit smoking [22]. Further research is required to confirm this initial finding.

Second-hand tobacco smoke restrictions

Smoke-free laws that ban smoking in workplaces and indoor public areas not only protect the health of nonsmokers by reducing potential exposure to second-hand tobacco smoke but also have a statistically significant impact on reducing tobacco use frequency for a general population from 1.4 to 6.3% with a median of 3.4% [23]. Smoke-free laws increases tobacco cessation by 6.4% [23]. Like tobacco tax increases, very few studies have focused on second-hand smoke restrictions in public areas with respect to inducing older adults to quit smoking [24]. In once recent case study of Fort Collins, CO, a smoke-free ordinance induced the general population to quit smoking by 4.5% while the ordinance induced people 50 and older to quit smoking by 2% [24]. Further research is required to confirm this finding.

Tobacco warning labels

Cigarette warning labels provide an important public health approach to inform smokers of all ages of the dangers of tobacco use and provide information on resources such as quit lines for help quitting smoking. Recent research has concluded that the most effective cigarette package warning labels for promoting cessation cover 30% or more of the front of the cigarette pack, are in colour with graphic depictions of health and disease due to smoking and contain clear messages about the direct health dangers due to smoking [13, 25–27]. Effective anti-tobacco warning labels have a significant impact on smoking frequency and quitting rates [28]. A recent study of Canadian smokers found that effective cigarette warning labels decreased the odds that a person would be a smoker by 12.5% and a daily smoker by 13.2% [29]. Additionally, the odds that all smokers would attempt to quit increased to 33% for smokers and 33.1% for daily smokers [29]. So far, no peer-reviewed articles have examined the impact of warning labels on adults 50 and older. Further research is required to ascertain the impact of warning labels on adults in this age group.

Anti-tobacco counter-marketing campaigns

Anti-tobacco counter-marketing messages used in recent years have been a valuable means to counter tobacco use among minors and young adults [30]. In particular, commencing in the mid-1990s, in California and later elsewhere, de-normalization, painting the tobacco industry as exceptional, a pariah and even evil, as well as causing significant health problems, has manifested itself as a counter-marketing approach to induce smokers to quit or consider quitting [31–44]. The de-normalization effort against the tobacco industry is also part of a larger effort to de-normalize and stigmatize societal norms affirming the social acceptability of smoking [45–47]. A small number of recent studies have confirmed that adults were more likely to consider quitting smoking or quit smoking if they held high social de-normalization or anti-tobacco industry beliefs [46, 48]. As noted in 2011, of all peer-reviewed articles covering tobacco de-normalization, most studies focused on youth while a few addressed younger adults [49]. No studies to this date have focused on adults aged 50 and older [49].

Tobacco cessation programmes

Effective smoking cessation efforts are comprehensive in nature. Cessation efforts should include a combination of proven nicotine replacement therapies, including drug or cold turkey interventions and counselling and therapy [50, 51]. Ending smoking is very difficult due to highly addicted nicotine dependence and may include several relapses [4]. A majority of smokers quit without evidence-based interventions [4]. However, for those smokers that do not quit on their own, a combination of counselling and drug treatment approaches, such as over-the-counter patches, gum or lozenges or prescription nasal spray or nicotine inhalants, leads to the greatest level of tobacco cessation [4, 52]. A number of studies have also determined that smoking cessation for older adults can be a very beneficial approach to increase life expectancy and counter major incidents of disease, such as cardiovascular disease [53–56].

Recent anti-tobacco proposals

In the fourth phase, from 2001 to 2013, several anti-tobacco policies have been advanced to reduce the current adult smoking rate even further [57]. The following are the current policy proposals.

Product modification and 'safer' cigarettes

Since 1999, there has been a considerable effort in the United States to require the Food and Drug Administration (FDA) to make cigarettes purportedly safer [58]. In a culmination of these efforts, Congress passed the *Family Smoking Prevention and Tobacco Control Act* of 2009 (P.L. 111-31), which empowered the FDA to approve safer tobacco products by assessing a possible reduction of health risks [58]. However, prior to the *Family Smoking Prevention and Tobacco Control Act*, there was no scientific consensus and little evidence that removing one or more ingredients from cigarettes will make them safer [56, 59]. Since the 1950s, the tobacco industry as well as the federal government have spent millions of dollars to create a marketable and less risky cigarette [59]. None have ever been manufactured. A key problem is determining, in a scientifically conclusive fashion, short-term as well as long-term (up to 20 years) health effects on smokers based on the removal of one or more ingredients [59]. Compounding this significant problem of determining health impacts, from 2009 to 2013, the FDA has never approved the removal of one cigarette ingredient or additive, including menthol, from cigarettes.

Harm reduction

A market-based proposal that has surfaced since 2000 is the substitution of cigarette smoking with smokeless tobacco or e-Cigarettes. The primary motivation is that chewing tobacco and e-Cigarettes cause substantially less harm in the form of disease and deaths than regular cigarette smoking. However, smokeless tobacco is not a totally safe alternative to smoking because smokeless tobacco contains about 30 cancer-producing substances [60]. Among the complications that can occur from smokeless tobacco are addictions, oral, pancreatic and kidney cancer, tooth decay, gum disease, heart attacks, strokes and pre-cancerous mouth lesions [60]. According to the FDA, the safety of e-Cigarettes has not been determined. This includes the possible harm of inhaling nicotine and other ingredients from an e-Cigarette and any possible benefits [61].

Cigarette neo-prohibitionism

Recently, cigarette neo-prohibitionists have argued that a cigarette ban can be reached by phasing out cigarettes through effective anti-tobacco regulations and high taxes in conjunction with aggressive application of nicotine replacement therapies [62]. Critics of the neo-prohibition approach have argued that this idea is not politically viable, causes tobacco smuggling and creates black markets, and would not end tobacco use [62]. Early evidence from Bhutan, where cigarette sales has been banned since 2004 while allowing the importation of small amounts for personal consumption, indicates there is robust cigarette smuggling, a thriving black market and continued consumption of tobacco products, particularly among youth [62].

Smoke-free movies

A recent proposal to counter tobacco use by minors includes: rating new movies 'R' if smoking is shown or implied, no payments from the tobacco industry for tobacco promotions, no tobacco brand identification and strong anti-tobacco smoking advertisements [63]. However, no research findings, to date, have concluded whether this would be effective in inducing older adults to quit or consider quitting [64–66].

Policy proposals to further reduce tobacco prevalence

Based on current best practices and scientific research the anti-tobacco policies and approaches that should be employed include proper warning labels on cigarette packs, higher tobacco taxes, restrictions on second-hand tobacco smoke in public areas and effective counter-marketing using de-normalization of smoking and the tobacco industry. More scientific research needs to be funded and conducted for each of these anti-tobacco approaches to determine the specific impact and efficacy in reducing tobacco use for older adults. Further research is also required regarding smoke-free movie restrictions that may impact tobacco use by older adults.

Additionally, another effective anti-tobacco approach includes, when appropriate, continuing individual suits as well as class action suits that particularly award damages which fund or require public anti-tobacco efforts. Another approach that research has found effective in reducing disease and death for older Americans is effective tobacco cessation programmes and outreach.

Policy efforts that should be currently de-emphasized for the time being due to insignificant information on effectiveness and possible or actual safety issues are product modification, cigarette neo-prohibitionism and e-Cigarettes. Further, harm reduction by substituting smokeless tobacco with cigarettes, which still harms the individual user, should not be pursued [67].

Current scientific research and best practices provide a clear course of action for further policymaking with respect to reducing tobacco use among older adults. The link between rational policy alternatives and effective advocacy, enactment and implementation of anti-tobacco policies requires astute advocacy and mobilization of resources, financial and otherwise. Putting health organizations engaging in insider lobbying on the same footing as the tobacco industry quite often produce no results [68]. Anti-tobacco organizing should also include, when warranted, outsider advocacy approaches such as media coverage and advertising, forums or public demonstrations [68]. One key strategy that is central to these efforts is holding politicians at all levels of government publicly accountable for their pro-tobacco actions, including voting them out of office [68].

References

1. Centers for Disease Control and Prevention (2012) Smoking and Tobacco Use: Adult Cigarette Smoking in the United States: Current Estimate. http://www.cdc.gov/tobacco/data_statistics/fact_sheets/adult_data/cig_smoking/ (last accessed 18 April 2014).
2. Centers for Disease Control and Prevention (2012) Smoking and Tobacco Use: Tobacco-Related Mortality. http://www.cdc.gov/tobacco/data_statistics/fact_sheets/health_effects/tobacco_related_mortality/index.htm (last accessed 18 April 2014).

3. Substance Abuse and Mental Health Services Administration (2011) *Results from the 2010 National Survey on Drug Use and Health: Summary of National Findings.* NSDUH Series H-41, HHS Publication No. (SMA) 11-4658, United States Department of Health and Human Services, Rockville, MD.

4. Centers for Disease Control and Prevention (2012) Smoking & Tobacco Use: Smoking Cessation. http://www.cdc.gov/tobacco/data_statistics/fact_sheets/cessation/quitting/index.htm (last accessed 18 April 2014).

5. Studlar, D. (2002) *Tobacco Control: Comparative Politics in the United States and Canada.* Broadview Press Ltd, Peterborough, ON, Canada.

6. Brandt, A. (2009) *The Cigarette Century: The Rise, Fall, and Deadly Persistence of the Product That Defined America.* Basic Books, New York.

7. Kluger, R. (1996) *Ashes to Ashes: America's Hundred-Year Cigarette War, The Public Health, and the Unabashed Triumph of Philip Morris.* Alfred A. Knopf, New York.

8. Tate, C. (1999) *Cigarette Wars: The Triumph of The Little White Slaver.* Oxford University Press, New York.

9. Doll, R. and Bradford Hill, A. (1950) Smoking and carcinoma of the lung. *British Medical Journal,* 2(4682), 739–748.

10. Doll, R. (2002) Proof of causality: Deduction from epidemiological observation. *Perspectives in Biology and Medicine,* 45(4), 499–515.

11. Doll, R. (2004) Mortality in relation to smoking: 50 years' observations on male british doctors. *British Medical Journal,* 328(328), 1519–1533.

12. Surgeon General's Advisory Committee on Smoking and Health (1964) *Report of the Advisory Committee to the Surgeon General of the United States.* Public Health Service Publication No. 1103, US Department of Health, Education, and Welfare, Washington, DC.

13. Givel, M. (2007) A Comparison of the impact of U.S. and Canadian cigarette pack warning label requirements on tobacco industry profitability and the public health. *Health Policy,* 83, 343–352.

14. Hammond, D., Fong, G.T., McNeill, A. *et al.* (2006) Effectiveness of cigarette warning labels in informing smokers about the risks of smoking: Findings from the International Tobacco Control (ITC) four country survey. *Tobacco Control,* 15(Suppl III), iii9–iii25.

15. Blanke, D. (2002) Towards health with justice: Litigation and public inquiries as tools for tobacco control. In: *Tobacco Free Initiative,* World Health Organization, Geneva, Switzerland.

16. Givel, M. and Glantz, S. (2004) The global settlement with the tobacco industry: 6 years later. *American Journal of Public Health,* 94(2), 218–224.

17. United States of America v. Philip Morris, *et al.* (2006) In *449 F.Supp:* Federal District Court, District of Columbia. No. 1:99-cv-02496.

18. United States of America, Apellee v. Philip Morris, *et al.* (2012) United States Court of Appeals, District of Columbia. No. 04-5252.

19. World Health Organization (2011) *WHO Technical Manual on Tobacco Tax Administration.* World Health Organization, Geneva, Switzerland.

20. American Lung Association (2013) By Failing to Equalize Tobacco Taxes, States Lose Revenue and Fail to Reduce Tobacco Use. http://www.stateoftobaccocontrol.org/at-a-glance/state-governments/states-lose-revenue-dont-reduce-tobacco-use.html (last accessed 18 April 2014).

21. van Walbeck, C., Blecher, E., Gilmore, A. and Ross, H. (2012) Price and tax measures and illicit trade in the framework convention on tobacco control: What we know and what research is required. *Nicotine & Tobacco Research,* 15(4), 767–776.

22. DeCicca, P. and McLeod, L. (2008) Cigarette taxes and older adult smoking: Evidence from recent large tax increases. *Journal of Health Economics,* 27, 918–929.

23. Hopkins, D., Razi, S., Leeks, K. *et al.* (2010) Smokefree policies to reduce tobacco use: A systematic review. *American Journal of Preventive Medicine*, **38**(2S), S275–S289.

24. Prochaska, J., Burdine, J., Bigsby, K. *et al.* (2009) The impact of a communitywide smoke-free ordinance on smoking among older adults. *Preventing Chronic Disease*, **6**(1), 1–10.

25. Hammond, D., Fong, G.T., McDonald, P.W. *et al.* (2003) Impact of Canadian warning labels on adult smoking behavior. *Tobacco Control*, **12**, 391–395.

26. Chapman, S. and Carter, S.M. (2003) Avoid health warnings on all tobacco products for just as long as we can: A history of Australian tobacco industry efforts to avoid, delay, and dilute health warning on cigarettes. *Tobacco Control*, **12**(Suppl. III), iii13–iii22.

27. Thrasher, J.F., Carpenter, M.J., Andrews, J.O. *et al.* (2012) Cigarette warning label policy alternatives and smoking-related health disparities. *American Journal of Preventive Medicine*, **43**(6), 590–600.

28. Borland, R., Yong, H.-H., Wilson, N. *et al.* (2009) How reactions to cigarette packet health warnings influence quitting: Findings from the ITC four country survey. *Addiction*, **104**(4), 669–675.

29. Azagba, S. and Sharaf, M. (2012) The effect of graphic cigarette warning labels on smoking behavior: Evidence from the Canadian experience. *Nicotine & Tobacco Research*, **15**(3), 708–17.

30. Murphy-Hoefer, R., Hyland, A. and Rivard, C. (2010) The influence of tobacco countermarketing ads on college students' knowledge, attitudes, and beliefs. *The Journal of American College Health*, **58**(4), 373–381.

31. Asbridge, M. (2004) Public place restrictions on smoking in Canada: Assessing the role of state, media, science, and public health advocacy. *Social Science and Medicine*, **58**, 13–24.

32. Ashley, M. and Cohen, J. (2003) What the public thinks about the tobacco industry and its products. *Tobacco Control*, **12**, 396–400.

33. Bal, D., Lloyd, J. and Manley, M. (1995) The role of the primary care physician in tobacco use prevention and cessation. *California Cancer Journal for Clinicians*, **45**, 369–374.

34. Bal, D., Lloyd, J., Roeseler, A. and Shimizu, R. (2001) California as a Model. *Journal of Clinical Oncology*, **19**(18s), 69s–73s.

35. Balbach, E, Smith, E. and Malone, R. (2006) How the health belief model helps the tobacco industry: Individuals, choice, and information. *Tobacco Control*, **15**, iv37–iv43.

36. Bero, L., Montini, T., Byron-Jones, K. and Mangurian, C. (2001) Science in regulatory policy making: case studies in the development of workplace smoking restrictions. *Tobacco Control*. **10**, 329–336.

37. Chapman, S. (2004) Advocacy in action: Extreme corporate makeover interruptus: denormalizing tobacco industry corporate schmoozing. *Tobacco Control*, **13**, 445–447.

38. Chapman, S. (2007) *Public Health Advocacy and Tobacco Control.* Blackwell Publishing, Oxford.

39. Durrant, R., Wakefield, M., McLeod, K. *et al.* (2001) Tobacco in the news: An analysis of newspaper coverage of tobacco issues in Australia, 2001. *Tobacco Control,* **12**, 75–81.

40. Goldman, L. and S Glantz, S. (1998) Evaluation of antismoking advertising campaigns. *Journal of the American Medical Association*, **279**(10), 772–777.

41. Hirschhorn, N. (2004) Corporate social responsibility and the tobacco industry: Hope or hype? *Tobacco Control*, **13**, 447–453.

42. Ibrahim, J.K. and Glantz, S. (2006) Tobacco industry litigation strategies to oppose tobacco control media campaigns. *Tobacco Control*, 15, 50–58.
43. Ling, P., Neilands, T. and Glantz, S. (2008) The effect of support for action against the tobacco industry on smoking among young adults. *American Journal of Public Health*, 97(8), 1449–1456.
44. McDaniel, P., and Malone, R. (2005) Understanding Philip Morris's pursuit of U.S. Government regulation of tobacco. *Tobacco Control*, 14, 193–200.
45. Bell, K., Salmon, A., Bowers, M. *et al.* (2010) Smoking, stigma, and tobacco denormalization: Further reflections on the use of stigma as a public health tool. A commentary on social science & medicine's stigma, prejudice, discrimination and health issue. *Social Science and Medicine*, 70(6), 795–799.
46. Hammond, D., Fong, G., Zanna, M. *et al.* (2006) Tobacco denormalization and industry beliefs among smokers from four countries. *American Journal of Preventive Medicine*, 31(3), 225–232.
47. Thrasher, J. (2006) Clarifying the concept of denormalization in tobacco prevention efforts. Paper read at 13th World Conference on Tobacco OR Health, 14 July 2006, Washington, DC.
48. Netemeyer, RG, Andrews, J.C. and Burton, S. (2005) Effects of antismoking advertising based beliefs on adults smokers' consideration of quitting. *American Journal of Public Health*, 95, 1062–1065.
49. Malone, R.E, Grundy, Q. and Bero, L.A. (2011) Tobacco industry denormalisation as a tobacco control intervention: a review. *Tobacco Control*, 21, 162–170.
50. Black, J.H. (2010) Evidence base and strategies for successful smoking cessation. *Journal of Vascular Surgery*, 51(6), 1529–1537.
51. Stack, N.M. and Zillich, A.J. (2007) Implementation of inpatient and outpatient tobacco-cessation programs. *American Journal of Health and Systemic Pharmacy*, 1(64), 2074–2079.
52. Nayan, S., Gupta, M.K. and Sommer, D.D. (2011) Evaluating smoking cessation interventions and cessation rates in cancer patients: A systematic review and meta-analysis. *ISRN Oncology*, Epub 2011 Jul 10.
53. Jeremias, E., Chatkin, J.M. Chatkin, G. *et al.* (2012) Smoking cessation in older adults. *International Journal of Tuberculosis and Lung Disease*, 16(2), 273–278.
54. Gellert, C., Schottker, B., Muller, H. *et al.* (2013) Impact of smoking and quitting on cardiovacular outcomes and risk advancement periods among older adults. *European Journal of Epidemiology*, 28(8), 649–658.
55. Kriekard, O.P., Gharacholou, S.M. and Peterson, E.D. (2009) Primary and secondary prevention of cardiovascular disease in older adults: A status report. *Clinical Geriatric Medicine*, 25(4), 745–755.
56. Tait, R.J., Hulse, G.K., Waterreus, A. *et al.* (2007) Effectiveness of a smoking cessation intervention in older adults. *Addiction*, 102(1), 148–155.
57. Centers for Disease Control and Prevention (2013) Adult Cigarette Smoking in the United States: Current Estimate. http://www.cdc.gov/tobacco/data_statistics/fact_sheets/adult_data/cig_smoking/ (last accessed 18 April 2014).
58. Givel, M. (2008) Policy and health implications of using the U.S. Food and Drug Administration product design approach in reducing tobacco product risk. *Current Drug Abuse Reviews*, 1(2), 135–141.
59. Givel, M. (2011) In search of the less risky cigarette. *International Journal of Health Services*, 41(1), 77–94.
60. Mayo Clinic (2012) Chewing tobacco: Not a safe alternative to cigarettes. http://www.mayoclinic.com/health/chewing-tobacco/CA00019 (last accessed 18 April 2014).

61. United States Food and Drug Administration (2013) Electronic Cigarettes (e-Cigarettes). http://www.fda.gov/newsevents/publichealthfocus/ucm172906.htm (last accessed 18 April 2014).
62. Givel, M. (2011) History of Bhutan's prohibition of cigarettes: Implications for neo-prohibitionists and their critics. *International Journal of Drug Policy*, 22(4), 306–310.
63. Glantz, S. (2013) Smokefree Movies: The Solution. http://www.smokefreemovies.ucsf.edu/solution/index.html (last accessed 18 April 2014).
64. Glantz, S. and Polansky, J. (2011) Movies with smoking make less money. *Tobacco Control*, 21(6), 569–571.
65. Tickle, J.J., Sargent, J.D., Dalton, M.A. *et al.* (2001) Favourite movie stars, their tobacco use in contemporary movies, and its association with adolescent smoking. *Tobacco Control*, 10(1), 16–22.
66. Jamieson, P.E and Romer, D. (2010) Trends in US movie tobacco portrayal since 1950: A historical analysis. *Tobacco Control*, 19(3), 179–184.
67. Centers for Disease Control and Prevention (2010) Press Release: CDC Releases Data on Smokeless Tobacco Use Among Smokers. http://www.cdc.gov/media/pressrel/2010/r101104.html?s_cid=mediarel_r101104 (last accessed 18 April 2014).
68. Givel, M. and Glantz, S. (2001) Tobacco lobby political influence on US State Legislatures in the 1990s. *Tobacco Control*, 10, 124–134.

Chapter 27

RECOMMENDATIONS

Ilana B. Crome[1,2,3,4], Peter Crome[5], Rahul (Tony) Rao[6] and Li-Tzy Wu[7]

[1] Keele University, UK
[2] Queen Mary University of London, UK
[3] Imperial College University of London, UK
[4] South Staffordshire and Shropshire Healthcare NHS Foundation Trust, UK
[5] Research Department of Primary Care and Population Health, University College London, UK
[6] Department of Old Age Psychiatry, Institute of Psychiatry, UK
[7] Department of Psychiatry and Behavioral Sciences, School of Medicine, Duke University Medical Center, USA

Background

Throughout the evolution of this book, we have been struck by major – some recurring – challenges.

It is vital to try to establish agreement on what constitutes 'older' in the substance misuse field. What we have witnessed in the development of this book, is that there are a variety of age thresholds that have been applied. Different operational definitions have been used, which often relate to severity, intensity and duration of substance use. It would support research if there were internationally agreed definitions. On an international, national and certainly a more local level, organizations of various kinds need consensus.

Then it is essential to separate out what is specifically distinctive about older people, so that what can be applied from younger age groups to older people is undertaken with the major differences borne in mind, and specific approaches or interventions can be tailored or developed for the benefit of older age groups. This can only be done if older people are included rather than excluded from studies of all sorts: epidemiological, clinical, prevention and clinical trial studies.

Medical, psychological, biological, sociological and social sciences can continue to contribute to an improved knowledge base of substance misuse among older adults. This includes a better understanding of the reasons why older people use and misuse substances, such as what they self-report as their use levels, how they explain their use and what meaning the substance use has in their lives. It includes understanding the apparent links, associations or consequences between behaviours and symptoms and illnesses. It incorporates determining the risk factors which appear to be related to substance use behaviours and which may be susceptible to intervention or extend understanding. Delineation of clear mechanisms and processes that demonstrate how the condition is triggered and caused would enhance understanding of the potential associations, but this is still to be demonstrated in the case of addictive behaviours.

Substance Use and Older People, First Edition.
Edited by Ilana B. Crome, Li-Tzy Wu, Rahul (Tony) Rao and Peter Crome.
© 2015 John Wiley & Sons, Ltd. Published 2015 by John Wiley & Sons, Ltd.

Epidemiology

It is not only the prevalence of each substance that requires consideration but the risks and risk factors related to the use, and interaction, of multiple substances, including medications that are now so prevalent in older people. What determines vulnerability and indeed, resilience, need a closer examination.

This will undoubtedly strengthen our appreciation of what constitutes a 'safe' limit or recommendations for older people in terms of alcohol use, as well as other substances in the form of medications or over-the-counter medications.

Determination of the risk factors likely to lead to substance misuse is an important aspect, because this might provide a guide to preventive measures. Whilst there is a degree of knowledge in relation to alcohol use, this has not generalized to other substances of misuse, nor to misuse of psychoactive and other medically prescribed drugs.

The course of substance misuse and the potential deterioration in the condition of the older person with regard to severity, intensity and duration, likewise, has not been the subject of systematic research. Patterns of relationships between conditions need elucidation.

Intergenerational issues, too, have received fleeting reference, though we know there are genetic contributions to the development of dependence, and families with several generations of difficulties are often present in clinical services. We know that most of those who have addiction problems in later life, start using substances in their teens. Teasing out the interrelationships is yet to be carried out but the impact is crucial in terms of influencing management.

Listening to the patient experience – often extreme suffering and being shunted from pillar to post due to stigma and prejudice and the chronicity of their conditions – will further enlighten our capability to provide a compassionate, empathic, respectful, sensitive and dignified response. Understanding health (mental illness, cognitive dysfunction), life circumstance (poverty, family conflict, social isolation), behaviour (being labelled a 'druggie'), status (being older, a victim of abuse) and personal quality (low self-esteem, impaired functional life skills) will enhance both the clinical interaction and improve motivation for change, and the research agenda. Patients are sensitive to, amongst other issues, the stigmatizing nature of addiction, their socioeconomic status, difficulty in accessing and engaging with services, and the impact of culture and ethnicity. This needs high priority in the clinical situation as well as in research.

The socioeconomic impact of substance misuse in older people is also evident from carer burden and the arising opportunity cost, as well the public health burden, particularly from rising rates of alcohol misuse in successive cohorts.

Clinical presentations

Complex interrelationships need to be understood in order to best appreciate the myriad of problems to be managed. Different disciplinary approaches have to applied, for example biological, medical, psychological and even sociological, to fathom the nature and extent of complications which present in seemingly a protean fashion. That substance use, intoxication, harmful use and dependence lead to physical and psychological symptoms and syndromes as well as social instability, is well documented. Understanding in what way substance misuse triggers or exacerbates pre-existing mental or physical symptomatology or disorder, or how psychological or physical morbidity or disorders may precipitate substance use, in older people is germane to optimal treatment.

The complexity inherent in the use of multiple substances is that there will be multiple presentations which are sometimes subtle or atypical, a manifestation of drug interactions itself or with the illness. There may be psychiatric symptoms which may not be severe but can be debilitating in the older person who may have physical illness in a particular social context.

Much more needs to be known about these complex presentations, explicitly because these are usually mainstream rather than exceptional clinical issues, with an impact on mortality, re-hospitalization, increased severity of illness, poor compliance and, also, social dimensions such as violence, impoverishment and marginalization.

Clinical presentations may fluctuate with time due to substance use, intoxication and withdrawal, so may motivation for change. The challenge is to recognize the need to make a balanced assessment of needs based on clinical judgment, experience, expertise and intuition.

Education and training

Competence in assessment is a key challenge. Little systematic training is currently available for professionals engaged in clinical activities and research in this field. Without in-depth knowledge the trainee or working professional will not be in a position to undertake the comprehensive – often repeated – assessment that is required to formulate a clinical case and place the individual in her/his social context. There needs to be a pool of resources so that professionals can update their knowledge and skills, which is partly related to awareness raising and (change of) attitudes. New technologies and resources which are developing in other areas of medical education need to be applied to training about the older substance misuser.

As educators, we can challenge the stigma, stereotyping and the idea the substance misuse is a moral weakness by demonstrating a nonjudgemental and nonconfrontational approach. We can challenge the underreporting of substance problems by training colleagues how to take a comprehensive history. We can challenge the misattribution of symptoms and underdiagnosis by a high index of suspicion and awareness of the subtlety of presentation. However, all this demands the creation of a climate that is receptive to the notion that older people have rights to civilised services. Training can reverse therapeutic nihilism by improving attitudes and reducing stigma. Undergraduate, specialist postgraduate and continuing professional development courses can facilitate this change.

Who gets treatment – treatment interventions

Far fewer people with addiction problems receive the help they need compared with those with other conditions such as breast cancer, hypertension, asthma and diabetes. Even fewer older people get the treatment they deserve. It is critical to have access to appropriate services. That having been achieved, they become a robust base for research, training and feed into policy.

Exclusions should be minimal. Re-assessments should be priorities. It should be recognized that for some patients the treatment is a long haul. Every opportunity should be galvanized to make the service and interactions user friendly. Treatments should be tailored to the individual. Guidance for older people is limited by paucity of research. Much more is needed. What are appropriate treatment goals? Is medical advice credible to older people? How far has socioeconomic status been a barrier to treatment in a particular case? Has the patient's ethnicity or culture been taken account of? What social networks are in place? Are the techniques of assessment appropriate? Is there understandable ambivalence to medication, its effects and compliance? What happens to the patient post-treatment episode?

Although there are many treatment interventions available, relatively few have been evaluated in an older age group. Although the results are encouraging, we still do not know, for example, whether older people perform optimally in an elder-orientated treatment setting as compared with a mixed-age group. Many of the pharmacological agents for withdrawal, abstinence and relapse prevention, too, need investigating in older people.

Knowledge about what constitutes the optimal model for services remains to be clarified. It is helpful to think of the functions that a comprehensive service would need, and attempt to ensure that all relevant practitioners contribute. There is sufficient information about interventions that are likely to have a degree of effectiveness and, therefore, can be applied to the older substance misuser, which are not already being implemented. It is imperative to offer for each component what you would anyway, for example addiction, mental illness, physical disorder, social difficulties. Collaboration, by formal or informal means, with the patient, providers and other significant support is to be maximized. The usefulness of self -help and mutual aid is to be encouraged if it suits the individual. The use of new technologies, too, can be a stimulus for earlier detection and brief interventions. Finally, there is a need for research to inform the implementation of the Screening of substance misuse, Brief Intervention and Referral to Treatment (SBIRT) practice in medical settings to facilitate early identification and detection of substance misuse and to reduce and prevent healthcare costs and consequences from substance misuse related conditions.

Concluding remarks

This book has demonstrated that there is considerable interest and enormously talented clinicians, researchers, policy makers and educators who, often with little support, acknowledge the problems and are attempting to improve their domain.

However, research funding is sparse and it is difficult to undertake due to the fact that it is long-term and expensive. There is no national strategy in place, as far as we could discern, to prioritize this group. Moreover, this group of patients are not naturally easy research subjects to recruit, as they are often traumatized by having had a chaotic past and have multiple problems with which to cope. Clinicians need to be encouraged to participate in research, as do patients and their families, where there can be some reluctance. There is much heterogeneity and many subgroups of patients and, perhaps for this reason, specificity of treatment for the older substance misuser is still lacking.

Furthermore, the overall context in which treatment and research is taking place is constantly changing. National policies differ and change as does the availability of substances. While efforts in raising awareness may still be embryonic, there is also misinformation on the impact of substances on health and well-being. There are the differing philosophies, objective, models, languages in the addiction, mental health and medical services, where the roles and responsibilities of practitioners may be differently perceived. Often, due to the complexity of the patients, practitioners are working outside their comfort zone. But these are increasingly global problems that need national and local solutions. These can be variously through clinicians, with experience and intuition, who can provide insights for future research and much needed training, through updated reviews, guidance and guidelines, and working groups which can infuse policy, and where collaborative funding for research developments can answer some of the many questions posed through the course of the book.

INDEX

Note: Page numbers in *italics* refer to Figures; those in **bold** to Tables.

activities of daily living (ADLs),
    181–2
Addenbrookes Cognitive Assessment
    Revised (ACE-R), 187
addiction liaison services
    drug and alcohol problems, 256–7
    elements, 258–9
    fall-induced fracture, 260–261
    general hospitals, 256
    older adults, 257–8
    screening
        alcohol problems, 259–60
        drug use problems, 260
    substance misuse problems, 257
Advance Care Planning (ACP)
    advance decisions, provisions, 6, 7
    Lasting Power of Attorney
        (LPA), 6–7
    specific medical treatments, 6
Affordable Care Act, 367
age-segregated or mixed-age
    treatment, 329
age-sensitive psychosocial treatment
    baby boomers, 314–15
    characteristics
        client functioning, 318–19
        coping and social skills, 319
        cultural differences, 317–18
        flexible, 316–17
        gender differences, 317
        holistic approach, 319
        supportive and nonconfrontational,
            316

components
    biopsychosocial assessment, 320–321
    chronic pain, 323
    cognitive impairment or dementia,
        324–5
    empirically-supported psychosocial
        interventions, 325–8
    psychosocial interventions, 328–9
    referrals and care coordination, 325
    substance-related disorders, 325
    treatment planning, 321–322
    late life, 315
    psychosocial treatments, 315
    substance abuse, 315
alcohol
    abuse or dependence, diagnosis,
        83–4
    amount of drinking, estimation, 76–7,
        78, 79
    binge drinking
        Behavioral Risk Factor Surveillance
            System (BRFSS) data, 82, 83
        definition, 81
        demography, 82
        spinal cord trauma, 81
    demographic correlation
        general health status, 86
        higher education, 86
        income, 86
        racial differences, 86–7
    epidemiological estimation, 76, 81
    latent class analysis (LCA), 151
    mental disorder, 151

Substance Use and Older People, First Edition.
Edited by Ilana B. Crome, Li-Tzy Wu, Rahul (Tony) Rao and Peter Crome.
© 2015 John Wiley & Sons, Ltd. Published 2015 by John Wiley & Sons, Ltd.

National Survey on Drug Use and
Health (NSDUH) estimate, 149
problem use, threshold selection, 80
psychopharmacology, 153–4
survey, sample estimation, 150
Medicare population, 80
moderate drinking, 80–81
National Institute on Aging's Health
and Retirement Study sample, 80
treatment populations, 84–5
alcohol abuse
characteristics and treatment, 230,
231–3
clinical samples, 238
elders seeking alcohol treatment, 235
hazardous drinking, prevalence reports,
234–5
NHS Trust Community Alcohol Team
data, 234
older adults, 236–8
older women, 236
treatment, 237, 238, **239–41**
Veterans Administration (VA) evaluation
project, 235
withdrawal, 236
alcohol-drug interactions
CNS-acting medications, 158
comorbidity alcohol risk evaluation tool
(CARET), 157–8
cross-sectional survey, 157
health effects, 158
mechanisms, 156
National Council on Patient Information
and Education (NCPIE) report,
155–6
National Health and Nutrition
Examination Survey data
(1999–2002), 157
polypharmacy, 156
problem significance, 156–7
random sample study, 157
alcohol-related dementia, 23
alcohol-related policy development, United
States
driving policy questions, 365
legal policies
Affordable Care Act, 367
alcohol price and suicide, 367
behaviour problems, 365–6
drinking and driving laws,
367–8, 369

law, public support, 369
minimally intrusive, 368
reductions in targeted behaviours,
366–7
recommended low-risk alcohol
consumption levels, 364
traffic crash risks, 365
alcohol use and misuse, ageing and
development
biological hypothesis, 128
differences in use, 125
drinking patterns, sex and WHO region,
124, **125**
endogenous and exogenous
mechanisms, 127
epidemiological and demographic
aspects, 124
gender differences, 126
heavy and risk-full use or misuse,
123–4
heterogeneous process, 128
medicines, concomitant use, 124
morbidity hypothesis, 128
mortality hypothesis, 128
problem drinking, age and onset, 127
research results and community
programmes, 124
substance use within people,
developments, 126
trajectories, 126–7
alcohol use disorder (AUD), 83–5
Alcohol Use Disorders Identification
Test (AUDIT), 199, 200
biomarkers, 199, 201
brief intervention (BI), 207–8
Cut down, Annoyed by criticism, Guilt
about drinking, needing Eye-opener
(CAGE), 198
Phosphatidyl ethanol (PET), 197–9, 201
question screen, 197–8
Short Michigan Alcoholism Screening
Test-Geriatric Version (SMAST-G),
199, 201
symptoms, abuse or dependence, 199
time frame, 198
Alcohol Use Disorders Identification Test
(AUDIT), 182, 199, 200
alcohol withdrawal syndrome, 38, 45, 46,
275, 296
benzodiazepines, discontinuation, 46
clinical examination, 45

alcohol withdrawal syndrome (*cont'd*)
  elderly individuals, 46
  intake after excessive consumption, 45
  opiate, 46
  treatment
    acamprosate and naltrexone, 276
    benzodiazepines (oxazepam,
      lorazepam), 275
    sertraline-naltrexone combination,
      276–7
American Public Health Association and
    National Highway Traffic Safety
    Administration, 78–9
American Society of Addiction Medicines'
    (ASAM) Client Placement
    Criteria, 322
anti-ageing drugs, 45
anti-tobacco counter-marketing
    campaigns, 376
Assessing Care Of Vulnerable Elders
    (ACOVE), 298
Assessment of Underutilization of
    Medication (AUM) tool, 298
Australian National Health and Medical
    Research Council high risk
    criteria, 85

baby boomers (1946 to 1964), 18, 60, 285
  chronic medical disorders, 60
  marijuana use, 18
  substance misuse, ethical and legal
    aspects
    capacity, 21–4
    coercion, 24
    confidentiality, 19–20
    informed consent, 20–21
Beers criteria, 298, 309
Behavioral Risk Factor Surveillance System
    (BRFSS), 76–7, 79, 80, 84, 85–6
benzodiazepines
  chronic use, 278–9
  discontinuation studies, 279
  insomnia, treatment, 279
  sleep complaints, 279
binge drinking, 226, 227, 235, 237, 245
  Behavioral Risk Factor Surveillance
    System (BRFSS) data, 82
  definition, 81
  demography, 82
  spinal cord trauma, 81
blood alcohol concentration (BAC), 177

brief intervention (BI)
  5As
    ADVISE, 207
    ARRANGE, 208
    ASK, 207
    ASSESS, 207–8
    ASSIST, 208
    FRAMES, 326
    Motivational Interviewing (MI), 206–7
Brief Intervention and Treatment for Elders
    (BRITE), 282, 326 *see also* brief
    intervention (BI)

capacity *see also* The Mental Capacity Act
    2005 (MCA)
  assessment, 23
  clinical capacity evaluation, 21
  decisional capacity, elements, 21–2, **22**
  dementia, alcohol-induced, 23–4
  denial, 23
  medical and psychiatric conditions, 21
  mental capacity legislation, 4
  and substance misuse, 3–4
Center for Substance Abuse Treatment
    (CSAT), 77
Centers for Disease Control and
    Prevention (CDC) criteria, 79, 116
chronic obstructive pulmonary disease
    (COPD), 181
Cigarette Labeling and Advertising Act,
    373
cigarette neo-prohibitionism, 377
cigarette smoking
  adjusted odds ratios (2002 *vs.* 2011)
    adults aged ≥ 65 years, **69–70**, 71
    aged 45–64 years, 66, **69–70**, 71
  annual health care and labour costs, 59
  census data, 60
  current smoking prevalence,
    socioeconomic status (2002 *vs.*
    2011)
    adults aged 45–64 years, 66, **67–8**
    adults aged ≥ 65 years, 66, **67–8**
  demographic characteristics, 59
  Epidemiologic Transition Theory, 60
  evaluation methodology, 61
  Global Adult Tobacco Survey
    (GATS), 59
  multiple health conditions, 60
  national trend, current smoking
    prevalence (2002–2011)

current smoking, 65
daily smoking, 65, 66
nondaily smoking, 65, 66
preventable risk behaviours, 60
sociodemographic characteristics, older
adults (2002 *vs.* 2011)
adults aged 45–64 years, 62, **63–4**
adults aged ≥ 65 years, 62, 65
tobacco use *see* tobacco cessation
clinical medicine
ageing, 35
assumed/real physical limitations, 38
Cut down, Annoyed by criticism, Guilt
about drinking, needing Eye-opener
(CAGE), 37
drug-related mental health/behavioural
disorders, 36
healthcare interactions, 36
health effects, substance abuse
chronic, 39
'Geriatric Giants' *see* 'Geriatric
Giants'
identification tools, 47–8
importance, 36–7
issues, 38
misdiagnosis, health professionals, 37
polypharmacy and functional issues, 46
primary care practitioners, 37
professional awareness and service
provision, 35
research, 47
secondary care resources, 36
Short Michigan Alcohol Screening Test
(SMAST), 37
substance abuse issues, 36–7
symptoms, 37
training and support, 48–9
uncertainty, factors, 37–8
cocaine, 242
coercion
elder abuse, 24
emotional/financial dependence, 24
legally adjudicated incompetence, 24
cognitive behavioural therapy (CBT), 327
cognitive impairment
alcohol consumption, 40
benzodiazepines, 40
cerebral degeneration and eventual
dementia, 40
chronic, 41
extrapolation, 40

medications, 39–40
mental, physical and functional
consequences, 39
methodological incompatibilities, 41
psychomotor retardation, 42
Community Mental Health Team
(CMHT), 345
comorbidity alcohol risk evaluation tool
(CARET), 157–8
Comprehensive Geriatric Assessment
(CGA), 48, 307–8
alcohol withdrawal, 178
barriers, 176–7
blood alcohol concentration
(BAC), 177
British Medical Association, 177
cannabis and stimulant intoxication, 178
case presentations
alcohol and cognitive impairment,
186–7
driving and substance misuse, 184
frequent attender, 185–6
older women and alcohol, 184–5
pain, 187
polysubstance misuse, 185
collateral information, 178–9
high-risk groups, 177
principles
examination, 180–181
functional status, 181–2
history, 179–80
mini mental state examination
(MMSE), 183
psychiatric assessment, 183–4
screening, 182–3
problems, 177–8
setting, 176
SUD, diagnostic and statistical manual
criteria, **174–5**
computerized provider order entry with
clinical decision support (CPOE/
CDS), 309–10
confidentiality
health care professional's obligation, 19
primary care settings, 20
privacy regulations, 19, 20
consent
Advance Care Planning (ACP), forms,
6–7
granting permission, 6
informed, 20–21

COPD *see* chronic obstructive pulmonary disease (COPD)
Cut down, Annoyed by criticism, Guilt about drinking, needing Eye-opener (CAGE), 37, 182, 198, 234–5, 259–60

Diagnostic and Statistical Manual of Mental Disorders IV (DSM-IV), 3, 76, 83, 125, 212, 214
Driver and Vehicle Licensing Agency (DVLA), 184
drug abuse
  amphetamines, 205
  brief intervention (BI), 206–8
  chronic pain, 205
  illicit and nonmedical, 150
  medical and mental health disorders, 204
  methadone maintenance patients, 151–2
  muscle relaxants, 205
  psychopharmacology, 154–5
  screening, 205–6
  treatment use and outcomes, 243–5
The Drug Abuse Prevention, Treatment and Rehabilitation Act, 19
drug abuse screening tool (DAST), 182, 183, 260
Drug Abuse Warning Network (DAWN), 109, 110, 112, 113, 151, 245
drug–drug interactions
  alcohol and anticonvulsants, 45
  chronic alcohol misuse, 44
  CNS depressant effects, 45
  diabetics, 44
  elderly, 43–4
  'prescribing cascade', 44
  self-medicators, 44
drugs, policy development
  policy design and implementation, 359
  policy options, 356–9
  policy recommendations and guidelines, 357
  problem and arguments, 354–5
  'problem drug users', 353–4
DSM-III-R alcohol abuse/dependence, 237
DSM-IV Axis I mental disorders, 236

e-cigarettes, 377
elder abuse, 21
  ageism and ageist practices, 11
  alcohol and substance misuse risk factors, 12–13
  awareness, professionals, 16
  definition, 11
  domestic violence and crimes, 12
  effects, 14–15
  health and care professionals, 15
  practitioners and managers, 15
  risk factors, 13–14
  safeguarding, 12
  social services agencies, 12
  types, 12
Elder Abuse and Alcohol, WHO review, 14
elderly, substance use disorders
  clinical presentations
    alcohol dependence, depression, 159–60
    alcohol dependence, medical problems, 159
    benzodiazepine dependence, anxiety, 160–161
    opioid dependence, chronic pain, 160
  cognitive impairment, 163–4
  co-morbid medical conditions, 161
  evaluation, 162–3
  medications, 164–5
  safety assessment, 164
  screening, 161–2
English National Survey of Psychiatric Morbidity (ENSPM), 92
The European Convention of Human Rights (EUCR)
  human rights and freedom, 28
  Prohibition of Discrimination (Article 14), 29
  right of liberty, 28–9
  right to respect for private and family life, 29
European Monitoring Centre for Drugs and Drug Addiction (EMCDDA), 123, 356
European perspective
  'controlled drugs', UK law, 28
  crime, 28
  The European Convention of Human Rights (EUCR), 28–9
  legal and ethical aspects, 27
  penalizing use of drugs, 28

policy making, 31
research and development, 30
service providers, 27
services for elderly, 29–30
stigma, 32
treatment, ethical issues, 32
underprescribing controlled drugs, 32–3
and USA, 31–2

Family Smoking Prevention and Tobacco Control Act, 377
FRAMES, 252, 326

'Geriatric Giants', 36, 48
cognitive impairment, 39–41
iatrogenesis, 43–6
instability, falls and immobility, 41–3
urinary incontinence, 43
GET SMART, 356
Global Adult Tobacco Survey (GATS), 59
Guiding Older Adult Lifestyles (GOAL) project, 282

Harmful Interactions: Mixing Alcohol with Medicines (NIAAA), 364
healthcare models and clinical practices
ageing population
frailty, 266
long-term medical conditions (LTCs), 265
National Health Service, 265
care and workforce development, 267–9
community care, 269
service development and provision, 266–7
Health Insurance Portability and Accountability Act (HIPAA), 19, 20
Health Profiles Project, 282
Healthy Living as You Age (HLAYA) study, 283
heavy or high risk drinking, 77, 78, 226, 236

iatrogenesis, 39
alcohol withdrawal syndrome, 45–6
anti-ageing drugs, 45
drug–drug interactions, 43–5
ICD-9 alcohol-related diagnosis, 246
illicit drug, use and disorders
abuse/dependence, 203
brief intervention (BI), 206–8
health implications, 104
older adults, 202

psychiatric setting, 202
survey studies
marijuana and cocaine users, 98–100
race/ethnicity, 100
toxicology screening, 203–4
treatment-seeking or clinical patients, studies
drug use initiation, age, 103
methadone, 102
racial characteristics, 102–3
uses, 202
Impact, 281
inappropriate prescribing (IP)
alcohol abuse, 296–7
Comprehensive Geriatric Assessment (CGA), 307–8
computerized provider order entry with clinical decision support (CPOE/CDS), 309
definition, 295
dementia, 296
explicit IP criteria, 298–9
implicit IP criteria, 297–8
inappropriate psychotropic use, 296–7
opioids, 297
pharmacist review and intervention, 308
potential prescribing omissions, 299, *304*
prescriber education, audit and feedback, 308
STOPP/START criteria, randomized controlled trial, 305, *306*
Wernicke/Korsakoff syndrome, 297
independent decision makers, 6
legislation, 8
stipulations, 8, 9
substance misuse, 8
Independent Mental Capacity Advocate (IMCA)
stipulations, 8, 9
substitute decision maker, 8
infectious diseases, screening, 328
informed consent
Anglo-American ethics and law, 20–21
decisional capacity, enhancing, 21
integrated treatment models
development, 344–6
educational interventions, 283–4
Health Profiles Project, 282
Impact, 281
Pathways, 281

integrated treatment models (*cont'd*)
  primary care treatment, 282
  Project *MATCH*, 281
  Prospect, 281
  research evidence, 346–7
  Substance Misuse and Co-morbid
    Mental Disorder, 342–4
International Classification of Diseases,
  Tenth Revision (ICD-10), 114–15
International Classification of the Diseases
  (ICD), 31

Lasting Power of Attorney (LPA)
  behaviour, 7
  health and welfare decisions, 6
  provisions, 7
  substitute decisions, 7
latent class analysis (LCA), 151

mean corpuscular volume (MCV), 185
Medication Appropriateness Index
  (MAI), 297
medication use review (MUR), 308, 310
The Mental Capacity Act 2005 (MCA)
  assessment, 5–6
  best interest decisions, 8
  consent, 6–7, 20–21
  independent decision makers, 8–9
  principles, 5
  safeguard provisions and vulnerable
    rights enhancement, 4
  and unwise decisions, 6
Michigan Alcoholism Screening Test–
  Geriatric version (MAST–G), 48, 76
mini mental state examination
  (MMSE), 183
motivational enhancement therapy
  (MET), 327
motivational interviewing (MI), 206–7, 326

National Center for Health Statistics
  (NCHS), 109, 114, *115*
National Comorbidity Survey-Replication
  study, 83–4
National Council on Patient Information
  and Education (NCPIE), 155–6
National Drug Treatment Monitoring
  System (NDTMS), 92
National Epidemiologic Survey on Alcohol
  and Related Conditions (NESARC),
  92, **93–7**, 99, 364, 366

National Health and Nutrition
  Examination Survey, 157
National Health Interview Survey (NHIS)
  epidemiology, cigarette smoking, 61
  illness and disability, 61
National Household Survey on Drug
  Abuse (NHSDA), 98–9
National Institute on Aging's Health and
  Retirement Study sample, 80
National Institute on Alcohol Abuse and
  Alcoholism (NIAAA), 77, 92
National Longitudinal Epidemiologic
  Survey (NLAES), 84
National Survey of American Life
  (NSAL), 245
National Survey on Drug Use and
  Health (NSDUH) data, 82–3, 92,
  110–111
New Hampshire VA detoxification
  unit, 236
'New Ways of Working', 345
nonbinge drinkers, 233, 237
nonmedical prescription drug use
  ageing populations, characteristics,
    109–10
  benzodiazepines, 117–18
  drug poisoning deaths, 114–16
  emergency department cases, 112, **113**
  inappropriate prescribing, 117
  misuse, 117
  pain and insomnia, 116
  race/ethnic and gender distribution, 111
  treatment admissions, 113, **114**
Norwegian General Practice (NORGEP)
  Criteria, 298

opioids, treatment
  agonist substitution therapy, 277
  medical-psychiatric stepped care, 278
  methadone maintenance treatment,
    277–8
  naltrexone and buprenorphine, 278

Pathways, 281
pharmacological treatments
  age-specific programmes, 273–4
  alcohol, 275–7
  benzodiazepines, 278–9
  cannabis, 281
  low dose, 273
  opioids, 277–8

stimulants, 280–281
tobacco, 274–5
phosphatidyl ethanol (PET), 199, 201
polypharmacy, 46, 156
potentially inappropriate medications
    (PIMs), 295, 296, 299, 304
potential prescribing omissions (PPOs),
    299, 304
prescription drugs, misuse, 136
primary care
    Alcohol-Related Problems Survey
        (ARPS), 252
    benefit, 252
    co-morbidities and social context, 252
    FRAMES approach, 252
    implications, 249–50
    misuse, prescribed medication, 251
    populations at risk, 250–251
    'pseudo-addiction', 252
    psychoactive prescription medicine
        misuse, 251
    screening, 251–2
Primary Care Research in Substance Abuse
    and Mental Health for the Elderly
    (PRISM-E) study, 282–3
Project MATCH, 281, 327
Prospect, 281
PsychINFO, 123
psychoactive substances, misuse, 141
psychoeducation, 328
Public Health Cigarette Smoking Act, 373
PubMed, 47, 123
pulmonary emphysema, 280

recommendations
    clinical presentations, 384–5
    education and training, 385
    epidemiology, 384
    treatment interventions, 386
relapse prevention therapy (RPT),
    327–8

Scottish Drugs Forum, 359
screening
    alcohol, 197, 259–60
    breast cancer, 196
    drug abuse, 260
        aberrant drug behaviours, 205
        older adults, 204–5
        urine toxicology testing, 205–6
    illicit drugs, 202–4

mental health issues, 197
older adults, 195, 196
Screening of substance misuse, Brief
    Intervention and Referral to
    Treatment (SBIRT) practice, 386
SDDCARE project (Senior Drug
    Dependents and Care Structure
    Project), 359
second-hand tobacco smoke, 372, 375
self-medication hypothesis, 139
Short Michigan Alcoholism Screening
    Test-Geriatric Version (SMAST-G),
    37, 199, 201, 259
smoke-free movies, 377–8
Southeast London Community Health
    Survey (SLCHS), 92
South London and Maudsley NHS
    Foundation Trust, 346
START (Screening Tool to Alert to Right
    Treatment) criteria, 302–3
stimulants, 280–281
STOPP (Screening Tool of Older Persons'
    Prescriptions) criteria, 300–302
Substance Abuse and Mental Health
    Services Administration (SAMHSA),
    18, 77, 92, 109, 315
substance misuse/addiction see also The
    Mental Capacity Act 2005 (MCA)
    anxiety disorder and antisocial
        personality disorder, 151
    and capacity, 3–4
    clinical settings, 150–151
    decision making capacity, 3
    latent class analysis (LCA), 151
    lifetime disorders, prevalent rates, 152
    mental capacity legislation, 3–4
    mental disorder, 151
    opioid-dependent patients, 152
    past-year psychiatric and medical
        diagnoses, 152
Substance Misuse and Co-morbid Mental
    Disorder (SMCD)
    care for substance misuse and mental
        disorders, 341
    comprehensive assessment, 343
    integrated treatment models, 342–7
    service implications, 342
substances abuse
    alcohol, 153–4
    benzodiazepines and sedative-hypnotics
        (SH), 154–5

substances abuse (*cont'd*)
  cannabis, 155
  cocaine, 155
  dopamine (DA), 152–3
  opioids/opiates, 154
substance use progression process *see also*
      elderly, substance use disorders
  access, 135–6
  advances in medicine, 134
  alcohol use, 133
  cross-sectional surveys, 142–3
  environmental influences, 140–141
  individual factors
    early-onset abusers, 138
    heritable factors, 138
    influences, **137**
    late-onset abusers, 138
    pharmacokinetic/dynamic
      changes, 138
    prescribed medications, 138–9
    self-medication hypothesis, 139
  multiple substances, use, 136–7
  prescription drugs, misuse, 136
  psychoactive substance use spectrum,
      133, *134*
  regular use, 136
  severe consequences, 136
  substance properties
    miscommunication, 141
    policies and norms, 140–141
    prescribing practices, 141
    psychoactive substances, misuse, 141
  symptoms, **142**

tobacco cessation
  bupropion, 275
  community sample study, 212–13
  counselling and behavioural
      interventions, 217
  DSM-IV psychiatric disorders, 214
  evidence-based smoking cessation
      programmes, 274–5
  health status, 213
  intensive and multimodal interventions,
      219
  older adults, 214–17, **215**
  past-year cigarette smoking, 213

  physician-delivered interventions,
      217–18
  programmes, 376
  service use and characteristics
    health conditions, 229–30
    National Ambulatory Medical Care
      Survey data (2001–2102), 229
    older adults, 225, **277–8**
  telephone quit-lines, 218
tobacco, policy development
  anti-tobacco counter-marketing
      campaigns, 376
  anti-tobacco proposals
    cigarette neo-prohibitionism, 377
    harm reduction, 377
    product modification and 'safer'
      cigarettes, 376–7
    smoke-free movies, 377–8
  legal approach, 373–4
  past and present approaches, reduced
      consumption, 372–3
  policy proposals, reduced tobacco
      prevalence, 378
  regulatory and tobacco tax approaches
    second-hand tobacco smoke
      restrictions, 375
    tobacco taxes, 374–5
    tobacco warning labels, 375–6
Treatment Episode Data Set (TEDS), 18,
      84–5, 101–2, 109, 150–151, 238,
      239–41, 242–6

urinary incontinence
  alcohol, 43
  benzodiazepines, 43
  description, 43
  opioids, 43
US Census Bureau's 2011 American
      Community Survey, 79
US National Institute on Alcohol Abuse
      and Alcoholism (NIAAA), 364

Veterans Administration (VA) evaluation
      project, 235
VINTAGE, international projects, 284

Wernicke/Korsakoff syndrome, 297